Twenty-Seventh Hanford Symposium
on Health and the Environment

Multilevel Health Effects Research:
From Molecules to Man

Twenty-Seventh Hanford Symposium
on Health and the Environment

Multilevel Health Effects Research: From Molecules to Man

October 18-21, 1988
Richland, Washington U.S.A.

Edited by

James F. Park

and

Richard A. Pelroy

Sponsored by
the United States Department of Energy
and Battelle, Pacific Northwest Laboratories

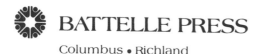 BATTELLE PRESS

Columbus • Richland

DISCLAIMER

This report was prepared as an account of work sponsored by an agency of the United States Government. Neither the United States Government nor any agency thereof, nor Battelle Memorial Institute, nor any of their employees, makes **any warranty, expressed or implied, or assumes any legal liability or responsibility for the accuracy, completeness, or usefulness of any information, apparatus, product, or process disclosed, or represents that its use would not infringe privately owned rights.** Reference herein to any specific commercial product, process, or service by trade name, trademark, manufacturer, or otherwise does not necessarily constitute or imply its endorsement, recommendation, or favoring by the United States Government or any agency thereof, or Battelle Memorial Institute. The views and opinions of authors expressed herein do not necessarily state or reflect those of the United States Government or any agency thereof.

PACIFIC NORTHWEST LABORATORY
operated by
BATTELLE MEMORIAL INSTITUTE
for the
UNITED STATES DEPARTMENT OF ENERGY
under Contract DE-AC06-76RLO 1830

Library of Congress Cataloging-in-Publication Data

Hanford Life Sciences Symposium (27th: 1988: Richland, Wash.) Multilevel health effects research: from molecules to man: proceedings of the Twenty-Seventh Hanford Life Sciences Symposium, October 1988/edited by R. A. Pelroy and J. F. Park.
p.   cm.
Includes bibliographical references.
ISBN 0-935470-55-7: $57.50
1. Pathology, Cellular—Congresses. 2. Pathology, Molecular—Congresses.
3. Carcinogenesis—Congresses. 4. Mutagenesis—Congresses.
I. Pelroy, R. A., 1938—   . II. Park, J. F., 1934—   . III. Title.
RB113.H25 1988   89-18083
616.07—dc20   CIP

Additional copies may be ordered through Battelle Press, 505 King Avenue. Columbus, Ohio 43201-2693.   614/424-6393.

CONTENTS

iii

Quantifying Molecular End Points in Differentiated Cells

Carcinogenesis and Developmental Studies with Multilevel Systems

Use of Multilevel Systems to Study Development

Molecular Markers for Cell Damage

Detection of DNA Adducts and Other Measures of Primary Cell Damage

PREFACE

The papers included in these proceedings represent the many disciplines (e.g., experimental pathology, epidemiology, molecular biology, and biophysics) that participated in the Hanford Symposium on Health and the Environment. Participants discussed an integrated approach to health effects research, emphasizing molecular studies in the intact animal. The premise underlying the multilevel theme of the symposium was that studies in cultured cells, in and of themselves, cannot be translated with certainty to the live animal because, for instance, complex systemic factors influence responses of cells in that animal. In these systems, damage is mediated by, for example, hormones, growth factors and receptors, and immunity. In addition, the various cell types found *in vivo* differ markedly in their ability to repair damage from exposure to agents such as ionizing radiation or carcinogenic and/or mutagenic chemicals; to undergo spontaneous or induced malignant transformation; or to demonstrate altered patterns of gene expression either during embryogenesis or in the mature adult. At the cellular level, there are tissue- and organ-specific differences in the capacity of cells to function and report damage that are the result of the separate developmental pathways followed by tissues during embryogenesis.

The study of molecular mechanisms in the intact animal poses a formidable challenge to the ingenuity of the experimenter from the point of view of experimental design and instrumentation for sensitive detection of molecular end points. Several approaches to this problem were illustrated during the symposium, including: (a) analysis of molecular end points in cells taken from the animal by direct cell counting and analysis of defined macromolecular structures, or physical and chemical separation of small molecules (e.g., DNA adducts, mutations in proteins on targeted DNA sequences; (b) transgenic insertion of DNA into the germline for genetic carcinogenesis or developmental studies; (c) use of movable genetic elements (e.g., shuttle vectors) to introduce genetic targets into a variety of mammalian cells to study mechanisms of mutagenesis and DNA repair; and (d) correlation of pathology with molecular analysis in tumor cell lines, in primary cultures that retain the specialized properties of the cells in the intact animal, and in preserved cells within archived tissues.

The scope of the symposium was necessarily broad. The general area of molecular genetics includes induced mutagenesis; structural and functional analysis of complex mammalian chromosomal loci; advanced molecular methods of physical genetic mapping; the exposure of experimental and computational strategies for physical chromosome mapping in mammalian models and humans; use of transgenic models to study gene expression during embryogenesis in mammalian systems; and use of sophisticated molecular systems such as shuttle vectors for detailed molecular analysis of the basic mechanisms of mutation in human cells. In addition, several presentations described nonmammalian systems that may be useful alternatives for studies of genetics and development.

Molecular cytogenetics was well illustrated by advanced techniques of instrumentation and molecular analysis capable of increasing the sensitivity and range of detectable genetic lesions in cells obtained directly from the animal. Use of flow cytometry for ultrarapid cell separation and molecular analysis figures prominently in this line of research, and interesting results were presented on the versatility of this device in the study of chromosome instability during cancer progression.

The importance of molecular genetics for elucidating the structural and functional organization and basic cellular mechanisms of intact animals is obvious and pervasive in biology today. In a sense it mirrors, albeit in a more difficult and complex organismic setting, decades of earlier work with much simpler unicellular systems where genetic analysis was integral in unraveling fundamental pathways of metabolism, biosynthesis, and repair of cell damage. The potential benefit to human health from multilevel research is readily apparent in regard to better diagnostics, genetic screening for birth defects and heritable mutations, and therapy. This research also provides a means for basic mechanistic studies in higher order animals.

H. M. Parker
Lecture

H. M. Parker Lecturer, 1988

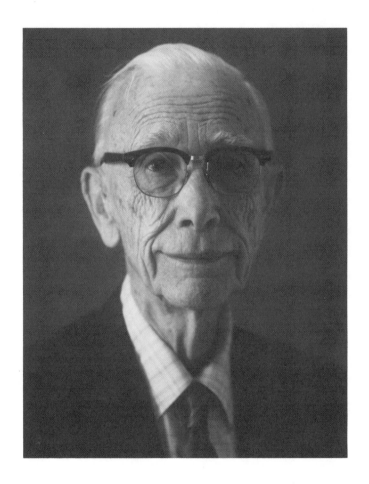

J. N. Stannard

INTRODUCTION

W. J. Bair

The H. M. Parker Lectures are presented each year, on the occasion of the Hanford Symposium on Health and the Environment. These lectures are sponsored by the Department of Energy; Battelle, Pacific Northwest Laboratories; and the Herbert M. Parker Foundation for Education in the Radiological Sciences.*

The objectives of the H. M. Parker lecture series are:

1. to memorialize H. M. Parker and his outstanding contributions to radiological sciences and radiation protection;

2. to honor contemporary scientists who evoke H. M. Parker's high technical standards and concern for protection of the health of workers and the public;

3. to enhance the public's understanding of radiological health issues.

For the third lecture of the series, our speaker is Professor J. Newell Stannard. Dr. Stannard's contributions to research on the health effects of ionizing radiation and to the education of students in both basic and applied aspects of radiation protection began in the 1940s at the University of Rochester during the days of the Manhattan Project. Through lectures, work on technical committees, consulting, and authoring papers and books, he continues to contribute, in the tradition of H. M. Parker, to the protection of workers and the public against possible biological effects of radiation. Thus, he is well qualified to help us honor Herb by presenting this lecture.

Newell received a bachelor of science degree in biology and chemistry at Oberlin College and earned an M.S. and a Ph.D. in general physiology and biophysics at Harvard University. From Harvard he went to the University of Rochester Medical School to teach physiology.

During World War II, Newell Stannard spent several years doing respiratory physiology research as a naval officer at the Bureau of Medicine and

---

*The Herbert M. Parker Foundation is incorporated in the State of Washington. As a nonprofit corporation, it can receive public donations to perpetuate the lecture series and support other educational activities.

1

Surgery in Washington, D.C., and in a civilian capacity at the National Institute of Health. After the war he returned to the University of Rochester School of Medicine to establish a graduate education program in the field of atomic energy as applied to health sciences. Under Dr. Stannard's leadership, this became the first Ph.D. program in the world to apply atomic energy to the life sciences and medicine.

Newell Stannard's educational and research activities have been vital to many programs related to atomic energy, including nuclear medicine, nuclear power, weapons, and space. Hundreds of graduates from the programs developed under Dr. Stannard can today be found in positions of responsibility in research and in radiation protection—in government agencies such as DOE, NRC, EPA, NIH; in the armed forces; in nearly all U.S. nuclear power plants; in national laboratories; in universities; and in hospitals.

Newell began his radiobiological research in two areas: effects of radiation on cell membranes, and the biological effects of alpha-emitting radionuclides. The first represented an early attempt to understand the mechanism of the interaction of ionizing radiation on living cells. The second was directed at developing information about the biological effects of polonium. Polonium, an alpha-particle emitter, is currently used in antistatic devices.

Dr. Stannard's work with polonium and his earlier work in respiratory physiology led to his being given responsibility at the University of Rochester for research on the inhalation of radioactive aerosols. This program was the first to involve highly radioactive alpha-emitting materials such as polonium and plutonium. In the program, many graduate students were trained who not only contributed to research on inhaled radionuclides at the University of Rochester, but carried the techniques to programs at other laboratories. The first of these was here at Hanford, where research was begun in 1954 on the inhalation of plutonium and fission products.

Dr. Stannard's publications, numbering well over 100, represent significant contributions to biomedical research. Throughout his career, Dr. Stannard has served with distinction on numerous national and international committees concerned with radiation protection. He has received many honors and awards. He is currently Adjunct Professor of Community Medicine and Radiology at the University of California in San Diego, and Professor Emeritus of Radiation Biology and Biophysics and of Pharmacology and Toxicology at the University of Rochester School of Medicine and Dentistry.

It is frequently lamented that major scientific endeavors are not documented while the principals are living. During the past 10 years, Dr. Stannard addressed this problem directly in authoring a book, *Radioactivity and Health: A History*. In researching this book, Newell personally interviewed nearly all the scientists who have done research on the health and environmental aspects of radioactive materials since the 1930s.

In addition to the personal interviews, Newell conducted a massive literature search and visited libraries throughout the country. The result is a magnificent, 2000-page volume. It tells a fascinating story of scientific research and of the people who provided leadership and those who made important discoveries. It is also a story of how science successfully dealt with the potential hazards of working with highly radioactive material: doing research to understand its biological effects in living organisms and the environment, and applying this knowledge to the establishment of radiation protection standards.

I hope Dr. Stannard will draw from his book in presenting the third H. M. Parker Lecture, because this book typifies much of what Herb espoused: scholarship, scientific achievement, and effective communication.

As one of his former students, I am especially pleased to present to you, Dr. Newell Stannard.

H. M. PARKER LECTURE

SOME HEALTH ASPECTS OF NUCLEAR ENERGY: WHO MINDED THE STORE, AND WHAT DID THEY DO?

J. N. Stannard

Professor Emeritus, University of Rochester School of Medicine and Dentistry
Adjunct Professor, School of Medicine, University of California, San Diego

Key words: *History, atomic and nuclear energy, radiobiology, health, medicine, environment*

The title I have chosen requires some comment. By "the store" I mean the biomedical research establishment that is devoted to learning and understanding the health aspects of nuclear energy or, more broadly speaking, those of ionizing radiation. It is more like a department store than a single entrepreneurial enterprise, for it involves a wide spectrum of scientific disciplines—pure biology, radiobiology, biophysics, medicine, pathology, chemistry and biochemistry, epidemiology, environmental sciences, and some newer departments such as health physics. The store is smaller now than it was in the decades of World War II and from the 1950s through the 1970s. It is still, however, an active and essential enterprise. The public knows far too little about it.

My title carries the implication that the regular operators of "the store" were into other things and that a skeleton, substitute crew was left in charge, that is, "to mind the store." This is not really an accurate portrayal, but it seems to exist in the minds of many in the general public, and therefore I use it. The picture is of the mainstream of the scientific and technical community going pell-mell down the road to the release of atomic energy from bombs and reactors with little concern for the possible health and environmental consequences. The cartoon in Figure 1 hints at this point of view.

The story of the development of the atomic bomb and the release of nuclear energy has been told over and over. The most recent and, perhaps, the most pertinent version for today's society is *The Making of the Atomic Bomb*, by Richard Rhodes (Rhodes, 1987). This book treats the people and events in the manner of a novel. The principal figures need no naming here; the sheer immensity of what they did has caused them to be remembered.

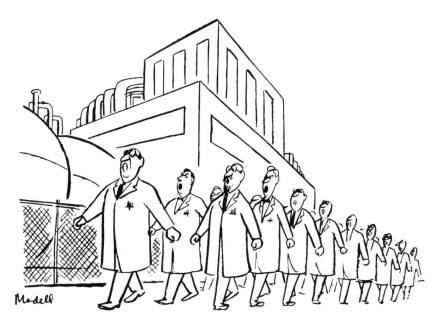

"From the cyclotron of Berkeley to the labs of M.I.T.,
We're the lads that you can trust to keep our country strong and free."

Figure 1. Cartoon illustrating one popular concept of the attitude of the scientific establishment toward release of atomic energy, published in *The New Yorker* 11-18-58. Drawing by Modell; ©1958, 1986, *The New Yorker* Magazine, Inc.

There are many who hold that the world would be better off if nuclear energy had never been released. I hear it from students at UCSD, and I get the impression that they feel the generation most involved wronged them terribly. Where were the guardians of health and morality? They were minding the store.

As an aside, it should be said that we had no choice concerning the release of atomic energy. Soon after the discovery of radioactivity, many eminent physicists said that someday the energy of the atom would be tapped. It was only a matter of time after Lise Meitner and her colleagues described the fissioning of uranium by neutrons. This was in Germany, just before the hostilities of World War II broke out. It was assumed that the Germans surely had the know-how to proceed with a bomb. It was not anticipated that Hitler's purges would drive off or destroy most of the keen minds who could have done the job for Germany. Not knowing that, we had to proceed. Do you think the world would be better off if Hitler had gotten there first?

Let us get back to "the store." I would like to say that I intend these remarks to lend perspective to events of several decades. I dare not say that. If I did, I would expect a sharp flash of lightning and a resounding peal of thunder, followed by Herb Parker's rich voice saying, "Don't be a pompous ass and think that you can bring perspective to matters where others have tried and failed." So I will not say it!

Herb Parker was a first-class physicist who turned to medical physics and fostered consideration of biology and health wherever he went. Like many great men, he could have strong opinions. He seemed to dislike, especially, pomposity in any form. He could always distinguish between simple enthusiasm and pomposity. I have often wondered how Herb regarded roosters.

However, I am getting ahead of my story. "The store" was founded long before atomic energy, bombs, or reactors. Soon after Roentgen's discovery of x rays, the fact that they could have biological effects became evident. However, their potential for imaging of tissues and for the treatment of cancer fired the imaginations of those concerned. It took the skin burns and, later, leukemias of British radiologists who used x rays extensively in field hospitals during World War I without adequate protective shielding to make it clear that these new radiations were a two-edged sword.

Radium was discovered very shortly after x rays, but it did not gain the immediate popularity that x rays did. It was used as another source of penetrating radiation and as a source of radon, which could be put into small seeds for internal application in the treatment of cancer. It was also ingested or injected as a therapeutic nostrum. The separation of radium from its ores has sometimes been termed "The First Nuclear Industry"; a picture of some of the extraction equipment is given in Figure 2 (Nauda, 1982).

The plight of the luminous-dial painters brought attention, in the mid-1920s, to the long-term effects of radium deposited in the body. The term "dial painters" refers to those individuals, largely young women, who were employed during World War I to paint numerals on dials for military instruments and, during that war and long afterward, to do likewise for clock dials. The paint was a mixture containing radium and compounds that would luminesce under bombardment by radiation from the radium. Thus, the painters were called "luminizers" or "luminous dial painters" or just "dial painters." A group of these women, at a clock plant in Ottawa, Illinois, in the 1920s, is shown in Figure 3.

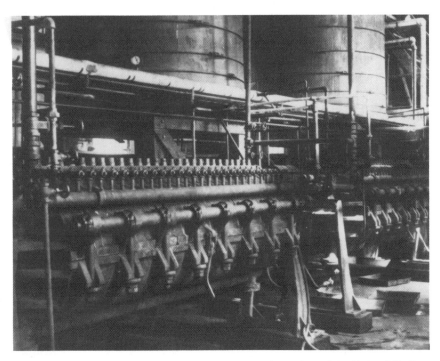

Figure 2. Radium extraction apparatus in 1915; part of the plant of the National Radium Institute in Denver. From Nauda (1982).

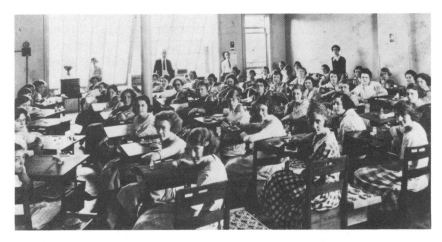

Figure 3. Luminous dial painters at their desks in an Ottawa, Illinois, plant in the 1920s (Stannard, 1988).

To make more precise numerals, these girls had the habit of "tipping" the brush with their lips and tongues, thus ingesting significant amounts of radium. It became evident that something was amiss when one of these girls (a large group worked at plants in New Jersey) was seen in the early 1920s by a perceptive dentist in New York for a stubborn kind of anemia and the beginnings of bone pathology in the jaw.

These cases multiplied and, later on, bone cancer developed. A picture of Dr. Harrison Martland, who did much to manage the continuing study of the dial painters, is shown in Figure 4. Martland was the medical examiner for Essex County, New Jersey; the medical school in Newark was, for many years, named after him.

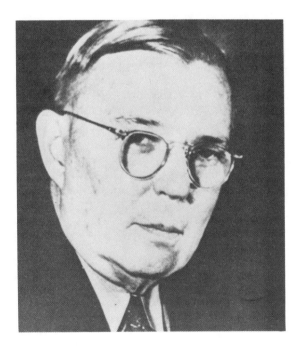

Figure 4. Dr. Harrison S. Martland, Medical Examiner, Essex County, New Jersey, who studied the clinical aspects of the work with the luminous dial painters for many years. Photograph courtesy of R. L. Kathren.

Further impetus was given to concerns about the biological effects of radium by the death of a prominent Pittsburgh industrialist named Eben Byers. Mr. Byers, a popular bachelor of the day, was sold, as were thousands of others, on the idea that radiation was good for you as a general stimulant and tonic. He took several bottles a day of a mixture known as "Radithor" and persuaded others to do likewise. He died of radium poisoning. A picture of Mr. Byers is shown in Figure 5.

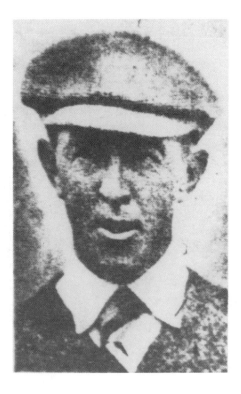

Figure 5. Eben M. Byers, Pennsylvania business tycoon, whose death from radium poisoning in 1932 helped to stimulate investigation of radium as a therapeutic nostrum. He was devoted to "Radithor" (NY Times, April 1, 1932).

The Byers incident brought to the scene Robley D. Evans, another of the greats, like Parker, in the marriage of physics and medicine. Evans and his colleagues, mostly working at MIT, developed methods for measuring the amount of radium in the body. These methods were the forerunners of our present-day whole-body counters. They and colleagues at other institutions kept track of a large and disparate group of people, many of whom didn't know they had radium poisoning until the symptoms forced them to seek medical help. These investigators kept accurate and complete clinical records, including a scoring system for the bone radiograms they took. They correlated the incidence of effects with the measured body burdens of radium and provided the basis for the first standard for a radioactive material.

The tradition of excellence established in these studies was embodied also at the Argonne National Laboratory in the "Argonne Radium Studies," which tapped new populations in the Chicago area in the postwar era. This included a group of patients in a mental hospital in Elgin, Illinois, who had been injected with radium in the 1930s.

In more recent years (after World War II), a population that received a different isotope (^{224}Ra instead of ^{226}Ra) was discovered in Germany. This group has been followed, particularly by Dr. Charles Mays at the National Cancer Institute and Dr. Heinz Spiess in Germany. Radium-224, a shorter-half-life radium isotope than ^{226}Ra, has both similarities to and differences from ^{226}Ra; it likewise produced bone cancer.

Another saga, one that I am sure is more familiar to this audience than some of the others I have mentioned, is that of the uranium miners. This goes back to at least the fifteenth century, but the malady, lung cancer, was not identified until toward the end of the nineteenth century. The causation, radon and its daughter products from the decay of radium in the uranium ore, was not identified until the 1920s. Even then there were scoffers, who persisted even into the 1950s. The miners do not constitute as large a population as the radium dial painters and patients treated with radium, but their deaths were even less necessary. Radon and its daughters have short half-lives, and, because its radioactivity does not linger in the body as does that from radium, instituting better mining practices as soon as the hazard was clearly identified could have saved many lives. However, our "storekeepers," although talented, were not numerous in those years, and they had to contend with a diffuse industry, part of an inherently dangerous trade scattered over large and inhospitable areas. Nevertheless, the word has now gotten around. Indeed, the saga of radon has done an about-face: People are now worried about radon in their homes. The scoffers have been replaced by the hand-wringers. It is ironic that the largest single source of radiation exposure to the general population in peacetime comes from natural sources, namely, radon and its daughter products.

Not all the storekeepers were looking at human populations, even in the early days. Many were busy in laboratories, quietly working to understand how ionizing radiations work. In the early 1900s, French workers realized that there were differences in the radiation sensitivity of different cell types in the body. Rapidly dividing cells and primitive cells were considerably more sensitive. Thus, the production of blood cells, development of the cells in the growing embryo and fetus, and cells in the germ line, such as the early stages of spermatozoa, would show effects sooner and at lower doses than others. This was just the beginning. Basic radiobiology, which can be regarded as a major department in our "store," has been very productive over seven decades both for pure science and for the understanding of health effects.

In the mid-1920s the geneticists became interested in radiation effects. The talented but somewhat irascible Hermann J. Muller, working then at the University of Texas in Austin, found that x rays could cause mutations in the fruit fly, *Drosophila*, as well as being lethal at high doses (Carlson, 1981). Furthermore, it appeared that the mutation rate was the same for a given total dose, whether delivered in small installments or as a single dose. In other words, the radiation effects were cumulative, and any radiation would thus add to the genetic load in the population—a worrisome prospect indeed. This created a considerable stir and brought possible genetic effects front and center. Muller continued his work while sojourning at several laboratories in Europe and, finally, at the University of Indiana. He received the Nobel Prize for this work in 1946 (Figure 6). The entire genetic fraternity began to use x rays to cause mutations, and people concerned with radiation protection began to base population exposure criteria, in part, on possible effects on future generations. What is frequently forgotten is that the x-ray doses required to produce significant increases in mutation rates in the fruit fly are quite large. It was only an assumption that effects at low doses would be directly proportional to the dose in mammalian species.

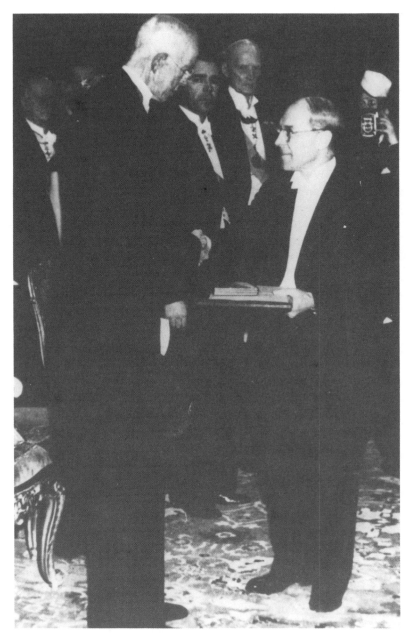

Figure 6. Dr. Hermann J. Muller (right), prominent geneticist, receiving the Nobel Prize in 1946 for his work on x rays and mutations. Nobel Foundation photo from Carlson (1981), p. 314.

The discovery that x rays could increase mutation rates had an interesting side effect. The American eugenics movement was already in full swing. Ideas for improving the human race by controlled breeding, even sterilization of certain "undesirable lines" (remember the Jukes and the Kallikaks?), were part of the movement. The finding that x rays speeded up mutation stimulated the eugenicists. Why not speed up evolution by x-ray-induced mutations?

It was a sad day for Muller when he had to blow the whistle on this idea. At a meeting, at Baylor University, of the Medical Society of Waco County, Texas, in 1928, Muller pointed out that x-ray mutations in man were an unknown area. Also, most mutations were from mildly to seriously deleterious. For every potential beneficial mutation there could be thousands of damaging ones. The certain damage to the race was not worth the uncertain chance of finding and selecting a beneficial mutation. He urged instead that the physicians put their efforts into protecting their patients, themselves, and the race from undesirable degradation of man's precious germ plasm.

The thanks that Muller got was to have many of the physicians in the hall stomp out; a planned future talk to a group of radiologists was canceled. Some of our "storekeepers" had to suffer considerable abuse.

The eugenics movement gradually waned, at least in the United States. But its demise was not in time to prevent the racial superiority ideas of Adolf Hitler from gaining credence and helping to plunge the world into World War II. So much for eugenics.

There were problems, of course, with basing policies concerning radiation protection of the population on information from fruit flies and plants. There was a perceived need to check out the genetic effects of radiation in a species more like the human. Considerable genetic work was done during World War II, using inbred strains of mice; some of it involved x rays. The real opportunity came, however, at the end of World War II, when both the will and the way developed. It was decided to undertake a project know as the "Megamouse Experiment," under the auspices of the newly founded Atomic Energy Commission. The project was so named because it was estimated that a million mice would be needed. (Actually, more than 7 million have been used to date.) An abandoned building dating from the Manhattan Project at Oak Ridge was pressed into service, and scientists began looking at a relatively few specific mutations in the mouse, a species that would allow an investigator to see results over several generations in a reasonable time. William L. Russell was in charge; he and his wife, Leanne (Lee), and their colleagues have done an outstanding job.

The results of the work with mice contrasted in important ways with those from *Drosophila*. Mutations were clearly produced by radiation, but there was a definite dose-rate effect. Recovery seemed to keep pace with damage at low doses, especially in the female. There was actually a region of no effect, at least for the mutations being observed.

This monumental project, covering a period of 30 years, actually downgraded the importance of genetic hazards in setting standards for radiation. Whereas these were considered the greatest hazard in the 1940s and 1950s, the effects on the irradiated individual (i.e., somatic effects such as leukemia, cancer, and other long-term changes) have gradually replaced genetic effects as the controlling hazard. Nevertheless, irradiation of the germ plasm was and is still discouraged. Genetic hazards cannot be termed nonexistent; it just seems that by controlling effects on the individual we can also control effects on the race. Work by this Oak Ridge group is continuing, as evidenced by papers at this meeting.

Several major enterprises helped to sharpen our knowledge of the somatic effects of radiation (i.e., effects on the individual). Some concerned radiation sources external to the body; others concerned the behavior and effects of radioactive materials deposited in the body.

A key enterprise in the external radiation field is the study of the Japanese survivors of the atomic bomb attack on Hiroshima and Nagasaki. This investigation included both somatic and genetic effects, but the latter were difficult to study because of the relatively small size of the population. The studies of leukemia induction and of other effects that are included have given us much of our information on the radiobiology of neutrons in man and have added significantly to our knowledge of gamma-radiation effects. There is currently a temporary hiatus while the exact doses are being revised, but the studies of effects are unchanged by this. It is to the everlasting credit of all concerned that the monumental tragedies of the atomic bombings have been used to advance our knowledge of radiation effects in humans. That applies especially to the Japanese, who not only permitted the study but have taken an active part in it.

Other data from man and external sources have been obtained as corollaries to the medical uses of radiation. Remember that the largest single source of exposure to man-made radiation is in medical uses. Special note should be taken of the groups in England treated with x rays for a painful disease known as ankylosing spondylitis; children in several countries who received x rays for treatment of ringworm of the scalp; radiologists, particularly fluoroscopists, who developed leukemia; and members of the general population who have had diagnostic radiographs. The latter include possible developmental or genetic effects in fetuses irradiated *in utero*. Most of these studies have difficulties with estimation of doses, but they have helped us "mind the store."

There were also some large experiments with animals exposed to x rays to determine the somatic effects of gamma rays. Primary players were Argonne National Laboratory, Colorado State University, the University of California, Davis, and the University of Rochester, where a study of fertility in male dogs took place.

Let us turn now to radiation from radioisotopes deposited in the body. New dimensions were added to the problem during World War II and after by the tremendous increases in the amounts of radioactive materials to be dealt with; by the development of whole new classes of elements, including plutonium; and by the nuclear weapons testing program. We must consider these, albeit briefly. Since it took several chapters in the 2000-plus-page book you have heard about (Stannard, 1988) to describe these efforts, you can imagine the degree of condensing we must utilize.

In the very early days of accelerator- (cyclotron-) produced radioelements, most of the work had to concern how the radioisotopes behaved in the body; there was not enough material to study effects. Pioneering in this was Joe Hamilton at the University of California, Berkeley (Figure 7). The production of larger quantities of the radionuclides in nuclear reactors allowed investigation of effects, largely in rodents but, to some degree, in larger animals. We should remember Miriam Finkel at Argonne National Laboratory Biology Division, then directed by Austin Brues, as the pioneer for the early, relatively long-term studies in the mouse. The work began before the end of World War II. She used a variety of radioisotopes of importance in nuclear energy. Radium was used as a benchmark because of human exposure to it.

Also, in several U.S. locations, a small number of patients deemed to have a short life expectancy were injected with tracer quantities of plutonium and other alpha-emitters to check for any major differences in the behavior of radionuclides in humans and animals. No major differences were evident.

As was the case in the genetic studies, there was a need to repeat the work with a longer-lived species, particularly since the important changes occurred mostly in later life. This resulted in a counterpart of the Megamouse experiment, although this study involved radioisotopes, and the end point was somatic effects, particularly cancer. I have termed these the "King-Sized Experiments." The principal groups involved were Argonne National Laboratory; University of California, Davis; Hanford (Battelle, Pacific Northwest Laboratories); Lovelace Foundation (Inhalation Toxicology Research Institute); and the Universities of Rochester and Utah. These studies required more than 30 years, 200 million dollars, and more than 5000 beagles, plus miscellaneous other animals, such as monkeys at Berkeley and Rochester, grasshopper mice and St. Bernard dogs at Utah, etc. A few of the principal scientists who are no longer with us are shown in Figures 8A through C. We should also pay tribute to the thousands of animals that took part in those studies; there was no other way in those days.

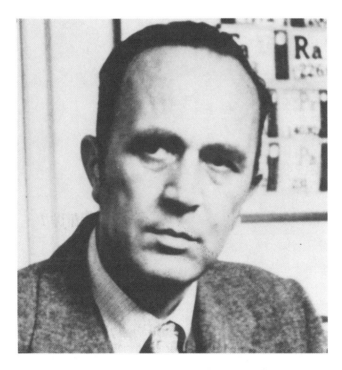

Figure 7. Dr. Joseph G. Hamilton, pioneer investigator and physician at the University of California, Berkeley, who did much of the early work with the cyclotron-produced radio-isotopes. Photograph courtesy P. W. Durbin, Lawrence Berkeley Laboratory.

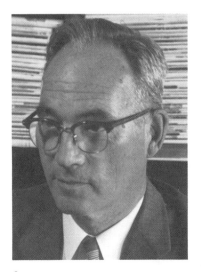

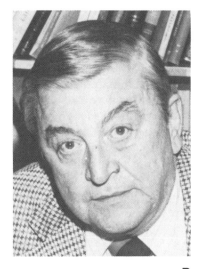

A   B

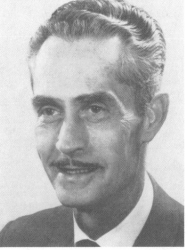

C

Figures 8A through 8C. A. Dr. Henry A. Blair (top left), Director, University of Rochester Atomic Energy Project; Member of Advisory Committee known as "The Founding Fathers" for the Utah project. Photograph courtesy of University of Rochester. **B.** Dr. Thomas Dougherty (top right), early director of the "King-Sized" beagle study at the University of Utah. Photograph courtesy of W. S. S. Jee, University of Utah. **C.** Dr. Wright H. Langham (bottom), Los Alamos Scientific Laboratory, a key figure in undertaking the "King-Sized Experiments" and frequently considered "Mr. Plutonium" in the biomedical realm. Photograph courtesy of Health Physics Society.

These experiments are probably familiar to many of you. The results of some were reviewed at the 22nd Hanford Life Sciences Symposium, held in 1983 and published in 1986 as a DOE Conference report (Thompson and Mahaffey, 1986). Keep an eye out also for the book-length summary of the dog experiments being readied by Roy Thompson under DOE sponsorship. What did all this work tell us? It would take a week to give details; let us consider only a few facts:

1. Plutonium and, to a lesser extent, the other actinides, such as americium, curium, neptunium, and so forth, rank as effective to potent carcinogens in bone or lung if sufficient time elapses. The acute toxicity of these elements is considerably lower than that of many chemical substances, such as botulinus and tetanus toxins, snake venoms, cyanide, strychnine, curare, and the like. This does not tally with the often-quoted remark that "Plutonium is the most toxic element known to man." It is not; it is a very effective, long-term carcinogen. This misconception about plutonium has had serious consequences.

2. Another finding is that radiostrontium is effective as a carcinogen only at relatively high doses.

3. In view of the importance of cesium in the Chernobyl incident and at Bikini, we wish more study had been devoted to it on a long-term basis. However, we are able to extrapolate from external radiation studies, since cesium localizes in the body to a lesser extent than the actinides, and its radiation distribution is more like that of whole-body irradiation.

4. Finally, we must consider the inhalation work. Much of it was done here at Battelle under the leadership of Bill Bair. These were difficult experiments to devise. The techniques for handling aerosols of radioactive materials with safety for the workers and the environment had to be developed from almost a standing start. These experiments taught us much about respiratory physiology and the long-term effects of radionuclides deposited in the lung, as well as about inhalation toxicology in general. This is an important department of our "store."

Along with these fairly practical and programmatic studies, it was possible, as mentioned earlier, to fit in considerable amounts of work bearing on the basic mechanisms of what was going on. This work influenced fundamental respiratory physiology, as just mentioned. The mechanistic aspects of radiobiological research were alluded to very briefly toward the beginning of this lecture. It is an exciting field.

Another area of great importance is the physiology and biochemistry of bone. Since many of the radioactive isotopes deposit in bone, it was possible to learn a great deal about the biology of bone and bone marrow; nearly everything except how the cancers started. Figure 9 shows a member of the group who worked in this field, William F. Neuman, University of Rochester, who died in midcareer. Neuman was a member of a group who called themselves "The Boneheads" because of their mutual interest in bone.

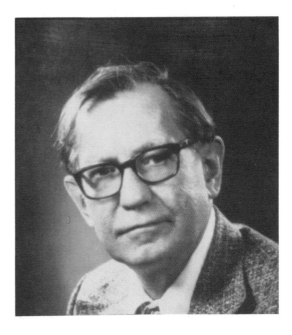

Figure 9. Dr. William F. Neuman, University of Rochester, noted for basic studies of biochemistry of bone using radioisotopes. Photograph courtesy of Margaret Neuman.

Let me close with a brief mention of two other departments in "the store." The first can be likened to the sporting-goods department; it concerns the environment. Its workers poke around in small boats or tramp through deserts, forests, and swamps to get samples of soil, and flora and fauna, or arrange to get samples of airborne radioactivity.

Did you know that major interest in the environmental impact of the atomic energy program began very early here at Hanford? Within a short time after the decision was made to build the plutonium production reactors along the Columbia River, Dr. Stafford L. Warren, medical director of the Manhattan Engineer District, took steps to measure and to ameliorate or prevent any effects of the reactor effluent on the fish or other biota in the Columbia River and its estuary. (Incidentally, Warren was an avid salmon fisherman himself.)

Fortunately, there was a group already at work at the University of Washington Applied Fisheries Laboratory that was studying the effects of x rays on salmon and trout, particularly in their developmental stages. This was under the direction of one of the "greats" in fisheries biology, Lauren Donaldson. Also, fortunately, there were two young men in his department doing thesis research on the subject; they were Richard Foster and Arthur Welander. Thus, this work could be financed and enhanced as an extension of these academic studies without betraying the highly classified fact that radiation had anything to do with what was going on at Hanford. The University of Washington group was later enhanced by the addition of Allyn Seymour, Kelshaw Bonham, and others.

After the reactors were operating, a concentrated and practical test program was set up at Hanford under the aegis of Richard Foster. Fingerlings of salmon and trout were exposed to pile effluent by having it run through troughs in a hatchery-style laboratory. An old picture of the inside of this laboratory is shown in Figure 10. The rest is history. Effects of the pile effluents were not radiation effects, at least over the short term of these studies, but were due to chemicals added to the cooling water to prevent corrosion.

Environmental concerns then multiplied everywhere, so that a new field, "radioecology," was born. It flourished here as both aquatic and terrestrial radioecology under the leadership of Burton Vaughan, Bob Gray, and their many predecessors and colleagues, including J. J. Davis, Joe Soldat, and others. It flourished, too, in the Pacific, in Alaska, at Oak Ridge, and at Savannah River, and is now a mature field. It is closely allied to parallel efforts against environmental pollution with chemicals and, to a degree, has led the way for them. Let it not be said that environmental concerns began with problems of fallout from nuclear weapons tests; the fallout problem merely magnified the efforts into a major challenge. Definite effects of radiation and radioactivity were found on the Pacific atolls as a result of the hydrogen bomb detonations. Also, some were found close to the tests in Nevada. However, it appears that effects of radiation or radioactivity in lower doses were not seen. The ecosystem has tremendous powers of recovery. It would be appropriate, someday, for a Parker lecturer to review these tremendous environmental efforts. Herb Parker always backed such work to the fullest.

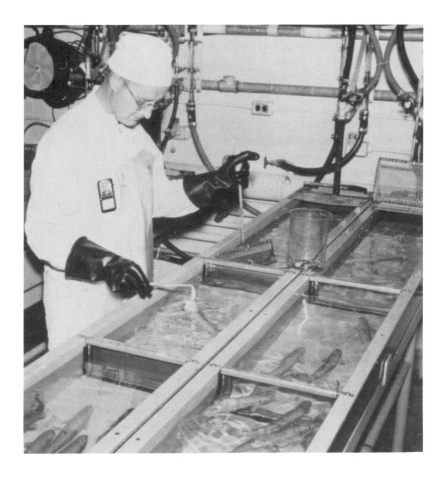

Figure 10. Interior of early laboratory at Hanford used to study effects of pile effluent on salmon and trout fingerlings.

Some of the prominent pioneers (now deceased) in the environmental studies are shown in Figures 11A through C.

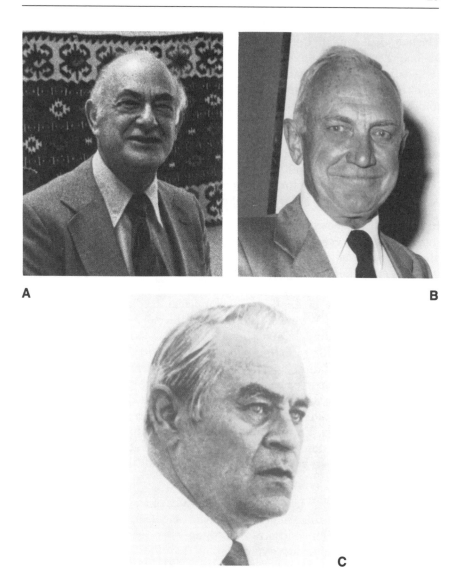

Figures 11A through 11C. A. Dr. Cyril L. Comar (top left), former director of the University of Tennessee-Atomic Energy Commission "Farm" at Oak Ridge and the Cornell University Department of Physical Biology. He devoted his career to studying the movement and effects of radioisotopes in organisms and the environment. Photograph courtesy of L. A. Sagan, Electric Power Research Institute. **B.** Dr. Harry Kornberg (top right), for many years director of the Biology operation at Hanford (later Battelle, Pacific Northwest Laboratories), which sponsored much environmental as well as laboratory research. **C.** Dr. John N. Wolfe (bottom), ecologist from Ohio State University, who spearheaded the development of radioecology as a field. From Cushing (1976).

The last "department" I wish to speak about has to be characterized as the glamour department of our store. I refer to "nuclear medicine." Soon after radioiodine was made available from the cyclotron (accelerator), the people at Berkeley and MIT thought of its possible use for treating hyperthyroidism and also, in tracer doses, to measure thyroid function in place of the old, clumsy, basal metabolism test. World War II delayed developments for both diagnosis and therapy because there was not much material available outside of the Manhattan District centers. All of that changed when isotopes by the dozens could be separated in quantity from the mixed fission products in a nuclear reactor. Large quantities were made available by the AEC, essentially free, to the medical profession and for research.

In the first two decades after World War II, there were high hopes for therapeutic uses, especially in cancer treatment. However, the problem of delivering a therapeutic dose to unwanted tissue while producing minimal damage to normal tissue haunted most efforts. We now have a few tried and true therapeutic uses for a few radioisotopes that work well. However, by far the majority of applications of nuclear medicine today are for diagnostic purposes. With the help of sophisticated detecting equipment and computer recording, both static and dynamic functions of many organs can be examined. The radiations from the injected radioisotopes make a picture on the scintillation screen. Bill Myers, a pioneer in nuclear medicine at Ohio State University, has termed the process "inside-out radiology," i.e., instead of using a radiation source outside the body and taking some sort of picture after the rays pass through, the source is inside the body and projects a picture out. Fortunately, the detecting equipment is so sensitive that only minuscule doses of radiation need be delivered to the body. Also, the isotopes used have very short half-lives and thus do not irradiate for very long.

It is now estimated that from a quarter to a third of all hospital admissions in the United States utilize some sort of nuclear medical procedure. This is a happy field, for it can concentrate on things that usually do some good, either in supplying diagnostic information or in therapy. It is glamorous and well-heeled; nevertheless, its practitioners are basically a part of "the store" devoted to guarding our health. Reducing patient doses is still an objective of much of their developmental work.

There is much more, but l think you get the picture. *The store has been tended.* Developments in nuclear energy have been continually monitored by a dedicated corps of biomedical scientists concerned with the health of people and the environment. In the early days, that is, 1900 to 1930, reaction was much delayed, and much damage was done before the whistle could be blown. Now, consideration of health and safety occupies a central position in most applications of nuclear science. Projects can be and have been stopped or prevented by considerations of health and safety. Some of the physicists connected with the development of the bomb have turned to biology; Leo Szilard, for example.

Nuclear power is considered moribund in the United States, even though nuclear medicine flourishes. Have we gone too far? In our zeal to mind the store have we forgotten that this is a world of checks and balances? Have we really balanced risk and benefit? Or do we have warring factions that do not listen to each other? We do, indeed, have problems with communication. They can be illustrated metaphorically by Figure 12. The man in the picture is a California State Senator who came all the way down to San Diego from Sacramento to investigate whether or not an elephant named Dunda, at the Wild Animal Park, had been abused. As you see, they are engaged in earnest conversation. However, the Senator couldn't get an answer. The elephant couldn't tell him. (Even if she could, would she spill the beans with the keeper right there?) Any direct evidence of mistreatment had disappeared by the time of his visit. Many of our problems in communication in the field of nuclear energy are not unlike this one, although I would not liken either the pros or the cons in the nuclear energy controversy to the elephant. Perhaps it is best to liken the elephant to Mother Nature: She gives up her secrets, particularly biological secrets, with great reluctance. Perhaps some real experts on elephants could extract an answer, but because they knew something about the subject, they would, very likely, be accused of conflict of interest.

I would like to quote from a recent address given at a medical meeting:

> "Whatever else we do, we must be sure that our historic opportunity is not lost. The glorious progress of biomedical science has given us a chance to face a major pandemic pathogen without panic and without resorting to draconian extremes of social reaction. We must insist that the firm basis of understanding provided by science is actually used to form the foundation of our policy making. I can think of no more profligate behavior than to abandon our hard-won progress to a public outcry of anachronistic fear."

The subject here was not nuclear energy but AIDS; the remarks were made by June E. Osborn, M.D., at the Association of American Medical Colleges' Council of Deans on November 8, 1987.

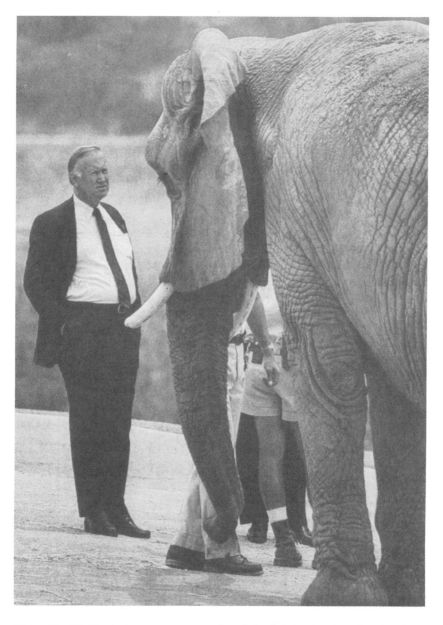

Figure 12. A California state senator meets alleged abuse victim, Dunda, at San Diego Wild Animal Park. From *San Diego Union*, June 18, 1988; published with permission.

The parallel to the dilemmas of nuclear energy is obvious, except that nuclear energy problems (except those of a nuclear war), although significant, pale by comparison to the problems of AIDS. Is it so nearly impossible to do the nuclear energy bit *right* that we should continue, unabated, our use of huge quantities of fossil fuels that spew out carbon dioxide and other gases and, by the greenhouse effect, might eventually make the earth uninhabitable? We must think this one through carefully without anachronistic fear.

One final point. In musing on the procession of dedicated and talented people who have taken part in understanding the effects of radiation and guarding our health, I got to thinking of how little recognition they and their work have received compared to the developers of bombs and reactors. However, they are not complaining, partly, I believe, because it is the nature of the human spirit to do what they have done. I was searching for words to say more about the spirit of these people when I found that someone else had already said just what I was thinking and probably said it better. Dr. Sherwin B. Nuland teaches surgery and the history of medicine at Yale University and has recently published a book entitled *Doctors—The Biography of Medicine* (Nuland, 1981). This is a history of medicine from Hippocrates to organ transplantation and is done as a series of selected minibiographies. The following is taken from the introduction to his book:

> "In these days, when it seems unrealistic to predict a future for mankind that is anything but bleak, I find something in the procession of characters that gives me hope. The reverence for life, the zeal for learning nature's secrets, the willingness to sacrifice for progress . . . are characteristics that I believe are inherent in our species, notwithstanding the mass self-inflicted tragedies to which our century has been witness. . . . I am convinced that there is a biologically determined characteristic that is the human spirit—that there is a gene or genes for it, just as surely as there is a gene or genes for the color of our eyes and the length of our fingers."

Let us give thanks. Gene or no gene, the procession of characters we have considered here fits the pattern. One of the chiefs among them is Herbert M. Parker (Figure 13). I cannot assure you that all is well with the world because of the spirit and the work of those who kept "the store." But I can assure you that it is considerably better than it would have been without them.

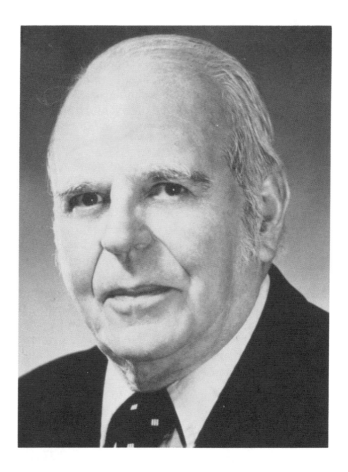

Figure 13. Herbert M. Parker, Battelle, Pacific Northwest Laboratories (Hanford), pioneer in radiation protection, in whose honor and memory this lecture was given.

REFERENCES

Carlson, EA. 1981. *Genes, Radiation and Society: The Life and Values of H. J. Muller*. Cornell University Press, Ithaca, NY.

Cushing, CE, Jr. (ed.). 1976. *Radioecology and Energy Resources*, Proceedings of the Fourth National Symposium on Radioecology, May 12-14, 1975, Oregon State University. Dowden, Hutchinson and Ross, Stroudsburg, PA.

Nauda, ER. 1982. The first nuclear industry. Sci Am 247:180-193.

Nuland, SB. 1981. *Doctors—The Biography of Medicine*. AA Knopf, New York.

Rhodes, R. 1987. *The Making of the Atomic Bomb*. Simon and Schuster, New York.

Stannard, JN. 1988. *Radioactivity and Health—A History*. DOE/RL/01830-T59 (DE88013791). NTIS, Springfield, VA. Available from Life Sciences Center, Battelle, Pacific Northwest Laboratories, Richland, WA 99352.

Thompson, RC and JA Mahaffey. 1986. *Life-Span Radiation Effects Studies in Animals: What Can They Tell Us?* CONF-830951 (DE87000491), NTIS, Springfield, VA.

Mutagenesis and Molecular Cytogenetics: A Multilevel Approach

ZYGOTE-DERIVED DEVELOPMENTAL ANOMALIES, A NEW END POINT OF MUTAGENESIS IN MICE*

W. M. Generoso[1] and J. C. Rutledge[2]

[1]Biology Division, Oak Ridge National Laboratory, Oak Ridge, TN 37831

[2]Department of Laboratories, Children's Hospital and Medical Center, Seattle, WA 98105

Key words: *Mice, mutagenesis, malformations, zygotes*

ABSTRACT

There are three generally known methods for the experimental induction of developmental anomalies in mammals. First, high frequencies of congenital anomalies are generated by exposing the embryo to teratogens *in utero*. The type of anomaly produced is closely related to the stage of development. In mice, the highest overall yield of anomalies occurs when exposures are given during the period of major organogenesis, between days 6 and 13 of gestation. Second, certain mutations that arise following premating exposure of parents to mutagens are expressed as congenital anomalies, but this type has been observed only rarely. Third, integration of transgenes (exogenous DNA sequences) into the mouse genome has proved to be a successful method of producing developmental mutants for basic studies.

We have discovered yet another effective method of inducing congenital anomalies. High frequencies of fetal malformations and death were induced when female mice were exposed to the mutagens ethylene oxide (by inhalation) or ethyl methanesulfonate (by intraperitoneal injection) near the time when their eggs were fertilized or during early stages of zygote development. The effects were absent or minimal when females were exposed either before copulation or after the fertilized eggs had progressed to the stage of precleavage DNA synthesis and beyond.

In studying the possible mechanisms for this phenomenon, we performed a reciprocal zygote transfer experiment, which showed that the effects were not mediated by the maternal environment, and a first-cleavage cytogenetic study, in which obvious numerical or structural chromosome anomalies were absent. Thus, while the evidence suggests a genetic basis for the fetal anomalies, the nature of

*This research was jointly sponsored by NIEHS under Interagency Agreement Y01-ES-20085 and the Office of Health and Environmental Research, U.S. DOE, under Contract DE-AC05-85OR21400 with Martin Marietta Energy Systems, Inc.

the damage has not yet been identified in mammalian mutagenesis. The zygote-derived developmental anomalies could be the result of changes in gene expression.

The fetal malformations produced in these studies are generally similar to sporadic common human defects, for which the etiology is usually unknown. Thus, the new phenomenon is of major interest both in chemical safety evaluation and in studying the etiology of congenital abnormalities. Not only does it raise questions regarding the vulnerability of human zygotes when the mother is exposed to environmental chemicals shortly after conception, but it may provide a model for the class of congenital malformations in humans for which the etiology is unknown.

INTRODUCTION

Induction of transmissible mutations in mice has been demonstrated for many chemicals to which certain groups of humans are exposed. Assessment of genetic risk to humans from these environmental mutagens requires identification and quantification, in experimental systems, of the types of mutagenic damage that they can produce in the germ line and transmit to the conceptuses. Conventionally, the types of genetic damage considered in this process are gene mutations (dominant, semidominant, and recessive), small deficiences, structural chromosomal anomalies (reciprocal translocations, inversions, duplications, etc.), and numerical chromosomal anomalies (whole chromosomes missing or in excess). This report presents yet another type of mutagenic response whose nature is still unknown.

A NEW PHENOMENON IN EXPERIMENTAL EMBRYOPATHY

Extensive experience in this and other laboratories in using the dominant lethal test in mice to study clastogenicity of chemicals and ionizing radiations in male and female germ cells has shown conclusively that induced dominant lethals are expressed no later than the periimplantation period, at which stage embryonic death is manifested as resorption bodies. However, in a preliminary experiment in which females were exposed by inhalation to a high concentration of ethylene oxide (EtO) for 1.5 hr, beginning 6 hr after mating, we observed a high frequency of mid- and late-gestation fetal deaths. It was clear that the response was a departure from the conventional clastogenic response. Follow-up EtO studies (Generoso et al., 1987, 1988) confirmed this observation and also revealed high frequencies of malformations among living fetuses; furthermore, they showed that the mutagen ethyl methanesulfonate (EMS) produced a similar response.

The response is highly stage specific. A high level of response occurred when females were exposed at 1 or 6 hr after mating, times that corresponded to prefertilization egg and sperm and early pronuclear zygote stages, respectively. In contrast, effects were absent or minimal when females were exposed at a later pronuclear stage (during DNA synthesis); at 1 day after mating when the embryos are at the two-cell stage; or before mating, when the oocytes were in maturing follicles.

FETAL PATHOLOGY

This new class of experimentally induced fetal anomalies was analyzed in detail by qualitative characterization of the defects and the progression of aberrant development (Rutledge and Generoso, 1989). Fetal death was multitemporal, ranging from mid- to late-gestation stages. Among living fetuses, malformations were varied and included hydrops, small size, cleft palate, and eye, cardiac, abdominal wall, and extremity and/or tail defects. The expression of most malformations did not become apparent until late gestation. Interestingly, many of the defects have analogies in humans, such as cleft palate, omphalocele, club foot, and hydrops. These defects are very frequent, and their etiology is largely unknown (Czeizel, 1985; Oakley, 1986).

FETAL ANOMALIES ARE A MUTAGENIC RESPONSE

Both EtO and EMS are well-known clastogens that produce dominant lethal mutations and reciprocal translocations in certain germ cell stages of male mice (Ehling et al., 1968; Cattanach et al., 1968; Generoso et al., 1980; Generoso, 1986). Nevertheless, because the mothers were exposed to these chemicals, the fetal anomalies might have resulted from maternal toxicity. That this new class of fetal anomalies is induced as a direct effect of the mutagens on the zygotes has been established by Katoh et al. (1989). Katoh et al. carried out a reciprocal transfer of pronuclear zygotes within hours after treatment, followed by cytogenetic analyses of pronuclear metaphases, early cleavage embryos, and midgestation fetuses. Results of the transplantation experiment ruled out maternal toxicity as a factor in the fetal maldevelopment; together with the strict stage specificity, this points to a genetic effect. The cytogenetic study failed to show structural or numerical chromosomal aberrations, however, and it was concluded (Katoh et al., 1989) that intragenic base changes and deletions could also be eliminated. Thus, it appears that the genetic lesions induced by EMS or EtO in zygotes are not the same as those that caused conventional chromosomal aberrations and gene mutations and may, therefore, be a new type of mutagenic event.

DIFFERENTIAL RESPONSE TO MUTAGENS

Mutagens other than EMS and EtO have been shown to produce developmental anomalies among fetuses after exposure of early pronuclear zygotes: these include ethyl nitrosourea (ENU), triethylene melamine (TEM), neutrons, and x rays (Generoso et al., 1988; Pampfer and Streffer, 1988). The striking observation is that, in contrast to EtO and EMS, these other mutagens did not increase the incidence of mid- and late-gestation fetal deaths. This difference suggests that the type of mutagenic events causing various types of fetal anomalies may differ from one mutagen to another. For example, conventional gene mutations and chromosomal aberrations are not the likely mechanisms for EMS- and EtO-induced fetal anomalies, but gene mutations might be involved in the case of ENU. Russell et al. (1988) observed that the zygotic stages were highly sensitive to ENU induction of presumed intragenic point mutations.

RELEVANCE TO PROBLEMS IN HUMAN PRENATAL DEVELOPMENT

Most human fetal malformations are of unknown etiology (Shepard, 1984). The observation that many of the anomalies produced in the mouse studies described here are similar to the human malformations in this class (Rutledge and Generoso, 1989) raises the possibility that one mechanism for human malformation is genetic, but of a type that is still unknown. Further, the new phenomenon implies vulnerability of the human conceptus to mutagenic damage during the stages from fertilization through zygote and, therefore, has important implications for developmental toxicology.

The nature of the underlying mutagenic damage and the molecular pathogenesis of the anomalies await investigation. The mouse experimental system presents an opportunity to carry out this investigation by virtue of the accessibility of the zygote and its descendant blastomeres. Studies on the molecular mechanisms of the zygotic response could contribute to the understanding of the etiology of certain sporadic but common human malformations, and provide the biological foundation for toxicological evaluation.

SUMMARY

High frequencies of fetal malformations and death were induced when female mice were exposed to the mutagens ethylene oxide or ethyl methanesulfonate near fertilization or during early stages of zygote development. The evidence suggests a genetic basis for the fetal anomalies, but the mechanism has not yet been identified. The fetal malformations produced in these studies are generally similar to sporadic common human defects, for which the etiology is also largely unknown.

ACKNOWLEDGMENTS

The submitted manuscript has been authored by a contractor of the U.S. Government under contract DE-AC05-84OR21400. Accordingly, the U.S. Government retains a nonexclusive, royalty-free license to publish or reproduce the published form of this contribution, or allow others to do so, for U.S. Government purposes. Research was sponsored by the Office of Health and Environmental Research, U.S. Department of Energy, under contract DE-AC05-84OR21400 with the Martin Marietta Energy Systems, Inc.

REFERENCES

Cattanach, BM, CE Pollard, and JH Isaacson. 1968. Ethyl methanesulfonate-induced chromosome breakage in the mouse. Mutat Res 6:297-307.

Czeizel, A. 1985. Teratoepidemiology, pp. 7-10. In: *Prevention of Physical and Mental Congenital Defects*, Part B, M Marois (ed.). Alan R. Liss, New York.

Ehling, UH, RB Cumming, and HV Malling. 1968. Induction of dominant-lethal mutations by alkylating agents in male mice. Mutat Res 5:417-428.

Generoso, WM. 1986. Relationship between alkylation sites and induction of dominant lethals and heritable translocation in mice, pp. 493-500. In: *Genetic Toxicology of Environmental Chemicals, Part B: Genetic Effects and Applied Mutagenesis*, C Ramel, B Lambert, and J Magnusson (eds.). Alan R. Liss, New York.

Generoso, WM, KT Cain, M Krishna, CW Sheu, and RM Gryder. 1980. Heritable translocation and dominant-lethal mutation induction with ethylene oxide in mice. Mutat Res 73:133-142.

Generoso, WM, JC Rutledge, KT Cain, LA Hughes, and PW Braden. 1987. Exposure of female mice to ethylene oxide within hours after mating leads to fetal malformations and death. Mutat Res 176:269-274.

Generoso, WM, JC Rutledge, KT Cain, LA Hughes, and DJ Downing. 1988. Mutagen-induced fetal anomalies and death following treatment of females within hours after mating. Mutat Res 199:175-181.

Katoh, M, NLA Cacheiro, CV Cornett, KT Cain, JC Rutledge, and WM Generoso. 1989. Fetal anomalies produced subsequent to treatment of zygotes with ethylene oxide or ethylene methanesulfonate are not likely due to the usual genetic causes. Mutat Res 210:337-344.

Oakley, GP. 1986. Frequency of human congenital malformations. Clin Perinatol 13:545-554.

Pampfer, S and C Streffer. **1988.** Prenatal death and malformations after irradiation of mouse zygotes with neutrons or x-rays. Teratology 37:599-607.

Russell, LB, JW Bangham, KF Stelzner, and PR Hunsicker. **1988.** High frequency of mosaic mutants produced by N-ethyl-N-nitrosourea exposure of mouse zygotes. Proc Natl Acad Sci USA 85:9167-9170.

Rutledge, JC and WM Generoso. **1989.** The fetal pathology produced by ethylene oxide treatment of the murine zygote. Teratology 39:563-572.

Shepard, TH. **1984.** Teratogenesis, pp. 499-527. In: *Mutation, Cancer, and Malformation*, EHY Chu and WM Generoso (eds.). Plenum, New York.

THE MOUSE MODEL FOR MUTATION IN LYMPHOCYTES: CELLULAR AND MOLECULAR STUDIES

I. M. Jones, K. Burkhart-Schultz, and C. Strout

Lawrence Livermore National Laboratory, P.O. Box 5507, Livermore, CA 94550

Key words: *Somatic mutation, hprt, molecular, lymphocytes, mouse*

ABSTRACT

We have developed a mouse model for analysis of somatic mutation, which enables us to study factors that affect the frequency and molecular nature of spontaneous and induced genetic changes affecting the HPRT gene of lymphocytes *in vivo*. We combine *in vivo* induction with *in vitro* isolation and analysis of mutations. The HPRT gene, the basis of a powerful mutant selection system, is a 34-kilobase (-kb) genetic target whose molecular biology has been well characterized. We have used ethyl nitrosourea (ENU) and gamma radiation as test mutagens for determining such cellular characteristics of mutants as expression time, persistence, and dose (rate) dependence of mutant frequency and to evaluate the spectrum of mutations that can be recovered in this system. Expression time in spleen lymphocytes was 3 wk; that for thymus lymphocytes was 1 wk. Both ENU- and gamma-radiation-induced mutants persisted *in vivo* for at least 1 yr.

Mutagen-specific characteristics of persistence, as well as the shapes of the dose-response curves and the effect of dose fractionation, have revealed the roles of repair and the repopulation kinetics of the mature lymphocyte compartment in *in vivo* mutagenesis of lymphocytes. We use Southern analysis to study the extent of major alterations affecting the HPRT gene.

Spontaneous mutations include partial and complete gene deletions, putative gene rearrangements, and putative gene mutations. Deletions of as many as 70 kb of flanking sequence have been detected both up and downstream of HPRT, using pulsed-field gel electrophoresis of DNA from mutants that have partially deleted HPRT genes. Point mutations are being identified by sequence analysis of enzymatically amplified DNA.

Substantial evidence from human epidemiology and rodent studies indicates that exposure of somatic cells to certain agents, including mutagens, increases the risk of cancer. In addition, steadily increasing chromosomal and molecular evidence indicates that particular mutations of the human genome are present in tumor cells. For example, rearrangement of DNA can lead to activation of genetic information, as in B-cell lymphomas and leukemias in which the *c-myc* oncogene comes under the control of an active immunoglobulin gene after a chromosome translocation that may have involved immunoglobulin gene recombinases (Haluska et al., 1986). Conversion of a heterozygote to a homozygous recessive, by point mutation, deletion, or other means, is involved in retinoblastoma (Cavenee et al., 1983; Dunn et al., 1988).

Our research effort focuses on understanding the mechanisms of somatic mutation *in vivo*. Our critical initial goal is to identify the characteristics of particular target sequences that affect the types of mutations that can occur and be recovered in them. Knowledge of the types of mutations induced by test agents in specific target sequences will help us identify patterns of mutation that predict the consequences of exposures. By comparing exposed and unexposed individuals, we may also be able to identify mutations that serve as indicators of genetically significant exposures and individuals at increased risk from particular exposures. Our mouse model system fills a major gap between work that can be performed *in vitro* and that performed in humans. By working *in vivo*, with mice, with cells analogous to those used in studies of humans, we are able to analyze the effects of factors such as tissue, dose rate, mutant persistence, and age. In addition, target cells can be studied in their normal histological and physiological context, in animals with genetically defined metabolic and repair capacities and under controlled conditions of exposure.

In our current studies we are using the hypoxanthine phosphoribosyltransferase gene (*hprt*) of mouse lymphocytes as the target for *in vivo* mutagenesis. By choosing the *hprt* gene, we start with a powerful selection system for cells with defective *hprt* function and a gene whose structure at the molecular level is well documented (Melton et al., 1984). By choosing lymphocytes, we can measure mutant frequencies *in vitro* after *in vivo* exposures to a mutagen and expand mutant lymphocyte clones for analyzing the molecular identity of mutations. At the same time we can gain insight into the molecular toxicology of hemopoietic tissues. The methods we use are similar to those first developed for studies of human lymphocytes by Albertini et al. (1982) and Morley et al. (1983), which are being used by their groups and others to study normal and exposed humans.

Our studies at the tissue and cellular levels have led to knowledge of characteristics of normal and mutant lymphocytes, and of their precursor cells, that has affected our approach to detailed molecular comparisons of spontaneous and exposure-induced mutations. In particular, we have learned that time elapsed since exposure is an especially important variable *in vivo*, one that reveals the interdependence of mechanisms of mutagen action and the normal events of lymphocyte ontogeny. Tissue-specific cell cycle distributions and DNA active enzymes affect cytotoxicity, repair, and mutability, and are subject to change as a function of age and exposure history. We have learned that repopulation of lymphocytes from precursor tissues leads to shifts in mutant frequencies, which could have associated shifts in the relative frequencies of different types of mutations (mutation spectra). Over time, mutant frequency and mutation spectrum can also be affected by expansion of immunologically active clones and by selection pressures. Nicklas et al. (1986) used T-cell receptor genes as markers of clonality to recognize clonal expansion of T lymphocytes. Analysis of mutation spectra is needed to detect mutation-specific selection pressures.

We have used two model mutagens, ethyl nitrosourea (ENU) and gamma radiation, to analyze characteristics of mouse T lymphocytes that have mutations at the *hprt* locus. Studies of the frequency of mutants induced with gamma radiation, which induces mutations independent of cell cycling, have revealed that the expression time of thioguanine-resistant, HPRT-deficient T cells is only 1 wk in the mitotically active thymus, but it is 3 wk in the spleen. Thus, one cannot expect to recover mutations induced in mature, noncycling lymphocytes until several weeks after an exposure. With ENU, a potent mutagen whose interaction with DNA requires no metabolic action, we also noted differences between target tissues. Maximal frequencies of mutated cells appeared in the thymus at 2 wk after exposure, whereas maximal frequencies of ENU-induced mutants appeared in the spleen after 10 wk of steadily increasing mutant frequencies (Jones et al., 1987a). For mutagens whose action requires cell cycling to convert adducts to mutations, maximal frequencies of mutated T cells apparently are recoverable from the thymus more quickly than from the spleen. We attribute the slow accumulation of mutants in the spleen to a combination of repopulation of the spleen with mutants originally induced in the thymus and bone marrow, and conversion of stable ENU adducts to mutations in long-lived cells of the spleen. It will be important to determine if there are differences in the mutations induced immediately after an exposure and those derived from stable adducts in long-lived cells. Persistence of mutant lymphocytes and the relationship of persistence to the molecular nature of the mutation may also be important to *in vivo* studies of induced mutations. We have determined that both ENU and gamma radiation induce elevated frequencies of mutant T lymphocytes that persist for at least 1 yr in the mouse. Because the induced elevated mutant frequencies varied over time, it will be important to determine whether the changes in mutant frequency were associated with selection against certain classes of mutations and if these changes were related to the dynamics of the hemopoietic system.

With both model mutagens we have detected agent-specific dose-rate effects on mutant frequency that may produce differences in the types of mutations induced by chronic and acute exposures. With five weekly doses of 11.7 mg ENU/kg, the frequency and persistence of mutants induced was the same as that induced by one dose of 58 mg ENU/kg (Jones et al., 1987a). This efficiency of induction of mutants was more than predicted by the response to a single fraction of 11.7 mg ENU/kg, suggesting that fractionated exposure to mutagens that induce stable adducts can lead to saturation of repair capacity and hence to efficiency of mutation induction similar to that of acute exposures. In contrast, fractionation of gamma radiation, eight daily doses of 50 cGy versus one dose of 400 cGy, resulted in less efficient induction of mutations (14×10^{-6} thioguanine-resistant spleen mutants at 3 wk after exposure versus 83×10^{-6}), presumably because of more effective repair with the fractionated dose.

We are applying powerful new techniques to the analysis of the DNA structure and sequence of mutations in the *hprt* gene of mouse lymphocytes to learn about mutation of this locus *per se* and to address questions about the induction and persistence of mutations in cells *in vivo* . It is critical to analyze mutations that occur spontaneously, both to determine the types of mutations that are recoverable in the mouse model system and to enable detection of changes in mutation spectrum associated with exposure and other variables. Using Southern blot analysis, we have determined that a high proportion of the mutant lymphocytes in unexposed, young-adult male mice have deletions or major rearrangements affecting the *hprt* locus (Jones et al., 1987b). Of 25 mutants studied, 7 had total deletions, 10 had partial deletions of the *hprt* locus, and 5 had no changes detectable by Southern analysis. We have used field inversion gel electrophoresis of high molecular weight, genomic DNA of mutants that carry part of the *hprt* locus, and Southern analysis with a cDNA probe, to determine that up to 70 kb of DNA can be deleted either upstream or downstream of the *hprt* gene. The high frequency of deletions demonstrates that there are no essential loci close to the *hprt* gene on the mouse X chromosome whose loss might prevent recovery of deletions. The high proportion of deletions is similar to that seen in human newborns (McGinnis and Albertini, 1988). Mutations that occur in the thymus during differentiation of T lymphocytes apparently are more likely to be deletions and rearrangements than are mutations that occur in mature T cells. T-cell receptor recombinases in thymus cells may in part be responsible for this distinction (Alt et al., 1987). Southern analysis of limited numbers of induced mutants (2 for ENU and 10 for gamma radiation) indicated that the spectrum of mutations can be shifted to either no changes detectable by Southern analysis, or more total deletions of the locus, respectively.

Enzymatic amplification of genomic DNA (Saiki et al., 1985, 1988), also known as polymerase chain reaction (PCR), allows us to selectively analyze the sequence of the exons of the 34-kb *hprt* locus (Melton et al., 1984). By synthesizing oligonucleotides with homology to the intron sequences that flank an exon, we have amplified exon DNAs of seven mutants that have no changes detectable by Southern analysis. We start with small amounts of either crude cell lysates or genomic DNA preparations in solution or agarose inserts and produce up to 300 ng of exon-specific DNA after 30 cycles of amplification of 0.1 µg of genomic DNA. At present we have PCR primers for exons 1, 3, 8, and 9; we will sequence additional flanking regions for the other exons and apply the method to them as well. We have detected no mutations in the amplified exon 8 of the five spontaneous and two ENU-induced mutants sequenced to date, although we have confirmed the mutation reported for a neuroblastoma cell line (NBR4) previously reported by Konecki et al. (1982). The PCR methodology will be invaluable in studies of the effect of tissue, dose, dose rate, persistence *in vivo*, and clonality. It will be used to simultaneously screen for deletions affecting exons of the *hprt* gene and synthesize exon-specific segments for sequencing of exons that are retained.

In summary, we are combining *in vivo* mutagenesis in the mouse with molecular analysis of mutations of a specific genetic target to increase our understanding of the mechanisms of somatic mutation. Techniques currently applied to the *hprt* gene may in the future be applied to other genetic sequences, thereby allowing us to extend our analysis of the role of genome structure in mutagenesis.

ACKNOWLEDGMENT

Work was performed under the auspices of the U.S. Department of Energy by Lawrence Livermore National Laboratory under contract W-7405-ENG-48.

REFERENCES

Albertini, RJ, KL Castle, and WR Borcherding. 1982. T-cell cloning to detect the mutant 6-thioguanine-resistant lymphocytes present in human peripheral blood. Proc Natl Acad Sci USA 79:6617-6621.

Cavenee, WK, TP Dryja, RA Phillips, WF Benedict, R Godbout, BL Gallie, AL Murphree, LC Strong, and RL White. **1983.** Expression of recessive alleles by chromosomal mechanisms in retinoblastoma. Nature 779:779-784.

Dunn, JM, RA Phillips, AJ Becker, and BL Gallie. **1988.** Identification of germline and somatic mutations affecting the retinoblastoma gene. Science 241:1797-1800.

Haluska, FG, S Finver, Y Tjujimoto, and CM Croce. **1986.** The t(8;14) chromosomal translocation occurring in B-cell malignancies results from mistakes in V-D-J joining. Nature 324:158-160.

Jones, IM, K Burkhart-Schultz, and CL Strout. **1987a.** Factors that affect the frequency of thioguanine-resistant lymphocytes in mice following exposure to ethylnitrosourea. Environ Mutagen 9:317-329.

Jones, IM, K Burkhart-Schultz, and TC Crippen. **1987b.** Cloned mouse lymphocytes permit analysis of somatic mutations that occur in vivo. Somatic Cell Mol Genet 13:325-333.

Konecki, DS, J Brennand, JC Fuscoe, CT Caskey, and AC Chinault. **1982.** Hypoxanthine-guanine phosphoribosyltransferase genes of mouse and Chinese hamster: Construction and sequence analysis of cDNA recombinants. Nucleic Acids Res 10:6763-6775.

McGinnis, MJ and RJ Albertini. **1988.** Deletions predominate in "spontaneous" *hprt* mutant T-cells of the human newborn. Environ Mol Mutagen (Suppl) 11:68.

Melton, DW, DS Konecki, J Brennand, and CT Caskey. **1984.** Structure, expression, and mutation of the hypoxanthine phosphoribosyltransferase gene. Proc Natl Acad Sci USA 81:2147-2151.

Morley, AA, KJ Trainor, R Seshadri, and RG Ryall. **1983.** Measurement of in vivo mutations in human lymphocytes. Nature 302:155-156.

Nicklas, JA, JP O'Neill, and RJ Albertini. **1986.** Use of the T cell receptor gene probes to quantify the *in vivo hprt* mutations in human T lymphocytes. Mutat Res 173:65-72.

Saiki, RK, S Scharf, F Faloona, KB Mullis, GT Horn, HA Erlich, and N Arnheim. **1985.** Enzymatic amplification of β-globin genomic sequences and restriction site analysis for diagnosis of sickle cell anemia. Science 230:1350-1354.

Saiki, RK, DH Gelfans, S Stoffel, SJ Scharf, R Higuchi, GT Horn, KB Mullis, and HA Erlich. **1988.** Primer directed enzymatic amplification of DNA with a thermostable DNA polymerase. Science 23:487-491.

QUESTIONS AND COMMENTS

Q: Jostes, PNL, Richland, WA
Did you use a heterozygous female or the functionally hemizygous male for this study?

A: The male (perhaps in the future we'll be able to avoid this chauvinistic circumstance), but for studies of genomic DNA, the hemizygous state is highly preferred.

Q: Brooks, Lovelace, ITRI, Albuquerque, NM
I am very interested in the persistence of the chemically induced mutations. The fact that these mutations are expressed for a long time after induction suggests that either the mutant cells have a very long life span or that the changes are induced in progenitor cells. These cells then continue to produce mutated cells over long time periods. Would you speculate on which of these options you think is responsible for the persistence of the mutations in the blood cells of the mouse.

A: I believe that both mechanisms contribute to the persistence of induced mutant lymphocytes. I have direct evidence at present only with respect to precursor tissues as a continuing source of induced mutants. In our study of persistence of ENU-induced mutants, we studied mutant frequency of both thymus and spleen cells. The thymus data, not presented here, suggest that mutants are initially induced very efficiently in the thymus, and that over time, as the thymus is successively repopulated by cells from thymic precursors (short term) and bone marrow (long term), elevated frequencies of thymus mutants can be seen up to at least 30 wk after exposure to ENU. Mutant frequencies in the thymus fluctuated dramatically at times later than 3 wk after exposure to ENU, suggesting that small cohorts of cells repopulate the thymus at any given time, and sample the mutant pool in bone-marrow precursor cells.

Q: Morgan, PNL, Richland, WA
Would you care to speculate about the apparent clustering of deletion breakpoints between exons 1 and 2?

A: Although an enriched number of deletion end points fall between exons 1 and 2, this region is a large one (almost 11 kb). Our precision in locating the precise breakpoint is low, as we are using a cDNA probe, and a unique probe from intron 1 that is close to exon 1, to probe our blots. Finer resolution mapping and inclusion of more mutants will be needed to determine if there are hot spots for deletion and rearrangement breakpoints.

CHEMICAL BINDING TO MOLECULAR TARGETS IN MAMMALIAN GERM CELLS AND ITS GENETIC CONSEQUENCES

G. A. Sega

Biology Division, Oak Ridge National Laboratory, P. O. Box 2009, Oak Ridge, TN 37831-8077

Key words: *Germ cells, molecular targets, protamine, DNA*

ABSTRACT

We have found that protamines, as well as DNA, are important molecular targets for chemical attack that may lead to chromosome aberrations. (The sperm protamines of both mouse and man are simple proteins that are intimately associated with DNA and found only in late-spermatid and mature-sperm stages.)

Experiments in which mice were exposed to ethylene oxide (EtO) or acrylamide (AA) showed large increases in chemical binding to late-spermatid and early-spermatozoa stages. Alkylation of DNA within these stages generally amounted to less than 1% of the total germ-cell alkylation; the remaining adducts were found to be bound to protamine. Furthermore, the pattern of both EtO- and AA-binding to protamine paralleled the pattern of genetic damage produced by these chemicals in the spermiogenic stages, while DNA alkylation showed no correlation with genetic damage.

Amino acid analysis of protamine recovered from AA-treated animals showed that the sulfhydryl groups of cysteine were being alkylated. Coupled with the results described above, this observation has been used to suggest a model of how chemicals like EtO and AA induce genetic damage in late-spermatid to early-spermatozoa stages of the mammal. Both can alkylate the free sulfhydryl groups of cysteine residues contained in the "immature" protamine of late spermatids and early spermatozoa, thus blocking normal disulfide bond formation. (Alkylation gradually diminishes in later stages as the number of free sulfhydryl groups decreases.) This would prevent normal chromatin condensation in the sperm nucleus, leading to stresses in the chromatin structure that eventually result in breakage and dominant lethal events.

Environmental chemicals can damage chromosomes in germ cells, which pass traits from one generation to the next. Sufficiently severe damage to the germ-cell chromosomes can result in dominant lethal mutations, in which case the embryos die before birth. Damage can also involve viable chromosome rearrangements (reciprocal translocation) that are passed on to the next generation, usually with some sort of detrimental effects; or the damage may involve a very small region (perhaps even a single-base site in the DNA) of chromatin, giving rise to a gene mutation.

GERM-CELL-STAGE SENSITIVITY TO MUTAGENS

In developing from stem cells to functional spermatozoa, the germ cells of all mammals progress through similar stages (Figure 1). Because germ-cell development is similar between mouse and man and because the genetic data base available for the mouse is extensive, this animal has proved to be an excellent experimental model for projecting how various external agents (such as radiation or chemicals) may affect human germ cells. Many studies carried out in mice have indicated that differential genetic sensitivity in the various germ-cell stages depends on the chemical agent being tested.

In studies of the genetic effects of chemical agents in mice, the amount of chemical given to the animals (by injection, inhalation, skin application, etc.) is accurately known. However, in general nothing is known about the molecular dose of the chemical that actually reaches the different germ-cell stages (Figure 2). The variability in genetic sensitivity among different germ-cell stages could result from the amount of chemical reaching the different stages, the molecular targets with which the chemical inter-acts in different stages, and the possibility of repair of lesions in specific germ-cell stages.

RADIOLABELED MUTAGENS

Part of our study of the molecular events that occur within mouse germ cells exposed to chemical mutagens has used radioactive labeling. Thus, we have studied a number of chemical mutagens in which a radioactive atom, either ^{3}H or ^{14}C, has replaced a corresponding nonradioactive atom (^{1}H or ^{12}C) in the molecule. The amount of radioactive chemical reaching the germ cells can then be traced by techniques such as liquid scintillation counting, which monitors the β-particles (electrons) emitted from the labeled atoms.

These techniques have been used to investigate ethyl methanesulfonate (EMS) (Sega and Owens, 1978), methyl methanesulfonate (MMS) (Sega and Owens, 1983), ethylene oxide (EtO) (Sega and Owens, 1987), which is widely used in industry in the manufacture of other chemicals and as a sterilant in hospitals, and acrylamide (AA) (Sega et al., in press), which is widely used in paper processing and water treatment. Genetic studies had shown that these chemicals were especially active in inducing dominant lethal mutations in late spermatids and early spermatozoa, and we wanted to determine the reasons.

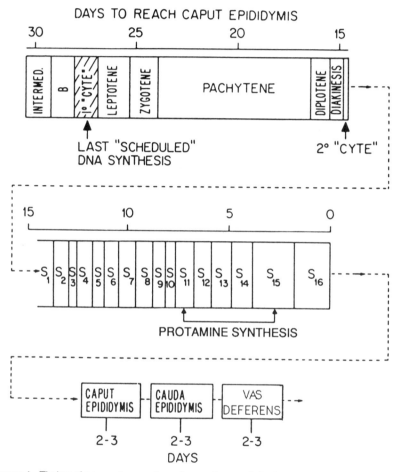

Figure 1. Timing of spermatogenesis and spermiogenesis in the mouse. Last "scheduled" DNA synthesis takes place in preleptotene primary spermatocytes. Spermatid stages are labeled from S1 (early) to S16 (late). Protamine is synthesized in mid- to late-spermatid stages.

MEASUREMENTS OF CHEMICAL BINDING

After mice were exposed to radioactively labeled mutagens, sperm were recovered at different intervals after exposure and assayed for the amount of bound chemical (alkylation). For chemicals that are powerful mutagens in late spermatids or early spermatozoa, we found a dramatic increase in the amount of mutagen bound to these stages (at least one order of magnitude more binding than in other stages). Thus, there was a correlation between increased genetic damage and increased levels of chemical binding to the sensitive germ-cell stages.

To further characterize the molecular nature of the lesions in the germ cells, DNA extracted from the different germ-cell stages was assayed for the amount of chemical mutagen bound to it. Surprisingly, binding of chemicals to DNA represented only a very small fraction of the total chemical that bound to the germ cells. Further, no increase in DNA alkylation occurred in the most sensitive stages, the late spermatids and early spermatozoa.

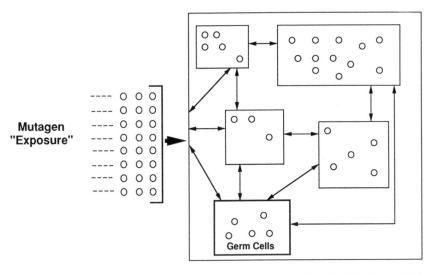

Figure 2. External exposure versus molecular dose: The amount of chemical (circles) to which an animal is exposed can be accurately established, but its distribution within molecular targets in different tissues is more difficult to analyze. Smaller boxes shown within the "mouse" (large box) represent different tissues. Levels of chemical binding in each tissue can vary, depending on such factors as transport and metabolic conversion to more (or less) potent chemical species. Chemical binding to targets within germ cells is our principal interest.

MUTAGENS BIND TO PROTAMINE

These results suggested we look for alternative molecular targets for mutagenesis within the germ cells. It was already known that, in mid- to late-spermatid stages of mammals, the usual chromosomal proteins (histones) are replaced with small, very basic proteins (protamines) that contain more than 50% of the amino acid arginine. Mammalian protamines also contain cysteine, and it is the cross-linking of the cysteine amino acids in protamine (through disulfide-bond formation) that gives mammalian spermatozoa their keratin-like properties (similar to some of the properties of fingernails and hair). Because protamine contains nucleophilic sites (e.g., the -SH group in cysteine), we reasoned that it might be a target for attack by EMS, MMS, EtO, AA, and other chemicals.

When we purified protamine from sperm recovered at different times after chemical treatment, we found that the amount of mutagen bound to protamine increased greatly in the most sensitive germ-cell stages (late spermatids to early spermatozoa). The amount of mutagen binding to protamine exactly paralleled the total amount of binding to the sperm. In fact, with chemicals that have their greatest effect in late spermatids or early spermatozoa, we have found that almost all the binding in the sensitive stages can be attributed to interaction with protamine.

To determine where the chemicals were binding on the protamine, we hydrolyzed samples recovered from animals exposed to different agents. Hydrolysis breaks down the protamine into its constituent amino acids and the radioactive adducts formed by exposure to the labeled mutagens. By analyzing the protamine hydrolysates with an amino acid analyzer and thin-layer chromatography, we have been able to show that these chemicals do, in fact, bind to the sulfur groups in cysteine.

MODEL FOR MUTAGEN BINDING AND GERM-CELL-STAGE SENSITIVITY

These findings have led us to postulate a model for the binding of certain chemicals to mouse chromatin in germ-cell stages that are sensitive to the induction of chromosome breakage and dominant lethality. In our model (Figure 3), the pairs of solid lines represent double-stranded DNA, and the dashed, spiraling line represents the associated germ-cell protamine (which replaces the histones in mid- to late-spermatid stages). The sulfhydryl (-SH) groups are part of the cysteine residues in the protamine, and chemical binding is represented by -Alk (alkyl group). In normal nuclear condensation (A), the sulfhydryl groups of cysteine cross-link to form disulfide bridges in the chromatin. However, if chemical binding to a nucleophilic sulfhydryl group occurs before a disulfide bond has formed (B), cross-linking of the sulfhydryl groups may not take place. Stresses in the chromatin structure could then occur, eventually producing either a single- or double-strand DNA break. The end result would be a dominant lethal mutation or chromosome translocation.

A

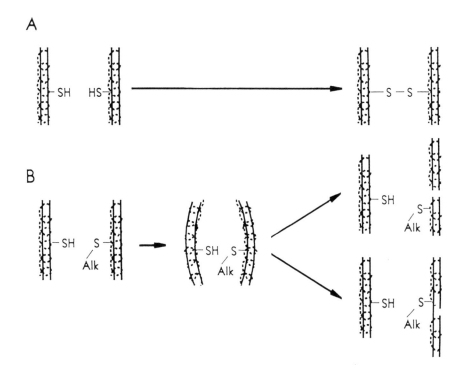

Figure 3. Model for chemical alkylation of chromatin in late-spermatid and early-spermatozoa stages, leading to breakage and dominant lethality. See text for explanation of model. A, normal; B, chemically treated.

It is unlikely that all mutagenic chemicals act by this mechanism, and other molecular targets may be important in other germ-cell stages. However, our observations of the strong binding of some chemicals to sperm protamine in mammals give a new dimension to our understanding of mutational processes in mammalian germ cells.

ACKNOWLEDGMENTS

This research was jointly sponsored by the Office of Health and Environmental Research, U.S. Department of Energy, under Contract DE-AC05-84OR21400 with Martin Marietta Energy Systems, Inc., by the Reproductive Effects Assessment Group of the U.S. Environmental Protection Agency under IAG No. DW930141-01-1, and by the National Institute of Environmental Health Sciences under IAG No. 222Y01-ES-10067.

REFERENCES

Sega, GA and JG Owens. 1978. Ethylation of DNA and protamine by ethyl methanesulfonate in the germ cells of male mice and the relevancy of these molecular targets to the induction of dominant lethals. Mutat Res 52:87-106.

Sega, GA and JG Owens. 1983. Methylation of DNA and protamine by methyl methanesulfonate in the germ cells of male mice. Mutat Res 111:227-244.

Sega, GA and JG Owens. 1987. Binding of ethylene oxide in spermiogenic germ-cell stages of the mouse after low-level inhalation exposure. Environ Mol Mutagen 10:119-127.

Sega, GA, RP Valdivia-Alcota, CP Tancongco, and PA Brimer. Acrylamide binding to the DNA and protamine of spermiogenic stages in the mouse and its relationship to genetic damage. Mutat Res (in press).

DEVELOPMENT OF MOLECULAR APPROACHES TO THE ESTIMATION OF THE GERMINAL GENE MUTATION RATE IN HUMAN POPULATIONS

B. A. Perry and H. W. Mohrenweiser

Biomedical Sciences Division, Lawrence Livermore National Laboratory, Livermore CA 94550

Key words: *Germinal genes, mutation rates, human population, health costs*

ABSTRACT

Estimation of human genetic risk associated with exposure to suspected mutagenic agents has been limited by the scarcity of relevant human data on germinal (heritable) gene mutation rates. One of the impediments, given the rarity of gene mutations, has been the small number of offspring available for study and the low level (by experimental standards) of parental exposure. Therefore, estimation of germinal mutation rates and the associated health costs requires new technologies that maximize the information obtained from each offspring of exposed parents.

Emerging DNA technologies appear to have promise in this respect, since it is possible, in principle, for a small number of individuals to provide sufficient information to detect changes in germinal mutation rates. Gene mutations may occur as insertion, deletion, and/or rearrangement (I/D/R) events or nucleotide substitutions. A modified restriction fragment-length polymorphism strategy, using many probes and only one or two restriction enzymes, can efficiently screen for I/D/R events. This is the class of mutational event expected after radiation exposure and, if it involves functional genes, it is physiologically significant. Utilizing this approach, two rare variant classes and three rare alleles were detected per 1000 fragments screened in a survey of 130 individuals. This approach also detected induced mutations in ethyl nitrosourea-treated somatic cells. The effectiveness of this approach in estimating mutation rates may be enhanced by using probes for repetitive DNA sequences, if the recombination rates in regions of repeat sequences are increased following exposure to mutagenic agents.

The techniques of genomic hybridization and heteroduplex mapping, using RNase digestion or gradient denaturant gel electrophoresis, could provide useful approaches for detecting nucleotide substitutions. These methods are being modified to enhance their usefulness in screening for germinal gene mutations. A combination of molecular approaches may constitute an effective strategy for monitoring induced mutation rates in individual humans.

INTRODUCTION

Mutational events are generally categorized as either "germinal" or "somatic," depending on the cell or tissue in which they occur. Those occurring in somatic cells (e.g., events potentially leading to carcinogenesis) have impact on only the immediate carrier. Conversely, germinal mutations may hold profound, potentially deleterious consequences for offspring, whose genetic constitution is derived from the parent. For example, it is estimated that 3% of all liveborn infants are affected with monogenic or polygenic genetic disorders and that 20% of these gene defects are caused by *de novo* mutations (Office of Technology Assessment, 1986). Once established in the germline, these mutations inextricably diminish the fitness of the gene pool and are passed to subsequent generations, magnifying the associated health cost burden.

In view of this potential for germinal mutations to result in genetic disease, it is important to establish a basis on which to estimate the rate of occurrence of *de novo* gene mutations and the impact of mutagenic agents in increasing the frequency of these events. Estimates based on a variety of approaches place the "spontaneous/background" germinal gene mutation rate in humans in the neighborhood of 0.4×10^{-5} events per locus per generation, or a nucleotide substitution rate of approximately 10^{-8} (Neel et al., 1988a) (70 substitutions/genome/generation). This rarity of events makes it difficult to establish a data base upon which to estimate the rate at which mutations occur. This is a reflection of our inability, with current techniques, to derive a significant amount of information from each subject and the unavailability of large cohorts for study (see Neel et al., 1988b). Thus, new approaches are required to derive the statistically significant data bases necessary to detect an increase in (or absence of) germinal gene mutation rate caused by exposure to known or suspected mutagenic agents.

Mutations that occur at the level of the gene, "point" mutations, include base substitutions and insertions, deletions, and rearrangements (I/D/R). These alterations in DNA structure appear to occur spontaneously as a result of errors in DNA replication and repair, or as a consequence of exposure to mutagenic agents. Nucleotide substitutions are the primary lesion following exposure to alkylating agents (Batzer et al., 1988); I/D/R are the predominant detectable lesion following exposure to ionizing radiation (Russell, 1983). The loss of base sequence integrity can result in genetic disease by interfering with any process required to convert genetic information into a protein product. Examples of human genetic diseases caused by *de novo* mutations resulting from a range of molecular alterations have been identified (reviewed by Mohrenweiser and Jones, in press).

METHODOLOGICAL DEVELOPMENTS

In the last few years, molecular biological techniques have been developed that could allow, at least theoretically, each of the 7×10^9 nucleotides in the human genome to be screened for mutational events (Delehanty et al., 1986). Our laboratory is currently developing these techniques as components of an efficient germinal gene mutation screening effort.

Restriction Analysis to Detect I/D/R Mutations

In the first approach, one assumes that either a base substitution has occurred within a particular restriction site, thereby negating the efficacy of that site, or that an I/D/R event has occurred between two restriction sites, thereby altering the size of that fragment. In either case, the result would be a change in the restriction pattern between the wild-type and mutant DNA. Because the ability of restriction analysis to detect base substitutions depends on the alteration of a particular restriction sequence, a restriction assay for base substitutions would require that the genome be screened with a large number of restriction enzymes. Clearly, restriction analysis would *not* be the method of choice for efficiently detecting base substitution mutations.

Restriction enzyme mapping may be an efficient approach for detecting I/D/R events if only a few enzymes but many probes are employed (Mohrenweiser et al., 1989). In this approach, only a few blots need be generated, because each could be stripped and reprobed with a number of different gene-specific sequences. A sufficiently large number of probes (e.g., 100-200) would allow a large portion of the genome and many clinically significant loci to be screened for the presence of I/D/R mutations. Detailed restriction mapping would allow the I/D/R to be characterized further, and, if necessary, isolated, cloned, and sequenced. Subsequent work might involve the determination of the functional significance, if any, of these alterations.

Additionally, probes for nonexpressed regions of the genome might be used. Jeffreys (1987), for example, has used probes for repetitive sequence elements; preliminary data suggest a mutation rate as high as 10^{-3} to 10^{-4} per "locus" for some probes. However, these mutations appear to occur via a recombinational mechanism, and it is possible that their rate of occurrence is not influenced by exposure to mutagenic agents. Also, because these mutations involve noncoding regions, they may not be physiologically significant.

Heteroduplex Analysis to Detect Nucleotide Substitutions

RNase A Cleavage. This technique relies on the ability of RNase A to cleave at single-stranded regions of duplex molecules (Winter et al., 1985; Myers et al., 1985a). To screen for putative base substitutions within a subject's DNA sample (either cloned or genomic), a fragment encoding the "wild-type" sequence is cloned within a vector that allows the production of radiolabeled "run-off" RNA transcripts. This radiolabeled transcript is then annealed to the complementary DNA (or RNA) strand that harbors the mutation, and the duplex is subjected to RNase A digestion. Base mismatch occurring at the site of the substitution results in a region of RNA that is not hydrogen bonded to the adjacent DNA/RNA strand. This single-stranded RNA portion can then be cleaved by the RNase A, generating two radiolabeled RNA fragments that are sized by electrophoresis. If the complementary DNA is restricted before annealing and RNase A treatment, a determination can be made concerning the position of the substitution relative to each end of the transcript (Myers et al., 1985a). Subsequent sequence analysis would provide more detailed information regarding the exact position and nature of the base substitution and, perhaps, evidence of potential functional significance.

Denaturing Gradient Gel Electrophoresis (DGGE). This technique, originally described by Fischer and Lerman (1979), involves the electrophoretic separation of duplex nucleic acids as a function of difference in base composition rather than in size. Specifically, a duplex molecule is subjected to electrophoretic migration through a polyacrylamide gel along a concentration gradient of denaturants such as urea and formamide. As the duplex encounters increasingly higher concentrations of the denaturants, relatively unstable areas termed "domains" begin to deanneal, resulting in a structure composed of single-stranded regions interspersed with helical regions. The progressive generation of single-stranded regions within an alpha-helical duplex results in a structure that becomes increasingly resistant to electrophoretic migration. At some point, migration ceases completely. In short, the duplex cannot "decide" whether to migrate as an alpha-helical duplex or as two single strands.

The propensity of a particular base to deanneal within a domain appears to be influenced by the collective interaction of all the bases comprising that domain. It is this interbase dependency which serves as the premise for using DGGE to detect base substitutions. The substitution of even one base within a domain is sufficient to alter its melting characteristics and therefore the electrophoretic migration profile of the entire duplex (Myers et al., 1985b; Noll and Collins, 1987). By comparing the relative migration distances of radiolabeled wild-wild versus wild-mutant duplex fragments, one can discern the presence of a base mismatch caused by a base substitution or small I/D/R.

SUMMARY

All the techniques discussed here allow the DNA to be evaluated at the level of finesse required to detect base substitutions and I/D/R. Restriction analysis should provide a useful method for the detection of I/D/R mutations over a large portion of the genome. In the approach described by Mohrenweiser et al. (1989), the genome could be screened for I/D/R with a minimum number of restriction enzymes and a large repertoire of probes. Development of nonradioactive and direct-probing methods will provide more versatility and expediency in the use of restriction analysis to determine the frequency of I/D/R events. Implementation of these techniques would allow the genome to be screened in a much less labor-intensive manner, thereby simplifying the assay and expediting the acquisition of data. Techniques such as these are currently employed to determine the induced mutation rate in somatic cells exposed to N-ethyl-N-nitrosourea (ENU) or radiation, and isolated without the intervention of selective criteria (a "proof-of-principle" experiment).

In contrast to restriction analysis, heteroduplex analysis would be most useful in delineating the presence of base substitutions (or small I/D/R). Either RNase A cleavage or DGGE would be used to delineate the presence of a base substitution within cloned or genomic DNA samples. Again, the objective of our developmental effort is to refine heteroduplex methods sufficiently to acquire enough data to estimate germinal gene mutation rates.

The polymerase chain reaction (PCR) technique could enhance the utility of both restriction and heteroduplex analysis (Saiki et al., 1988). Using this technique, experimentally useful quantities of a particular DNA sequence can be generated from even a single molecule of starting material, and could promote simpler methods of detection.

The approaches described represent significant advances in the ability to detect germinal mutations, but each is still somewhat limited in utility and applicability. Therefore, it seems likely that no single method will prove adequate in rendering the amount of information required to allow valid estimations of germinal mutation rates. Used collectively, however, techniques such as these should provide us with the tools required to estimate the germinal gene mutation rate in selected (control and exposed) human populations.

ACKNOWLEDGMENTS

This work was performed under the auspices of the U.S. Department of Energy, Office of Health and Environmental Research, by the Lawrence Livermore National Laboratory under contract number W-7405-ENG-48.

REFERENCES

Batzer, MA, B Tedeschi, NG Fossett, A Tucker, G Kilroy, P Arbour, and WR Lee. 1988. Spectra of molecular changes induced in DNA of *Drosophila* spermatozoa by 1-ethyl-1-nitrosourea and x-rays. Mutat Res 199:255-268.

Delehanty, J, RL White, and ML Mendelsohn. 1986. Approaches to determining mutation rates in human DNA. Mutat Res 167:215-232.

Fischer, SG and LS Lerman. 1979. Length-independent separation of DNA restriction fragments in two-dimensional gel electrophoresis. Cell 16:191-200.

Jefferys, AJ. 1987. Highly variable minisatellites and DNA fingerprinting. Biochem Soc Trans 15:309-317.

Mohrenweiser, HW, and I Jones. Review of the molecular characteristics of gene mutations of the germline and somatic cells of the human. Mutat Res (in press).

Mohrenweiser, HW, RD Larsen, and JV Neel. 1989. Development of molecular approaches to estimating germinal mutation rates. I. Detection of insertion/deletion/rearrangement variants in the human genome. Mutat Res 212:241-252.

Myers, RM, Z Larin, and T Maniatis. 1985a. Detection of single base substitutions by ribonuclease cleavage at mismatches of RNA: DNA duplexes. Science 230:1242-1246.

Myers, RM, N Lumelsky, LS Lerman, and T Maniatis. 1985b. Detection of single base substitutions in total genomic DNA. Nature 313:495-498.

Neel, JV, HW Mohrenweiser, and H Gershowitz. 1988a. A pilot study of the use of placental cord blood samples in monitoring for mutational events. Mutat Res 204:365-377.

Neel, JV, C Satoh, K Goriki, J Asakawa, M Fujita, N Takahashi, T Kageoka, and T Hazama. 1988b. Search for mutations altering protein charge and/or function in children of atomic bomb survivors: Final report. Am J Hum Genet 42:663-676.

Noll, WW and M Collins. 1987. Detection of human DNA polymorphisms with a simplified denaturing gradient gel electrophoresis technique. Proc Natl Acad Sci USA 84:3339-3343.

Office of Technology Assessment. 1986. Technologies for detecting heritable mutations in human beings. OTA-H-298. U.S. Government Printing Office, Washington, DC.

Russell, LB. 1983. Qualitative analysis of mouse specific locus mutations: Information on genetic organization, gene expression, and the chromosomal nature of induced lesions. Environ Sci Res 28:241-258.

Saiki, RK, S Scharf, F Faloona, KB Mullis, GT Horn, HA Erlich, and N Arnheim. 1988. Enzymatic amplification of β-globin genomic sequences and restriction site analysis for diagnosis of sickle cell anemia. Science 9:1350-1354.

Winter, E, F Yamamoto, C Almoguera, and M Perucho. 1985. A method to detect and characterize point mutations in transcribed genes: Amplification and overexpression of the mutant *c-Ki-ras* allele in human tumor cells. Proc Natl Acad Sci USA 82:7575-7579.

GENETIC AND DEVELOPMENTAL EFFECTS OF HIGH-LET RADIATION ON THE NEMATODE *CAENORHABDITIS ELEGANS*

G. A. Nelson, T. M. Marshall, and W. W. Schubert

Jet Propulsion Laboratory, California Institute of Technology, Pasadena, CA 91109

Key words: *Nematode, high-LET radiation, mutation, radiation-sensitive mutants, C. elegans*

ABSTRACT

Caenorhabditis elegans is being used as a model system for the evaluation of high and low linear-energy-transfer (LET) radiation effects on cell reproduction, differentiation, and mutation *in vivo*. Fluence/dose versus response and relative biological effectiveness (RBE) versus LET relationships have been constructed for the following end points using accelerated ions, gamma rays, and fission spectrum neutrons.

Cell inactivation. Radiation damage to a four-cell gonad primordium interferes with the developmental program that constructs a functional adult gonad whose normal function is to produce 282 offspring by self-fertilization.

Mutation. Recessive lethal mutations are being isolated in a large region corresponding to 15% of the nematode's genome using a strain (JP10) containing the reciprocal translocation *eT1(III;V)* as a balancer. A set of 29 mutants generated by ions is being characterized to determine the relative abundances of point mutations, deletions, and chromosomal rearrangements.

Nucleoplasmic bridge formation. When newly hatched larvae are irradiated, defects in karyokinesis of intestinal cells arise; we propose that these defects are derived from events that lead to formation of polycentric chromosomes, which prevent completion of nuclear division and are seen in adult worms as nucleoplasmic bridges.

Duplications of unc-3. The production of duplications of the right arm of the X chromosome has been quantified with interesting kinetics, which suggests that particles are very efficient in producing chromosome breaks but also are likely to produce second-site lethals.

Radiation-sensitive mutants. Rad mutants *rad-1,2,3,4* and *7* are being characterized with respect to the foregoing end points. Hypo- and hypermutability have been documented as well as inability to repair chromosome breaks.

High linear-energy-transfer (LET) ionizing radiation is characterized by structured patterns of energy deposition quite unlike the more uniform ionization patterns of gamma rays and x rays. This feature results in relative biological effectiveness (RBE) values greater than 1 for many end points, and may generate certain unique end points such as cataracts and postulated "microlesions" (Todd, 1983). An understanding of these features is essential for controlling certain tumor treatment protocols based on accelerated particles and for developing accurate risk assessments for spaceflight crews encountering cosmic rays during spaceflight.

Using the nematode *Caenorhabditis elegans* as a model eukaryote, we are attempting to characterize the kinetics of production and to identify any unique qualitative features of genetic lesions induced *in vivo* by accelerated particles and neutrons. Cell inactivation and effects of putative DNA repair-defective *rad* mutants are also being investigated in this context.

Caenorhabditis elegans possesses several features that make it a convenient system for investigation of developmental and genetic processes. It is a small, transparent, self-fertilizing hermaphrodite with a fixed cell number and a fixed mosaic developmental program that allows adult abnormalities to be directly traced to defects in progenitor cells. It is a diploid animal with six pairs of chromosomes and a genome size of 8×10^7 base pairs (per haploid genome); thus, it is intermediate in scale between *Drosophila* and *Saccharomyces*. Males can be used to perform crosses, and more than 700 genes have been identified and mapped. Its 3-day generation time and ease of handling by growth on *Escherichia coli*-seeded Petri plates combine to facilitate conventional genetic manipulation, and a large fraction of the genome has been cloned into a cosmid library for molecular analysis. The organism has been extensively reviewed; the most comprehensive summary is that of Wood (1988).

We have concentrated our efforts on five end points that result from exposure to radiation. These are (1) induction of mutations in a set of 400 essential autosomal genes; (2) induction of mutations in a single structural gene, *unc-22*; (3) induction of X-chromosome duplications; (4) formation of stable karyoplasmic bridges in the syncytial intestine; and (5) inactivation of gonad blast cells leading to sterility. After studies using ^{60}Co gamma rays and 254-nm ultraviolet (UV) light, worms were irradiated with accelerated particles at the Lawrence Berkeley Laboratory's BEVALAC accelerator and fission spectrum neutrons from the Argonne National Laboratory's JANUS reactor.

RECESSIVE AUTOSOMAL LETHAL MUTATIONS

The reciprocal translocation $eT1(III;V)$, which exchanges portions of chromosomes 3 and 5, can be used as a balancer chromosome for capturing lethal mutations in a 40-map unit or 1.2×10^7 base-pair region (Rosenbluth et al., 1983). Using this assay, linear mutation rates were observed for gamma rays out to 25 Gy (2500 rad); UV light kinetics exhibited a plateau above 120 J/m^2 (Coohill et al., 1988). Accelerated particles induced mutations linearly with fluence in the range of 10^5 to 10^{10}/cm^2. The RBE values (normalized to ^{60}Co) were maximal (RBE = 1.6) at an LET of about 130 to 150 keV/μm. The measured inactivation cross sections were found to be substantially smaller (0.1 μm^2 at LET = 100 keV/μm) than the geometric cross sections for gamete nuclei (12 μm^2). Ions of relatively low velocity were more effective than fast-moving particles of equal LET. Neutrons (0.8 MeV) showed linear kinetics out to 25 Gy with an RBE of 1.6. The relative proportions of point mutations, deletions, and chromosomal rearrangements are currently being assessed for a set of 29 mutants. They differ from the spectrum of gamma-induced mutations in a way that suggests that chromosomal rearrangements [duplications of $unc-36(+)$] are selected against in particle-cell interactions, possibly because strong interactions frequently result in the death of target gametes.

When *rad-1*, 3, or 7 were built into the tester strain it was found that *rad-3* was hypermutable to UV but not to gamma rays; *rad-1* was hypomutable to both UV and gamma, whereas *rad-7* was hypomutable to UV but resembled wild type in its response to gamma rays. This suggests the presence of at least two DNA-repair pathways, one error free and one error prone.

Mutations in *unc-22*

The *unc-22* is a gene that codes for a large (>500-kdalton) protein with a repeating domain structure that is tolerant of mutation (Moerman and Baillie, 1979). The gene is 20 kb in size, and lambda vectors containing the region are now available for hybridization analysis. We have isolated more than 90 *unc-22* mutants using a drug selection technique to recover Unc-22 heterozygotes. A large proportion of these are not recovered because of associated lethality and many appear to contain deletions that extend into flanking lethal *let* genes. The proportions of associated lethals are lower than those found with gamma-ray-induced *unc-22*s. Gamma-ray kinetics are linear to 60 Gy with a rate of 7.5×10^{-7} per chromosome per gray using wild-type fourth-larval-stage animals as targets and screening for F_1 generation Unc-22 using 1 mM levamisole.

X-Chromosome Duplications

The gene *unc-3* is located on the right arm of the X chromosome (LG X), and *unc-3* mutants are semiparalyzed. Because *C. elegans* males have only one LG X, outcross male progeny of *unc-3/unc-3* hermaphrodites and *unc-3(+)/0* males are all expected to be *unc-3/0* semiparalyzed animals. The appearance of rare wild-type F_1 males from matings of irradiated P0 males to Unc-3 hermaphrodites indicates the presence of a duplicated *unc-3(+)* gene on an autosome or as a free fragment (Herman et al., 1979). Accelerated ions varied systematically in their efficiency of inducing *unc-3(+)* duplications. Heavy ions were effective at the lowest fluence, but maximal rates were below the values for lighter ions at somewhat higher fluences. This suggests that the relative probability of killing a sperm, versus induction of a duplication, is greater for a heavy ion than for a lighter ion. Most animals bearing a duplication were not recoverable, suggesting that lethal mutations or epigenetic damage in *unc-3(+)*-bearing animals was common.

Intestinal Karyoplasmic Bridges

Newly hatched nematodes possess a syncytial intestine with precisely 20 nuclei (Wood, 1988). Just before the first larval molt, 14 of these nuclei divide once to generate a 34-nucleus tissue. When irradiated with ionizing radiation, the 14 dividing nuclei may be arrested, with the formation of a DNA stain-positive bridge. This is postulated to result from ring or polycentric chromosome formation following strand breakage. *Caenorhabditis elegans* chromosomes are too small for current methods of karyotyping, but are thought to be holocentric (polycentric) on the basis of the stability of free duplications and electron microscopy of nuclei: This condition would favor polycentric formation. In further support of this interpretation is the observation that UV light does not induce bridges (or many DNA strand breaks). Accelerated ions induced bridges in a fluence- and LET-dependent fashion with an RBE_{max} of approximately 2.5 over a broad LET range. Neutrons had an RBE of 1.7, based on an extrapolation of a partial dose-versus-response curve. Both *rad-2* and *rad-7* mutants were hypersensitive to neutrons for bridge formation; *rad-2* was hypersensitive to heavy ions.

Gonad Blast Cell Inactivation

The hermaphrodite ovotestis of *C. elegans* is generated from four blast cells, Z1, Z2, Z3, and Z4, which are present in newly hatched larvae. Z1 and Z4 generate the somatic structures of the anterior and posterior arms and Z2 and Z3 populate the gonad arms with gonia. It is known from laser microbeam ablations that the four cells reproduce and differentiate independently (Wood, 1988). When the cells are irradiated with gamma rays, a D_{37} dose of 84 Gy is obtained as measured by the fertility of individual self-fertilizing hermaphrodites. Heavy ions show LET-dependent inactivation-versus-fluence curves and combine to give an RBE-versus-LET relationship with a broad RBE peak of 2.5. By the D_{37} criterion, smooth inactivation-versus-dose/fluence behavior is indicated, which is at odds with laser micro-surgery results if complete inactivation of Z1 to Z4 by ions occurs. However, when populations of hermaphrodites are analyzed for their relationships of brood size versus frequency versus fluence, a different story emerges. Two stepwise inactivation events are detected, each corresponding to the inactivation of one gonad arm. Morphologically, the gonads were not absent or grossly deformed even at high fluence, indicating that loss of developmental potential was not accompanied by loss of reproductive integrity.

ACKNOWLEDGMENT

The work described in this report was carried out by the Jet Propulsion Laboratory, California Institute of Technology, supported under contract NAS 7-918 with the National Aeronautics and Space Administration.

REFERENCES

Coohill, TP, TM Marshall, WW Schubert, and GA Nelson. 1988. Ultraviolet mutagenesis of radiation-sensitive (*rad*) mutants of the nematode *Caenorhabditis elegans*. Mutat Res 209:99-106.

Herman, RK, JE Madl, and CK Kari. 1979. Duplications in *C. elegans*. Genetics 92:419-435.

Moerman, DG and DL Baillie. 1979. Genetic organization in *Caenorhabditis elegans*: Fine-structure analysis of the *unc-22* gene. Genetics 91:95-103.

Rosenbluth, RE, C Cuddeford, and DL Baillie. 1983. Mutagenesis in *Caenorhabditis elegans*. I. A rapid eukaryote mutagen test system using the reciprocal translocation, *eT1(III;V)*. Mutat Res 110:39-48.

Todd, P. 1983. Unique biological aspects of radiation hazards—An overview. Adv Space Res 3:187-194.

Wood, WB (ed.). 1988. *The Nematode Caenorhabditis elegans*. Cold Spring Harbor Laboratory, Cold Spring Harbor, NY.

QUESTIONS AND COMMENTS

Q: Is there unequivocal evidence for specific-ion effects on RBE for the various end points, i.e., does RBE depend on factors other than LET?

A: We have preliminary evidence that, for lethal mutation in our balanced autosomal region, LET is not sufficient to explain the efficacy of the particles. Specifically, argon at an LET of about 200 keV/μm was more effective than iron or niobium ions at LET = 200 and 560 keV/μm, respectively, and more than four times as effective as argon at LET = 100. All irradiations were in the plateau regions of the associated Bragg peaks. The major differences between particles (other than charge) were their velocities, which in turn determine the maximum ranges of scattered electrons (delta rays). In a nutshell, the slower-moving, high-LET argon ions had a more radially compact track structure than the other species. We believe that the details of the pattern of energy deposition must be considered, and we are pursuing this with particles of constant charge but lower and lower velocities.

NONRANDOM DISTRIBUTION OF MUTATIONS INDUCED BY X RAYS IN A PLASMID TARGET IN HUMAN CELLS

S. Mitra,[1] M. O. Sikpi,[2] R. J. Preston,[1] and L. C. Waters[1]

[1]Biology Division, Oak Ridge National Laboratory, Oak Ridge, TN 37831-8077

[2]University of Tennessee Graduate School of Biomedical Sciences, Oak Ridge National Laboratory, Oak Ridge, TN 37831-8077

Key words: *Shuttle plasmid, mutagenesis, ionizing radiation, alkylating agents*

ABSTRACT

The *supF* gene of *Escherichia coli,* incorporated in the recombinant human plasmids pZ189 and pZ190, was used as a target for mutagenesis induced by x rays and *N*-methyl-*N*-nitrosourea (MNU). Human lymphoblastoid cells were transfected with the mutagen-treated plasmid, and the progeny molecules carrying mutations in the target sequence were isolated and sequenced. An analysis of these mutations indicates the following: (1) Plasmid DNA treated with 40 Gy of x rays yielded 2-3 times more mutants than the unirradiated control. In contrast, MNU treatment of the target gene fragment alone yielded 15- to 80-fold more mutants than the control. (2) Multiple point mutations were more common in both control and x-irradiated plasmids than in MNU-treated DNA. (3) A significant fraction of mutants in all cases had deletions of as many as 100 or more nucleotides that included part of the target sequence. (4) Most of the point mutations in all cases involved guanine · cytosine (G · C) pairs and included both transitions and tranversions. (5) Single-base mutations were nonrandom; G at position 123 (G_{123}), the middle G of a GGG sequence, and C_{109} of the nontranscribed strand stood out as hot spots for both MNU- and x-ray-treated DNA, but not in the control. On the other hand, mutations in another run of G's (G_{102}-G_{105}) were observed in control DNA but not in x-irradiated samples. (6) C's of 5'-thymine · cytosine (5'-TC) doublets in the nontranscribed but not in the transcribed strand were the most common targets for change in x-irradiated DNA. This strand bias was not observed in the control DNA.

Recent advances in recombinant DNA methodologies and DNA sequencing techniques make it possible, for the first time, to investigate the mechanisms of mutagenesis at the molecular level. Nevertheless, in the case of mammalian systems *in vivo* or at the cellular level *in vitro*, the technical difficulties in locating the mutations in the whole genome and in identifying the nature of DNA sequence alterations are formidable. Because mutagens, as a rule, induce a variety of lesions in DNA, not all of which are mutagenic, it is essential to screen a large number of mutant sequences in a particular target before a pattern can be discerned. Such a pattern should lead to an understanding of the basis of mutation induction for a particular mutagen.

An interesting strategy that is being increasingly adopted is the use of a mutation target in a recombinant shuttle plasmid vector that replicates in mammalian cells. The rationale for this approach is that both chromosomal and plasmid DNA are exposed to the same intracellular environment and subject to similar metabolic processes, including DNA replication and repair. Thus, the mutational yield and spectrum in the surrogate plasmid target should be indicators of these processes in the cellular genome. The exquisite advantage of the plasmid system, however, is the ease and speed of identification of the mutants in the target with the availability of a phenotypic screen for mutants in bacteria, and isolation and subsequent sequencing of the mutant DNA. Hence, a large collection of mutants can be characterized in a reasonable length of time.

There is legitimate concern that the extrachromosomal plasmid targets may not faithfully represent the chromosomal targets because the plasmid replication is not under stringent control, both with respect to its temporal relation to the cell cycle and to the number of rounds per cell division. Further, the plasmid minichromosome structure may be significantly different from that of the cellular chromosomes. It should also be obvious that the plasmid systems cannot be used for screening mutations with large-scale DNA sequence changes, including deletions and insertions. Finally, recombinational repair and DNA sequence rearrangements resulting from double-strand breaks induced in chromosomal DNA by ionizing radiation could not be detected in the plasmid systems. Nevertheless, it is generally accepted that the information collected for mutations in a plasmid would provide at least a preliminary basis for prediction of mutations in cellular genomes.

It is becoming more and more evident that the nature and yield of induced mutations, including both single-base and large-sequence changes, are dependent on a number of factors in addition to the nature of the mutagen itself. These include the frequency and distribution of various specific lesions, repair or misrepair of these lesions, and misreplication of unrepaired lesions. All these factors may be affected by the tertiary structure of the target DNA so that the neighboring base sequence may modulate both the probability of lesion formation and its repair (Glickman et al., 1987; Topal et al., 1986).

MUTATIONAL TARGET IN A HUMAN SHUTTLE PLASMID

During the last few years, a number of laboratories have developed recombinant plasmid vectors that can replicate both in bacteria (usually *Escherichia coli*) and mammalian (mostly human) cells. These composite plasmids contain the two origins of replication (*ori*) sequences that can function in these diverse cell types. The genes for the unique proteins required for replication are either present in the plasmid itself or are provided by the cell. The mammalian replication systems are usually derived from viruses, for example, *ori* sequences of papovaviruses or Epstein-Barr virus (Seidman et al., 1985; Drinkwater and Klinedinst, 1986). These plasmids also carry a bacterial selection marker, for example, a drug-resistance gene. The target sequence for mutagenesis studies is usually a gene selectable in bacteria. The standard procedure for plasmid mutagenesis involves (1) incorporation of the plasmid in an appropriate mammalian cell before or after mutagenic treatment; (2) recovery of the plasmid after its replication, which is needed for the fixation of mutations; (3) removal of unreplicated plasmid molecules; (4) screening in bacteria for isolation of plasmids carrying a mutated target sequence; (5) recovery of the plasmid; and (6) characterization of the mutation at the nucleotide level.

Seidman et al. (1985) constructed a shuttle plasmid, pZ189, that contains the SV40 *ori* and T-antigen gene needed for its replication in human cells in addition to the β-lactamase gene providing resistance to ampicillin and the *ori* sequence of the *E. coli* plasmid, pBR327. The plasmid also contains the *supF*-tRNA gene of *E. coli* (Brown et al., 1979) as the target gene. The screening for mutations in the target is based on the fact that functional *supF*-tRNA produced from the plasmid suppresses the amber mutation of the β-galactosidase gene in the *E. coli* host, which will form blue colonies in the presence of a chromogenic β-galactosidase substrate, X-gal. *E. coli* cells lacking a functional β-galactosidase, that is, with an inactive or weakly active *supF*-tRNA, will yield white or pale blue colonies. The plasmids are recovered from these colonies for characterization of the mutant *supF* gene sequence. The rather high frequency of spontaneous mutations, often with large-scale sequence changes, has posed major problems in using the shuttle plasmid for mutagenesis studies. The strategic placement of the target between the *ori* and the drug-resistance gene reduces the frequency of spontaneous mutants in the viable plasmids recovered from the human cells (Seidman et al., 1985).

The synthetic *supF*-tRNA gene originally constructed by Khorana's group (Brown et al., 1979) consists of about 200 nucleotides (nt), starting with an

*Eco*RI site at the 5' end of the nontranscribed strand. Following the protocol developed by Seidman, Kraemer, and their colleagues (Bredberg et al., 1986), we routinely sequence the complete gene starting with the 5' end of the coding strand. However, as observed by us and others, most mutations occur in the region of the sequence corresponding to the mature tRNA sequence (nt 99-183). Although both *in vivo* studies in *E. coli* and induced mutations in the shuttle plasmid studies indicated mutations in both the 5' pre-tRNA region and the 3' flanking sequences, many of these are not single mutations and thus by themselves may not cause inactivation of the tRNA. On the other hand, only 12 nucleotide sites among the 85 nucleotides of the mature tRNA sequence have no known mutations (Kraemer and Seidman, 1989). Thus, base changes within this sequence should almost invariably be scored as mutations.

For both *in vivo* and *in vitro* studies, the target to be selectively mutagenized is rather small compared to the rest of the chromosome; for each mutagenic lesion in the target itself, other such lesions are introduced elsewhere in the genome, including in those genes essential for plasmid maintenance and replication. We therefore reasoned that it should be possible, at least for *in vitro* mutagenesis of the *supF*-tRNA gene, to mutagenize only this sequence before its reinsertion into the plasmid. To do so, we modified pZ189 by inserting an *Xho*I linker at position 250 (an *Xho*II site) beyond the 3' terminus of the nontranscribed strand of the *supF* gene. From this plasmid, called pZ190, the 250-bp *Eco*RI/*Xho*I fragment containing the tRNA gene can be isolated and mutagenized. After mutagen treatment of the fragments, the whole plasmid was reconstituted using the unique *Eco*RI and *Xho*I sites. We should point out, however, that this approach will not work when mutagen treatment leads to fragmentation of the target sequence or damages its cohesive ends.

PROTOCOL FOR MUTAGENESIS

We have followed the protocol developed in Kraemer's laboratory (Bredberg et al., 1986). Briefly, mutagenized plasmids, pZ189 or pZ190, are introduced into human lymphoblastoid cells, GM606, by the DEAE-dextran procedure (McCutchen and Pagano, 1968). After incubation for 48 hr to allow for their replication, the plasmid DNA molecules were recovered by the procedure of Hirt (1967) or by alkaline lysis (Kraemer, unpublished method). The plasmid DNA, after phenol extraction and alcohol precipitation, was treated with *Dpn*I to degrade unreplicated (parental) DNA (Seidman et al., 1985) and was then used to transform *E. coli* MLB100, a *lacZ*am mutant. Plasmid DNA was recovered from the β-galactosidase-negative (white or pale blue) *E. coli* clones and sequenced according to Zagursky et al. (1985), mostly using a primer for the nontranscribed strand synthesis with the 3' end at nt-5493.

Several other laboratories have employed different human cell lines, mostly fibroblasts, for the study of mutagenesis of pZ189 (Hauser et al., 1986; Yang et al., 1988). Because the different host cells may have different repair capacities for distinct DNA lesions, it may be difficult to compare the data from different laboratories with respect to yield and spectrum of mutations induced by a particular mutagen. For example, our data on the location of N-methyl-N-nitrosourea- (MNU-) induced mutations in pZ190 after its replication in Mex⁻ (L33) lymphoblastoid cells that are deficient in O^6-methylguanine repair show small but significant differences in the yield of mutants and location of hot spots from those in repair-proficient Mex⁺ cells (Sikpi et al., submitted for publication).

NATURE OF MUTATIONS INDUCED BY X RAYS

Both high and low linear-energy-transfer (LET) ionizing radiations induced strand breaks in DNA (Teebor et al., 1988). Exposure of plasmids pZ189 and pZ190 to increasing doses of x rays up to 40 Gy showed a dose-dependent conversion of form I supercoiled plasmid to form II nicked molecules. It is well documented that a large fraction of the form II molecules would not have simple phosphotriester bond cleavage, with 5' phosphate and 3' OH ends, but would contain nonligatable ends, often with sugar and base damage (Ward, 1988). A number of bases are also damaged without associated DNA strand cleavage. These base damages invariably result not from direct energy deposition of low-LET ionizing radiation such as x rays, but from reaction with OH radicals produced by radiolysis of water (Ward, 1988; Teebor et al., 1988). In fact, each base may be altered in a variety of ways. Even though some of the lesions are rather well characterized, for example, thymine glycol and 8-hydroxyguanine (reviewed by Teebor et al., 1988; Ward, 1988), the relative contributions of the single-strand nicks and the damaged bases in induction of various mutations are not known.

Attempts have recently been made to establish the mutagenic potential of the damaged bases by *in vitro* replication of DNA containing these lesions (reviewed by Breimer, 1988; Teebor et al., 1988). It appears that even though thymine glycol is one of the most abundant products of x-irradiation of DNA, it may not be a miscoding base. In contrast, 8-hydroxyguanine, another abundant lesion induced by x rays and oxidative damage, was clearly established as a mutagenic lesion without any base-pairing specificity (Kuchino et al., 1987). Although the approach of shuttle plasmid mutagenesis does not directly identify the mutagenic lesion induced after x-irradiation, it does provide a way to test whether, regardless of the nature of these damages, mutations are induced nonuniformly in the target DNA with some base specificity, and whether they show a unique pattern for each type of radiation, as with different LET characteristics.

Early *in vivo* experiments clearly established that ionizing radiation induces large-scale DNA sequence changes that include large deletions (see Breimer, 1988, for a review). It is not possible to analyze such changes in the pZ189 plasmid system, but it is possible to isolate and to characterize mutant plasmids containing point mutations as well as deletions, insertions, and sequence rearrangements involving from one to a few hundred bases flanking the *supF* gene.

X-irradiation of pZ190 with 40 Gy increases the mutation frequency in the *supF*-tRNA gene to 2-3 times the spontaneous rate. The observed spontaneous frequency of 0.036% is comparable to that observed by others using the parent plasmid, pZ189 (Bredberg et al., 1986; Hauser et al., 1987). As already discussed, the absolute frequency of both spontaneous and induced mutations that contain deletions, insertions, and other DNA rearrangements will be underestimated because they can involve sequences outside the tRNA gene that are vital for plasmid replication. The characteristics of mutations in the *supF*-tRNA gene of pZ190 that we have observed, both spontaneous and x-ray-induced, are shown in Table 1.

INDUCTION OF MULTIPLE MUTATIONS BY X RAYS

Unlike MNU, x rays appear to induce multiple point mutations. Table 1 shows the frequency of these multiple mutations in our studies. In contrast, MNU-induced mutants of the plasmid contained less than 6% multiple mutations in the *supF* target in the same (GM606) lymphoblastoid cells (Sikpi et al., submitted for publication). Similar results were observed by others with ultraviolet (UV) light (Hauser et al., 1986; Bredberg et al., 1986). It appears possible that low-LET radiation is unique in inducing multiple mutagenic lesions in each DNA molecule. We need to point out here that mutants with identical multiple base changes were presumed to arise from multiplication of one parent mutant plasmid, and that only distinct mutants from each plasmid preparation were scored as independent events. However, our results should be taken with some reservation because the spontaneous mutants in the control plasmid in both our studies and that of Hauser et al. (1987) also showed multiple mutations. Because x-ray exposure increased the mutation frequency by only a factor of 2-3, as many as half the mutations in the x-irradiated sample might be spontaneous.

Table 1. Characteristics of x-ray-induced mutations in the *supF*-tRNA gene of pZ190.

	Dose (Gy)						All
	0	3	5	10	20	40	Doses[a]
Number of mutants sequenced	13	8	28	13	20	17	86
Deletions[b]	1	0	3	0	3	1	7
Insertions[b]	0	0	0	0	0	1	1
Multiple base changes[b,c]	3	2	11	5	4	6	28
(%)	(23)	(25)	(39)	(38)	(20)	(35)	(33)
Type and number of base changes observed							
Transitions							
$G \cdot C \rightarrow A \cdot T$	16	12	46	31	23	26	138
(%)	(61)	(71)	(73)	(86)	(60)	(67)	(71)
$A \cdot T \rightarrow G \cdot C$	0	0	0	0	0	0	0
Transversions							
$G \cdot C \rightarrow T \cdot A$	9	2	9	2	8	7	28
(%)	(35)	(12)	(14)	(6)	(21)	(18)	(14)
$G \cdot C \rightarrow C \cdot G$	1	3	8	3	7	5	26
(%)	(0.4)	(18)	(13)	(8)	(18)	(13)	(13)
$A \cdot T \rightarrow T \cdot A$	0	0	0	0	0	1	1
(%)						(3)	(0.5)
$A \cdot T \rightarrow C \cdot G$	0	0	0	0	0	0	0

[a]3-40 Gy.
[b]Number of sequenced mutants with deletions, insertions, or multiple base changes.
[c]Number of sequenced mutants with more than two base changes per tRNA gene.

Sequence Specificity of X-Ray-Induced Mutations

Sequencing of the tRNA gene of nearly 100 mutant plasmids obtained from x-irradiated DNA has shown that although DNA lesions induced by ionizing radiation may be randomly distributed, the mutations are localized at a few selected sites. For single-base changes, the guanine · cytosine (G · C) pairs are the almost exclusive targets. Of some 86 mutants, many with multiple base changes, only one $A \cdot T \rightarrow T \cdot A$ transversion and one adenine · thymine (A · T) insertion was observed (Table 1). We should stress, however, that a similar trend was also observed among spontaneous mutants.

The most frequent change of G · C base pairs was transition to A · T pairs although both types of transversion were also often observed (see Table 1). It is interesting to note that the mutation spectrum induced by UV light is qualitatively similar to this distribution, although UV, as anticipated, induced a significant number of mutations at the A · T sites (Hauser et al., 1986; Bredberg et al., 1986; Brash et al., 1987). Polynuclear aromatic hydrocarbons

(PAH) such as benzo[a]pyrene (BaP) and 1-nitropyrene, on the other hand, induced mostly $G \cdot C \rightarrow T \cdot A$ transversions (Yang et al., 1988). A recent report indicates that gamma rays induced predominantly $G \cdot C \rightarrow C \cdot G$ transversions in a target sequence in duplex DNA of an M13 recombinant plasmid (Hoebee et al., 1988). Because this transversion was not observed at nearly such a high frequency in other studies after exposure to ionizing radiation in other bacterial systems, this may be an exception to the general trend.

Surprisingly, the $G \cdot C$ alterations produced in x-irradiated DNA were distributed among discrete sites. More remarkably, the common underlying feature of these $G \cdot C$ hot spots was the dinucleotide sequence, 5'-TC, in the coding strand of the target (corresponding to 3'-AG of the complementary strand). It is especially interesting that some 90% of all mutations sequenced so far involve the 5'-TC sites. However, not all 5'-TC sequences are equally susceptible to mutagenesis. This is partly because some of these sequences are located outside the mature tRNA region, for example, between nucleotides 40 and 100, so that changes in these sequences may not be scored as mutations. Nevertheless, C's in some 5'-TC sequences within the mature tRNA region, for example, nt 172, are known to be mutable by other mutagens (Kraemer and Seidman, 1989), yet these exhibited very few base changes among the mutants from both control and x-irradiated plasmids screened so far.

Classification of Mutational Hot Spots

Most of the x-ray-induced mutations (with more than 5 independent mutants per site) were clustered at 12 sites (Figure 1). Most (9) of these sites, as already mentioned, involved C's of 5'-TC sites in either strand. The remaining three sites involved two C's (nt 109, nt 110) within a run of 3 C's and the middle G, nt 123, in a run of 3 G's. However, all runs of several G's (or C's) were not equally mutable, because nt 102-105 (4 G's) and nt 172-176 (5 G's) in the coding strand are potential sites for mutation and because spontaneous mutants with changes in these sites have been isolated (Hauser et al., 1987). Nevertheless, mutations in these sites were rarely observed in DNA treated with x rays and MNU. Thus the probability of mutations at these sites must have been modulated by other unknown structural factors. This observation also provides a strong argument for the contention that the mutants derived from x-irradiated plasmids were not generated spontaneously from undamaged DNA molecules.

The sites of nt 109 and nt 123 are extremely interesting because they are highly mutable by diverse agents, including UV light, PAH, MNU, and x rays (Hauser et al., 1986; Bredberg et al., 1986; Yang et al., 1988; Sikpi et al., submitted for publication). In contrast, most other mutational hot spots are unique for each specific mutagen. For example, nt 163 and nt 185 are highly mutable by x rays by not by MNU or other mutagens. These patterns lead us to speculate that, at least in the case of the *supF*-tRNA gene, mutational hot spots arise from two phenomena: (1) the tertiary structure of the target, which makes certain nucleotides highly sensitive to modification by diverse mutagens, and (2) the specificity of mutagen reaction and repair of the resulting lesions. In the case of the first phenomenon, the hot spots are unlikely to result from simple replication error because this would also make these sites hot spots for spontaneous mutations. Accumulated evidence from several laboratories does not support this possibility. For example, C_{110} of the coding strand was a hot spot for mutations in x-irradiated DNA, but no spontaneous mutation was observed at this site.

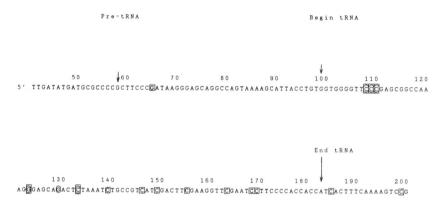

Figure 1. Sequence of *supF*-tRNA gene (nt 41-200 are shown). Termini of mature tRNA sequence are indicated. Hot spots for mutation after MNU and x-ray exposure are shown by circles and squares, respectively.

The observation that not only nt 123 and nt 109 but also nt 122 and nt 124 as well as nt 108 and nt 110 showed a higher-than-expected frequency of mutations with a number of mutagens (Yang et al., 1988; Hauser et al., 1986) has been related to the tertiary folding of the tRNA in which the G's of positions 122-124 are paired to the C's of positions 108-110 in loop I (Yang et al., 1988; Kraemer and Seidman, 1989). However, whether these hairpin base pairings are unique, and whether the unreplicated single-stranded DNA at the replication fork assumes a structure similar to that of mature tRNA, are not known.

Several attempts have recently been made to determine if the bases neighboring an altered base can influence the site of hot spots or conversely can result in cold spots. Following treatment with alkylating agents or ionizing radiation, Glickman and his colleagues observed that N-ethyl-N-nitrosourea treatment of $E.$ $coli$ results in an overabundance of mutations in the middle base of sequences 5'-GGG(or C) and 5'GTG(or C) (Burns et al., 1988). In another study in $E.$ $coli$, the second G in 5'-G(or A)G was shown more likely to be mutated than the G in 5'-C(or T)G with both methylating and ethylating N-nitrosamides and N-nitrosoureas (Burns et al., 1987; Glickman et al., 1987). Richardson et al. (1987) also observed that the second G of 5'-GGA (or T) was highly sensitive to mutation after N-methyl-N-nitro-N-nitrosoguanidine exposure of $E.$ $coli.$ Our results also show the preference of mutation of the middle G at position 123 in the 5'-GGG sequence and of the middle C at position 109 in the 5'-CCC sequence in the nontranscribed strand of the tRNA gene, and we have already pointed out that not all GGG(CCC) sequences are hot spots for x-ray- or MNU-induced mutations. Further, the high susceptibility of the C in 5'-TC doublet observed in our studies with x-ray mutagenesis in human cell systems has not been reported for other mutagens.

STRAND BIAS OF MUTATIONAL HOT SPOTS

Because the majority of point mutations were observed at the C's of 5'-TC sequences, we wondered whether the hot spots were distributed equally in both strands. In the sequence from nt 99 to nt 200, encompassing the mature tRNA sequence and the 3' flanking region, there are 12 5'-TC sequences in the coding strand and 6 5'-TC sequences in the complementary strand. Multiple (more than five) and independent point mutations, including all possible changes, and base loss were observed at C's in 9 such doublets in the coding and in none of the doublets in the complementary strand, respectively. More remarkably, the sum of all mutants in these sequences totaled 96 for the coding strand and 5 for the noncoding strand. The ratio expected from equal probability of conversion of a base change into a mutation is 2:1 for the coding to noncoding strand.

Hauser et al. (1987) observed from analysis of spontaneous point mutants in this plasmid grown in monkey fibroblast (CV1) cells that almost all mutations were in C's of 5'-TC and 5'-CC doublets. Our limited data on the mutations obtained from the control plasmid support their data. Thus, the preferred sites for mutations appear to be similar in control and x-irradiated plasmids. However, these data for spontaneous mutations do not indicate a strand bias for change in C's of the 5'-TC sequences. For example, only two mutations were observed in C_{111} and none in C_{156} of 5'-TC's of the transcribed strand in x-irradiated DNA, yet these appear to be hot spots for spontaneous mutations (Hauser et al., 1987).

There are two possible reasons for this nonuniform distribution of the induced mutations in the 5'-TC sequences in the two strands. Because the construction of the plasmid predicts that the tRNA gene is correctly transcribed in the human cell (Figure 2) (as is obviously true in *E. coli*), it appears likely that while the x-ray-induced lesions are probably distributed randomly, the lesions are repaired preferentially in the transcribed strand. Such a possibility is strongly supported by the elegant studies of Hanawalt and his colleagues (Bohr et al., 1985), which showed that transcriptionally active regions of mammalian genomes are preferentially repaired for UV-induced lesions and that the transcribed strand in these regions is more efficiently repaired than the nontranscribed strand (Mellon et al., 1987).

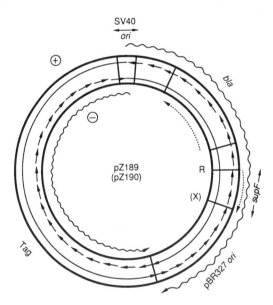

Figure 2. Structure, replication, and transcription of pZ189 (pZ190). Location of different components of the 5.5-kb double-stranded DNA represented by heavy lines are indicated (not to scale). Abbreviations: Tag, T antigen; *bla*, β-lactamase. (+) and (-) signs correspond to nontranscribed and complementary strands of early (T-antigen) transcription; R denotes the *Eco*RI site of the pZ189; pZ190 has additional *Xho*I site (X) at the 3' end of tRNA sequence of *supF* gene. Solid and broken lines between DNA strands represent nascent leading and lagging strands during DNA replication; *arrows* show directions of synthesis. Wavy lines outside circle indicate transcription in primate cells; dotted lines represent transcription in *E. coli*. (Adapted from Seidman et al., 1985; DePamphilis and Wassarman, 1982; Acheson, 1980.)

Alternatively, the strand bias of mutation may result from the distinct modes of replication of the two strands. As shown in Figure 2, the bidirectional replication of the plasmid pZ189 directed by the SV40 replicon dictates that the transcribed strand of the tRNA gene is replicated continuously. The nontranscribed strand is replicated discontinuously as Okazaki fragments that are normally 100-200 nucleotides long (DePamphilis and Wassarman, 1982). Although we do not know whether the priming of these fragments occurs within the tRNA gene, it is likely that there is a significant delay in replication of the lagging strand. Thus, if the damaged G's (e.g., 8-hydroxyguanine) of 3'-AG sequences in the transcribed strand are not repaired as efficiently as in the nontranscribed strand, they would be more susceptible to mutation fixation than those in the nontranscribed strand. However, the explanation for selective mutations at the G's of 3'-AG sequences is not obvious. Assuming that the OH-induced G lesions are randomly distributed, we may speculate that either the lesions other than those located 5' to A's are preferentially repaired, or mispairing of the lesions during DNA replication is favored only after incorporation of thymine at the growing fork.

ACKNOWLEDGMENTS

This research is supported by the Radon and Health Effects Programs, Office of Health and Environmental Research, U.S. Department of Energy, under Contract DE-AC05-84OR21400 with the Martin Marietta Energy Systems. We thank Ms. P.C. Gooch, Mr. H. Luippold, and Mr. W. C. Dunn for expert technical assistance. We also thank Dr. M. Seidman of Otsuka Pharmaceuticals, Gaithersburg, MD, for the plasmid pZ189 and Dr. K. H. Kraemer of the National Cancer Institute, Bethesda, MD, for providing laboratory facilities and technical guidance to one of us (M.O.S.) during the early phase of this work.

REFERENCES

Acheson, NA. 1980. Lytic cycle of SV40 and polyoma virus, pp. 125-204. In: DNA Tumor Viruses, J Tooze (ed.). Cold Spring Harbor Laboratory, Cold Spring Harbor, NY.

Bohr, VW, CA Smith, DS Okumoto, and PC Hanawalt. 1985. DNA repair in an active gene: Removal of pyrimidine dimers from the DHFR gene of CHO cells is much more efficient than the genome overall. Cell 40:359-369.

Brash, DE, S Seetharam, KH Kraemer, MM Seidman, and A Bredberg. 1987. Photoproduct frequency is not the major determinant of UV base substitution hot spots or cold spots in human cells. Proc Natl Acad Sci USA 84:3782-3786.

Bredberg, A, KH Kraemer, and MM Seidman. **1986**. Restricted ultraviolet mutational spectrum in a shuttle vector propagated in xeroderma pigmentosum cells. Proc Natl Acad Sci USA 83:8273-8277.

Breimer, LH. **1988**. Ionizing radiation-induced mutagenesis. Br J Cancer 57:6-18.

Brown, EL, R Belagaje, MJ Ryan, and HG Khorana. **1979**. Chemical synthesis and cloning of a tyrosine tRNA gene. Methods Enzymol 68:109-151.

Burns, PA, AJE Gordon, and BW Glickman. **1987**. Influence of neighboring base sequence on N-methyl-N'-nitro-N-nitrosoguanidine mutagenesis in the *lacI* gene of *Escherichia coli*. J Mol Biol 194:385-390. .

Burns, PA, AJE Gordon, K Kunsmann, and BW Glickman. **1988**. Influence of neighboring base sequence on the distribution and repair of N-ethyl-N-nitrosourea-induced lesions in *Escherichia coli*. Cancer Res 48:4455-4458.

DePamphilis, ML and PM Wassarman. **1982**. Organization and replication of papovavirus DNA, pp. 37-114. In: Organization and Replication of Viral DNA, AS Kaplan (ed.). CRC Press, Boca Raton, FL.

Drinkwater, NR and DK Klinedinst. **1986**. Chemically induced mutagenesis in a shuttle vector with a low-background mutant frequency. Proc Natl Acad Sci USA 83:3402-3406.

Glickman, BW, MJ Horsfall, AJE Gordon, and PA Burns. **1987**. Nearest neighbor affects G:C to A:T transitions induced by alkylating agents. Environ Health Perspect 76:29-32.

Hauser, J, AS Levine, and K Dixon. **1987**. Unique pattern of point mutations arising after gene transfer into mammalian cells. EMBO J 6:63-67.

Hauser, J, MM Seidman, K Sidur, and K Dixon. **1986**. Sequence specificity of point mutations induced during passage of a UV-irradiated shuttle vector plasmid in monkey cells. Mol Cell Biol 6:277-285.

Hirt, B. **1967**. Selective extraction of polyoma DNA from infected mouse cell cultures. J Mol Biol 20:365-369.

Hoebee, B, J Brouwer, P van de Putte, H Loman, and J Retel. **1988**. ^{60}Co α rays induce predominantly C/G to G/C transversions in double-stranded M13 DNA. Nucleic Acids Res 16:8147-8156.

Kraemer, KH and MM Seidman. **1989**. Use of *supF*, an *Escherichia coli* tyrosine suppressor tRNA gene, as a mutagenic target in shuttle vector plasmids. Mutat Res 220:61-72.

Kuchino, Y, F Mori, H Kasai, H Inoue, S Iwai, K Miura, E Ohstuka, and S Nishimura. **1987**. DNA templates containing 8-hydroxydeoxyguanosine are misread both at the modified base and at adjacent residues. Nature 327:77-79.

McCutchen, JA and JS Pagano. **1968.** Enhancement of the infectivity of SV40 deoxyribonucleic acid with diethylaminoethyldextran. J Natl Cancer Inst 41:351-357.

Mellon, I, G Spivak, and PC Hanawalt. **1987.** Selective removal of transcription-blocking DNA damage from the transcribed strand of the mammalian DHFR gene. Cell 51:241-249.

Richardson, KK, RM Crosby, FC Richardson, and TR Skopek. **1987.** DNA base changes induced following *in vivo* exposure of unadapted, adapted or Ada$^-$ *Escherichia coli* to N-methyl-N'-nitro-N-nitrosoguanidine. Mol Gen Genet 209:526-532.

Seidman, MM, K Dixon, A Razzaque, RJ Zagursky, and ML Berman. **1985.** A shuttle vector plasmid for studying carcinogen-induced point mutations in mammalian cells. Gene 38:233-237.

Teebor, CW, RJ Boorstein, and J Cadet. **1988.** The repairability of oxidative free radical mediated damage to DNA: A review. Int J Radiat Biol 54:131-150.

Topal, MD, JS Eadie, and M Conrad. **1986.** O^6-methylguanine mutation and repair is nonuniform. Selection for DNA most interactive with O^6-methylguanine. J Biol Chem 261:9879-9885.

Ward, JF. 1988. DNA damage produced by ionizing radiation in mammalian cells: Identities, mechanisms of formation and repairability. Prog Nucleic Acids Res Mol Biol 35:95-124.

Yang, J-L, VM Maher, and JJ McCormick. **1988.** Kinds and spectrum of mutations induced by 1-nitrosopyrene adducts during plasmid replication in human cells. Mol Cell Biol 8:3364-3372.

Zagursky, RJ, ML Berman, K Baumeister, and N Lomax. **1985.** Rapid and easy sequencing of large double-stranded DNA and supercoiled plasmid DNA. Gen Anal Tech 2:89-94.

Mutagenesis and Molecular Cytogenetics:
Libraries and Mapping

THE NATIONAL LABORATORY GENE LIBRARY PROJECT

L. L. Deaven[1] and M. A. Van Dilla[2]

[1]Los Alamos National Laboratory, Life Sciences Division, University of California, P.O. Box 1663, Los Alamos, NM 87545

[2]Lawrence Livermore National Laboratory, Biomedical Sciences Division, University of California, P.O. Box 5507, Livermore, CA 97550

Key words: *Gene library, chromosome mapping, phage vectors*

ABSTRACT

The aims of the National Laboratory Gene Library Project are to provide a series of human chromosome-specific DNA libraries to interested investigators for use in gene-mapping and chromosome-ordering studies. When the project was initiated in 1983, participants, in collaboration with an advisory committee, set priorities for the types of libraries to be constructed and the strategy to be used in library development. Our first priority was to prepare two sets of complete-digest libraries to meet the needs of the medical genetics community in the search for markers for genetic disease diagnosis. When construction of these libraries was finished, we planned to reevaluate the need for a set of partial-digest libraries for use in basic studies of the human genome at the molecular level. We have now constructed two sets of complete-digest libraries cloned into the *Eco*RI or *Hin*dIII site of the phage vector Charon 21A. These libraries are now available to user groups from a repository at the American Type Culture Collection in Rockville, Maryland.

The second phase of the project, the construction of large-insert (20- to 40-kb) libraries, is underway. New requirements, such as partial digestion of very small (microgram) amounts of sorted DNA and maintenance of long fragment-length (from 50 to 100 kb) before digestion, make these constructions more difficult than those for the small-insert, complete-digest libraries. Partial-digest libraries have been constructed for human chromosomes 16, 19, 21, 22, and X in phage vectors (17- to 20-kb insert size) and for chromosomes 16 and 19 in cosmid vectors (40-kb insert size).

The two National Laboratories at Livermore, California, and Los Alamos, New Mexico, have played a prominent role in the development and application of flow cytometry and sorting to chromosome classification and purification. In 1982, both laboratories began to receive numerous requests for specific human chromosomal types purified by flow-sorting for the

81

construction of DNA libraries, but these requests were difficult to satisfy because of time and personnel constraints. Through its Office of Health and Environmental Research (OHER), the U.S. Department of Energy (DOE) has a long-standing interest in the human genome in general and in the mutagenic and carcinogenic effects of energy-related environmental pollutants in particular. Thus, it was decided in 1983 to use the flow cytometric and molecular biological skills at both laboratories to construct chromosome-specific gene libraries to be made available to the genetic research community.

The National Laboratory Gene Library Project was envisioned as a practical way to handle requests for sorted chromosomes, and also as a way to promote increased understanding of the human genome and the effects of mutagens and carcinogens on it. Project strategy was developed with the help of an advisory committee as well as suggestions and advice from many other geneticists. The committee included P. Berg (Stanford), T. Maniatis and S. A. Latt (Harvard), A. G. Motulsky (University of Washington), W. J. Rutter (University of California, San Francisco), C. W. Schmid (University of California, Davis), T. B. Shows (Roswell Park), C. T. Caskey (Baylor), F. R. Blattner (University of Wisconsin), M. H. Edgell (University of North Carolina), and R. E. Gelinas (University of Washington).

Our first goal was the construction of small-insert (complete-digest) libraries for each of the 24 human chromosomal types. These were intended mainly for the medical genetics community to use in studying and diagnosing genetic diseases by the restriction fragment-length polymorphism method. For such studies, short DNA probes about 1 kb in size are ideal, and complete-digest libraries are the easiest to produce from the limited amounts of chromosomal DNA available from flow-sorting. We made two sets of libraries: one was cloned into the *Eco*RI site (Los Alamos), and one into the *Hin*dIII site (Livermore) of the bacteriophage vector Charon 21A. A listing of these complete-digest libraries, available from the American Type Culture Collection, Rockville, Maryland, is given in Tables 1 and 2.

The second goal is the construction of larger-insert (partial-digest) libraries in phage and cosmid vectors. These libraries will provide a rich source of DNA sequences for physical mapping and for studies of gene structure and function. Our strategy for these constructions is to divide the human karyotype between the two laboratories and produce one phage and one cosmid library for each chromosome. Our current vector choices include Charon 40 and sCos1 (Los Alamos) and λGEM11 and Lawrst5 (Livermore). These vectors

Table 1. Characteristics of 28 chromosome-specific DNA libraries cloned into the EcoRI site of Charon 21A.

Library ID No.[a]	Independent Recombinants	Frequency of Nonrecombinants	Chromosome Equivalents[b]	Chromosome Source[c]	Starting Chromosomes ($\times 10^6$)	Starting DNA (ng)
LA 01 NS01	1.3×10^6	<0.01	31	UV24HL10-12	0.5	250
LA 02 NS01	7.0×10^4	0.04	1.8	UV24HL5	0.5	260
LA 03 NS01	2.7×10^4	0.04	0.8	314-lb	0.4	160
LA 03 NS02	2.1×10^5	0.08	6.4	314-lb	0.4	180
LA 04 NS01	5.1×10^4	<0.01	1.6	UV20HL21-27	0.9	370
LA 04 NS02	7.4×10^4	<0.01	2.3	UV20HL21-27	0.9	370
LA 05 NS01	1.3×10^6	<0.01	43	640-12	0.4	130
LA 06 NS01	4.8×10^4	0.06	1.7	UV20HL15-33	1.9	700
LA 07 NS01	2.4×10^5	0.06	9.2	MR3.316TG6	0.1	40
LA 08 NS04	3.6×10^4	0.10	1.5	UV20HL21-27	0.5	150
LA 09 NS01	1.6×10^6	0.07	7	HSF-7	0.3	90
LA 10 NS01	4.0×10^5	<0.01	18	762-8A	0.3	90
LA 11 NS02	6.2×10^4	0.17	2.8	80H10	0.4	100
LA 12 NS01	6.0×10^5	<0.01	27	81P5d	1.5	210
LA 13 NS03	7.5×10^4	0.14	4.2	HSF-7	0.4	80
LA 14 NS01	6.1×10^5	<0.01	36	1634	0.5	115
LA 15 NS02	4.0×10^5	0.06	20	81P5d	0.3	71
LA 15 NS03	6.8×10^4	0.09	4	1634	0.4	82
LA 16 NS02	4.0×10^4	0.08	2	HSF-7	3.0	590
LA 16 NS03	3.3×10^5	0.03	21.7	HSF-7	0.5	100
LA 17 NS03	1.1×10^5	0.01	7.9	GM130A	0.6	110
LA 18 NS04	2.5×10^5	0.02	19	HSF-7	0.5	81
LA 19 NS03	1.1×10^6	0.16	11	HSF-7	0.5	65
LA 20 NS01	1.6×10^4	0.24	1.5	HSF-7	0.5	72
LA 21 NS01	1.1×10^6	<0.01	137	HSF-7	0.9	87
LA 22 NS03	9.3×10^4	0.19	11	HSF-7	0.5	55
LA 0X NS01	2.1×10^5	0.02	8.5	81p5d	1.2	380
LA 0Y NS01	1.1×10^5	0.10	11.5	HSF-7	0.5	64

[a] The ID Code consists of eight alphanumeric items. The first two items indicate which laboratory made the library, i.e., LL = Lawrence Livermore National Laboratory and LA = Los Alamos National Laboratory. The next two items are underlined and indicate chromosome type (in the one case of a mixed 14/15 library, chromosome type is designated as 45). The fifth item is a letter indicating chromosome status, i.e., N for normal, T for translocation, etc. The sixth item is either S (for small-insert, complete-digest libraries) or L (for large-insert, partial-digest libraries). The final two items represent library construction number.

[b] Number of recombinants for 1 chromosome equivalent = $\dfrac{(3 \times 10^9)\,(0.65)\,(f)}{4100}$

where 3×10^9 bp is the size of the human haploid genome; 0.65 is the clonable fraction; f is the fraction of cellular DNA in a particular chromosome; 4100 bp is the averge fragment size.

[c] Cell lines from which metaphase chromosomes were isolated:
1. Normal diploid human fibroblast lines 761, 811, HSF-7.
2. Apparently normal human lymphoblastoid line GM130A and multiple X lymphoblastoid line 1634 (49, XXX).
3. CHO x human lymphocyte lines (human chromosome content):

UV24HL5 (#2, X)	UV20HL 15-33 (#6, 9, 13, 15,17, 20, 21)
314 -lb (#3)	UV41HL4 (#6, 9)
UV20HL21-27 (#4, 8, 21)	762-8A (#10)
640-12 (#5, 9, 12)	UV24HL 10-12 (#1, 3, 11, 13)

4. E36 x human lymphocyte lines (human chromosome content) 81 P5d (X, 12, 15).
5. V79 x human lymphocyte lines (human chromosome content) MR3.316TG6 (7 x del).

Table 2. Characteristics of 28 chromosome-specific DNA libraries cloned into the
*Hin*dIII site of Charon 21A.

Library ID No.[a]	Independent Recombinants	Frequency of Nonre-combinants	Chromosome Equivalents[b]		Chromosome Source[c]	Starting Chromosomes ($\times 10^6$)	Starting DNA (ng)
LL 01 NS01	8.3×10^4	0.04	2.1		UV24HL10-12	0.5	270
LL 01 NS02	1.3×10^6	0.01	32	(20)	UV24HL6	0.5	270
LL 02 NS01	6.6×10^5	0.08	16	(5)	UV24HL5	0.5	270
LL 03 NS01	1.6×10^5	0.10	4.8		314-lb	0.5	220
LL 04 NS01	2.3×10^4	0.02	0.8		UV20HL21-27	1.0	400
LL 04 NS02	5×10^5	0.27	10		UV20HL21-27	0.5	210
LL 05 NS01	3.4×10^6	0.26	113	(30)	640-12	0.5	200
LL 06 NS01	7.6×10^5	0.06	27	(20)	UV20HL15-33	0.4	135
LL 07 NS01	3×10^5	0.01	11.5		GM131	0.9	310
LL 08 NS02	2.2×10^6	0.03	93	(20)	UV20HL21-27	0.7	210
LL 09 NS01	3.0×10^5	0.02	13		UV41HL4	0.4	120
LL 10 NS01	2.4×10^5	0.01	10.6		762-8A	0.5	150
LL 11 NS01	1.1×10^5	0.05	4.9		UV20HL4	0.2	50
LL 12 NS01	7.5×10^5	0.01	34	(20)	81P5D	0.4	120
LL 13 NS01	2.2×10^4	0.04	1.3		761	1.0	240
LL 13 NS02	8.5×10^5	0.03	47	(20)	GM131	0.5	120
LL 14 NS01	2.3×10^6	0.06	135		GM131	0.5	110
LL 45 NS01	2.6×10^6	0.02	152	(30)	811	1.0	210
LL 15 NS01	7.0×10^4	0.06	4.4		GM131	1.0	110
LL 16 NS03	7.6×10^5	0.02	51	(20)	HSF7	0.5	100
LL 17 NS02	3.4×10^5	0.02	24	(20)	HSF7	0.5	95
LL 18 NS01	8.9×10^5	0.13	72		761	1.0	170
LL 19 NS01	1.5×10^6	0.02	145	(10)	811	1.0	130
LL 20 NS01	3.9×10^6	0.01	354	(20)	811	1.0	140
LL 21 NS02	4.7×10^5	0.34	60	(20)	811	0.5	45
LL 22 NS01	6.1×10^5	0.05	71	(17)	811	0.5	50
LL 0X NS01	2.1×10^6	0.33	84	(30)	UV24HL5	0.5	170
LL 0Y NS01	2.5×10^5	0.02	27		811	1.0	115

[a] The ID Code consists of eight alphanumeric items. The first two items indicate which laboratory made the
library, i.e., LL = Lawrence Livermore National Laboratory and LA = Los Alamos National Laboratory.
The next two items are underlined and indicate chromosome type (in the one case of a mixed 14/15 library,
chromosome type is designated as 45). The fifth item is a letter indicating chromosome status, i.e., N for
normal, T for translocation, etc. The sixth item is either S (for small-insert, complete-digest libraries) or L
(for large-insert, partial-digest libraries). The final two items represent library construction number.

[b] Number of recombinants for 1 chromosome equivalent $= \dfrac{(3 \times 10^9)\,(0.65)\,(f)}{4100}$

where 3×10^9 bp is the size of the human haploid genome; 0.65 is the clonable fraction; f is the
fraction of cellular DNA in a particular chromosome; 4100 bp is the averge fragment size.
Numbers in parentheses refer to representation of amplified library; for very large libraries, only a fraction of
the packaging reaction was amplified.

[c] Cell lines from which metaphase chromosomes were isolated:
1. Normal diploid human fibroblast lines 761, 811, HSF7.
2. Apparently normal human lymphoblastoid line GM131.
3. CHO x human lymphocyte lines (human chromosome content):

UV24HL10-12 (#1, 2 del, 3, 11, 13, 19)	UV20HL 15-33 (#6, 9, 13, 15, 17, 20, 21)
UV24HL6 (#1, 2 del, 37, 11-13, 147, 187, 19)	UV41HL4 (#6, 9. 13, 16, 18, Y)
UV24HL5 (#2, X)	762-8A (#10, Y)
314 -lb (#3)	UV20HL4 (#1, 4-6, 11, 14-16, 19, 21)
UV20HL21-27 (#4, 8, 21)	81P5D (#12, 15, X).
640-12 (#5, 9, 12)	

were chosen on the basis of cloning efficiency, sequence preservation, and user convenience. As new and improved vectors become available, they will be considered for use in the project. Partial-digest libraries have been made for chromosomes 16, 19, 21, 22, X, and Y. The partial-digest libraries will also be available for general distribution through the American Type Culture Collection.

We expect to complete the partial-digest libraries in 1.5 to 2 yr. Our directions after these libraries are completed are speculative and to some extent depend on future changes in technology.

At present, a set of libraries for each mouse chromosome would be a valuable resource to the genetics research community. Our advisory committee had a difficult time deciding whether the large-insert human libraries or mouse libraries should be given first priority for the current work. Depending on changes in technology or activities in other laboratories, the need for mouse libraries may or may not exist 2 yr from now. We expect this need will continue to be a high priority, and although the sorting of mouse chromosomes is difficult, we believe it is feasible. Therefore, construction of mouse-chromosome-specific libraries is a likely future direction for the project.

A group of plant geneticists would like to see a national effort organized to begin sorting and preparing libraries for a plant species. This would require considerable preliminary work to develop adequate sources of isolated chromosomes for sorting.

We are also considering constructing sets of human chromosome libraries in one of the new large-fragment-accepting vectors (YAC, phage P1); such libraries will probably be necessary for closure of physical maps. Currently, cloning efficiencies do not permit the use of flow-sorted chromosomes as a source of target DNA; however, these efficiencies could improve markedly by 1990. Other possibilities for the construction of these libraries include the use of monochromosomal hybrids as a source of DNA and the selection of human clones after library construction. Our ability to monitor hybrids for specific chromosomal content by flow analysis would be advantageous if the latter approach had to be used.

BIBLIOGRAPHY

Deaven, LL, CE Hildebrand, JC Fusco, and MA Van Dilla. **1986.** Construction of human chromosome specific DNA libraries: The National Laboratory Gene Library Project. Genet Eng 8:317-332.

Deaven, LL, MA Van Dilla, MF Bartholdi, AV Carrano, LL Cram, JC Fuscoe, JW Gray, CE Hildebrand, RK Moyzis, and J Perlman. **1987.** Construction of human chromosome-specific DNA libraries from flow-sorted chromosomes. Cold Spring Harbor Symp Quant Biol 51:159-168.

Van Dilla, MA, LL Deaven, KL Albright, NA Allen, MR Aubuchon, MF Bartholdi, NC Brown, EW Campbell, AV Carrano, LM Clark, LS Cram, JC Fuscoe, JW Gray, CE Hildebrand, PJ Jackson, JH Jett, JL Longmire, CR Lozes, ML Luedemann, JC Martin, J Meyne, JS McNinch, LJ Meincke, ML Mendelsohn, RK Moyzis, AC Munk, J Perlman, DC Peters, AJ Silva, and BJ Trask. 1986. Human chromosome-specific DNA libraries: Construction and availability. Biotechnology 4:537-552.

Van Dilla, MA, LL Deaven, KL Albright, NA Allen, MF Bartholdi, NC Brown, EW Campbell, AV Carrano, M Christensen, LM Clark, LS Cram, PN Dean, P de Jong, JJ Fawcett, JC Fuscoe, JW Gray, CE Hildebrand, PJ Jackson, JH Jett, S Kolla, JL Longmire, CR Lozes, ML Luedemann, JS McNinch, ML Mendelsohn, J Meyne, LJ Meincke, RK Moyzis, J Mullikin, AC Munk, J Perlman, L Pederson, DC Peters, AJ Silva, BJ Trask, and G van den Engh. 1989. Chapter III B2. In: *Flow Cytogenetics*, JW Gray (ed.). Academic Press, New York, NY.

QUESTIONS AND COMMENTS

Q: Gantt, NCI
   What is the molecular weight of the DNA in isolated chromosomes?

A: There is some sample-to-sample variation in the molecular weight of DNA in sorted chromosomes; however, in many samples the bulk of the DNA is greater than 700 kb.

INSERTIONAL MUTAGENESIS IN TRANSGENIC MICE

R. P. Woychik,[1] B. R. Beatty,[2] and W. L. McKinney, Jr.[1]

[1]Biology Division, Oak Ridge National Laboratory, Oak Ridge, TN 37831-8077

[2]The University of Tennessee, Oak Ridge Graduate School of Biomedical Sciences, P.O. Box 2009, Oak Ridge, TN 37831-8077

Key words: *Genetic loci, nucleotide sequence, mouse genome, mutations*

ABSTRACT

Recent advances in gene-cloning and embryo-manipulation technologies are currently being used to probe the relationship between the basic structure of the genetic material and the physiological, biochemical, and behavioral characteristics of the developing and mature organism. Within the U.S. Department of Energy, strategies to physically map and sequence the entire mammalian genome will unquestionably contribute to this effort. However, nucleotide sequence and physical mapping data alone lack the information necessary for locating and determining the size and the temporal/spatial expression of the functional loci on the genome. Genetic approaches involving the analysis of individual mutations, on the other hand, have historically been the principal mechanism for establishing the position of genes on the genomes of several organisms, including those of the mouse and humans.

Accordingly, we are using our resources within the Mammalian Genetics Section to implement a large-scale insertional mutagenesis program using transgenic mice. Unlike most mutations that currently exist, mutations generated in transgenic mice are "tagged" with a molecular marker and can be readily cloned using the recombinant DNA technology. Cloned sequences from the transgenic animals can be used to study the molecular biology of the mutation, which, in turn, will allow us to draw a molecular connection between the mutant phenotype and a specific gene on the genome.

Additionally, we are using genomic sequences derived from transgenic mice as probes in the molecular studies of gene mutations and chromosomal rearrangements derived either spontaneously or from radiation and chemical mutagenesis experiments. This approach has proven valuable for studying the molecular nature and transcriptional consequences of genetic damage and also for the physical mapping and sequencing of specific regions of the mammalian genome.

The relationship between the basic structure of the genetic material and the physiological, biochemical, and behavioral characteristics of the developing and mature organism is currently an area of intense investigation in medicine and biology. Strategies to physically map and sequence the entire human genome will unquestionably contribute significantly to this effort. However, nucleotide sequence and physical mapping data alone lack the information necessary for studying functional loci within the genome. On the other hand, genetic approaches coupled with the molecular analysis of individual mutations are among the most efficient means of establishing the function and organization of genes of several organisms, including those in the mouse and man.

The analysis of mutations in the human genome is the most direct route for studying human genetic disease. The limitation of this approach follows from the infeasibility of performing certain experiments on humans. The mouse, with its extensive experimental genetic and embryological history, relatively short generation time, accessibility to experimental manipulation with the molecular tools to perform gene therapy, and, most importantly, its close biological similarity to humans, is a suitable alternative model system for studying the structure and function of the mammalian genome.

The study of mutations at the molecular level requires that a given mutant locus be identifiable and clonable with our present technology. For this reason, insertional mutagenesis approaches have proven extremely valuable because they "tag" the mutant locus with a molecular marker. Transposable elements in bacteria, yeast, maize, *Drosophila* spp., and *Caenorhabditis elegans* have been used as molecular "tags" for insertional mutagenesis experiments in these organisms. With the recent development of the transgenic mouse technology, it is now possible, using either retroviruses or the pronuclear microinjection procedure, to readily generate insertional mutations in the mouse. Numerous insertional mutations, with phenotypes ranging from embryonic lethalities to various types of limb deformities (Palmiter and Brinster, 1986), have been reported in transgenic mice. Moreover, many of these insertional mutations are proving to be alleles of existing mutations. Recent estimates that approximately 10% of all transgenic mice harbor insertion mutations (Palmiter and Brinster, 1986; Covarrubias et al., 1985) imply that this form of mutagenesis is a relatively efficient means of generating molecularly tagged mutations in the mouse.

We are using our resources at the Oak Ridge National Laboratory to implement a large-scale insertional mutagenesis program in transgenic mice. We have designed the program so that each transgenic animal will contain the chloramphenicol acetyl transferase (CAT) gene as the transgene. The biochemical assay for CAT activity is rapid and highly sensitive; therefore, performing CAT assays on tissues from individual animals should greatly facilitate the identification of transgenic offspring during the screening process. Additionally, the CAT gene construction is designed in a way that enables it to be used as a selectable marker in bacteria to simplify the cloning of the mouse genomic sequences flanking the inserted transgene.

The screening procedure we have instituted will allow us to maintain several hundred individual lines of transgenic mice and to test them for the expression of a wide variety of phenotypes. We expect that this mutagenesis program will enable us to generate a considerable number of insertional mutations expressing a wide range of phenotypes; many of these molecularly "tagged" mutations will be made available to interested investigators within the international scientific community for an in-depth molecular analysis.

Another aspect of our research program involves the utilization of genomic probes derived from transgenic mice to analyze major structural rearrangements produced in chemical- and radiation-mutagenesis studies at Oak Ridge National Laboratory. In one such experiment, the genomic probes derived from the transgenic insertional mutation ld^{Hd} (Woychik et al., 1985) are being used to characterize a complex structural DNA rearrangement in a line of mutant animals carrying a 2;17 chromosomal translocation. These animals express phenotypes corresponding to mutations in the limb deformity (ld) and nonagouti (a) loci in chromosome 2. We are using the probes from the transgenic mouse to study how this structural rearrangement in DNA affects the expression of genes within both the ld and the a loci. This work clearly demonstrates the usefulness of probes derived from transgenic mice for the analysis of mutations in the stock of mice currently being maintained at the Oak Ridge National Laboratory.

ACKNOWLEDGMENTS

The submitted manuscript has been authored by a contractor of the U.S. Government under Contract No. DE-AC05-84OR21400. Accordingly, the U.S. Government retains a nonexclusive, royalty-free license to publish or reproduce the published form of this contribution, or allow others do so, for U.S. Government purposes. Research was sponsored by the Office of Health and Environmental Research, U.S. Department of Energy under Contract No. DE-AC05-84OR21400 with Martin Marietta Energy Systems, Inc.

REFERENCES

Covarrubias, LY and B Mintz. 1985. Early developmental mutations due to DNA rearrangements in transgenic mouse embryos. Cold Spring Harbor Symp Quant Biol 50:447-452.

Palmiter, RD ånd RL Brinster. 1986. Germ-line transformation of mice. Annu Rev Genet 20:465-499.

Woychik, RP, TA Stewart, LG Davis, P D'Eustachio, and P Leder. 1985. An inherited limb deformity created by insertional mutagenesis in a transgenic mouse. Nature 318:36-40.

QUESTIONS AND COMMENTS

Q: Hankinson, Laboratory of Biomedical Environmental Science, University of California, Los Angeles
Have you considered microinjecting a plasmid containing a *cos* site to facilitate rescue of the tagged genes from the transgenic mice?

A: There are many ways to facilitate the rescue of transgenes. The method we prefer involves the use of bacterial selectable antibiotic resistance genes like the CAT gene because these genes can also be used as reporter genes to monitor the expression of the transgene.

Q: Nelson, Jet Propulsion Laboratory
Occasionally it is useful to produce mutations that leave residual gene activity. Does insertional mutagenesis always produce null alleles or can hypomorphic alleles also be generated?

A: It is conceivable that insertional mutagenesis may only partially inactivate the function of a complex gene. It is my prediction that many mammalian developmental genes will be found to be structurally complex and undergo transcriptional and posttranscriptional regulation to generate different forms of mRNA. Integration of a foreign fragment of DNA within the 5' or 3' regulatory regions or within an intron may not totally abolish the expression of a gene but rather may affect the level of expression and/or may redirect any tissue-specific and developmentally related posttranscriptional alternate processing of the mRNA.

SATURATION-MUTAGENESIS AND PHYSICAL-MAPPING STRATEGIES FOR REGIONS OF THE MOUSE GENOME

E. M. Rinchik,[1] D. K. Johnson,[2] M. L. Klebig,[2] R. Machanoff,[1] C. C. Cummings,[1] A. K. Jimmerson,[1] and D. A. Carpenter[1]

[1]Biology Division, Oak Ridge National Laboratory, Oak Ridge, TN 37831-8077

[2]The University of Tennessee-Oak Ridge Graduate School of Biomedical Sciences, P.O. Box 2009, Oak Ridge, TN 37831-8077

Key words: *Mouse germline deletions, physical and functional mapping, mutagenesis, molecular developmental genetics*

ABSTRACT

Our research program is currently exploiting the many spontaneous and agent-induced heritable mutations of the mouse, generated by years of germ-cell-mutagenesis experiments at Oak Ridge National Laboratory, to learn more about the genetic control of normal and abnormal mammalian development. Much of our emphasis is on the analysis of radiation-induced lethal mutations that have been identified within specific regions of the genome. These types of mutations, which are usually chromosomal deletions of varying lengths, are proving to be unique and extremely useful reagents for this type of integrated molecular and functional study of the mouse genome.

Genetic analyses of panels of such overlapping germ-line deletions have resulted in gross functional maps of specific genomic regions, and have identified a host of hitherto undefined genes that not only expand the genetic map but also are critical for normal development. We are currently using the largest deletion available for each of several "model" regions to select region-specific DNA clones from appropriately enriched genomic libraries. These clones (and derivative larger clones) are being mapped and ordered with respect to chromosomal breakpoints within each panel of overlapping deletions. Because the gross functional map is based on the location of these same breakpoints within each deletion complex, DNA clones are automatically mapped to specific genomic functional units.

An important complement to this deletion-facilitated molecular mapping of genomic regions is our program to "saturate," with presumed point mutations, specific regions of the mouse genome associated with the same long, radiation-induced deletion mutations that are the targets of our molecular-mapping analyses. These germ-line-mutagenesis experiments, which employ the supermutagen

N-ethyl-*N*-nitrosourea, are designed: (1) to estimate the minimum number of genes within a region that are mutable to specific, biologically significant phenotypes; (2) to provide, for several regions of the genome, a *fine-structure functional map* that is based on a series of heritable intragenic mutations with characteristic phenotypes, which can subsequently be correlated with detailed molecular/ physical maps; and (3) to provide fundamental genetic, logistical, and statistical information on which to base strategies for subsequent large-scale expansion of the functional maps of mammalian genomes.

INTRODUCTION

Our research program is currently exploiting the many spontaneous and agent-induced heritable mutations of the mouse, generated by years of germ-cell-mutagenesis experiments at Oak Ridge National Laboratory (ORNL), to learn more both about the physical and the functional composition of the mammalian genome and about the genetic control of normal and abnormal mammalian development. Much of our emphasis is placed on the analysis of radiation-induced lethal mutations that have been identified within specific regions of the genome associated with loci employed in the mouse specific-locus germ-cell mutagenesis test (Russell, 1951). These types of mutations, which are often chromosomal deletions of varying lengths, are proving to be both unique and extremely useful reagents for detailed integrated molecular and functional studies of approximately 1% to 2% of the mouse genome.

Genetic analyses of panels of such overlapping germline deletions have resulted in gross functional maps of specific genomic regions, and have identified a host of hitherto undefined genes that not only expand the genetic map but also are critical for normal development (Russell, 1971; Russell et al., 1982; Rinchik et al., 1985, 1986; Russell and Rinchik, 1987). Large multilocus deletions can also be used to identify, from appropriately enriched genomic DNA libraries, DNA probes that map to a specific region of interest, completely bypassing laborious standard transmission linkage experiments that map such probes with respect to visible or biochemical marker loci. Once clones are obtained for a large region (defined, for example, by the longest deletion available for that region), panels of nested, smaller deletions can be used to map and order clones rapidly with respect to each other. Moreover, because the gross functional map is based on the location of these same breakpoints within each deletion complex, DNA clones are automatically mapped to specific genomic functional units within each regional functional map.

MOLECULAR GENETICS OF DELETIONS OF SPECIFIC LOCI

Our continuing analysis of the albino- (c-) locus region of chromosome 7 associated with the 6- to 11-centimorgan (cM) germline deletion $Df(c\ sh\text{-}1)^{Fq1}$ provides one example of these mapping strategies. Complementation analyses of independent, radiation-induced lethal c mutations [including $Df(c\ sh\text{-}1)^{Fq1}$] resulted in a linear map of this region surrounding c that was composed of at least eight functional units (Russell et al., 1982). Some phenotypes associated with these mutations include: embryonic lethality at preimplantation or implantation stages (Lewis et al., 1976; Lewis, 1978; Russell and Raymer, 1979; Russell et al., 1979, 1982; Niswander et al., 1988); neonatal lethality, accompanied by abnormalities in the regulation of certain metabolic enzymes (reviewed in Gluecksohn-Waelsch, 1979; Schmid et al., 1985; Loose et al., 1986); juvenile lethality and male sterility (Lewis et al., 1978; Russell et al., 1982); and structural abnormalities in the ear labyrinth (Deol, 1956; Mikaelian and Ruben, 1964). Not surprisingly, the $Df(c\ sh\text{-}1)^{Fq1}$ deletion, which may encompass 6- to 20-megabase pairs of DNA, is lethal (at the preimplantation-embryo stage) when homozygous.

Using a series of genetic crosses and progeny tests, we have placed the very large $Df(c\ sh\text{-}1)^{Fq1}$ *Mus musculus*-derived deletion (and 28 smaller, lethal deletions) opposite a *Mus spretus* chromosome 7. These genetic constructions have been useful as mapping reagents because they allow molecular marking [by *spretus-musculus* restriction fragment-length polymorphisms (RFLP) (Robert et al., 1985)] of homologous chromosomes 7 in each F_1. DNA clones can be mapped rapidly by testing in genomic Southern analysis whether a given probe maps within a given deletion (*musculus*-specific fragment absent) or outside the deletion (*musculus*-specific band present). We have used DNA prepared from these balanced-deletion *musculus/spretus* F_1 to identify a DNA probe (defining the locus *D7OR1*) that maps distally to c near chromosomal subregions associated with survival of the preimplantation embryo and with inner-ear development. [This probe was obtained from a library constructed from flow-sorted, long $T(X;7)$ translocation chromosomes.] This mapping panel of DNA, based on the *musculus/spretus* balanced-deletion F_1, will be very useful when higher purity libraries (such as those obtained from two-variable chromosome sorting or from chromosome microdissection and microcloning) become available.

We have also exploited a different mapping panel of DNA that is based on smaller, homozygous-viable or complementing, overlapping c deletions, to map a DNA clone associated with the site of integration of an ecotropic murine leukemia provirus (Rinchik et al., 1989). Silver (1985) reported tight linkage with c of such a provirus (which we have designated Emv-23). By cloning Emv-23 plus flanking chromosome-7 sequences from the DNA of C58/J mice, we have demonstrated by both standard transmission-genetics and deletion-mapping experiments that the viral integration site maps less than 0.5 cM distal to c, between the tyrosinase locus (c) itself and a subregion associated with sterility in males, spontaneous mid-gestation "abortion" in females, and reduced fitness in both sexes. A 1.4-kb unique-sequence chromosome 7 probe derived from the 5' end of this integrated provirus is being used to develop a long-range restriction map of this particular subregion of the albino deletion complex.

SATURATION MUTAGENESIS OF DELETION-ASSOCIATED REGIONS

An important complement to deletion-facilitated molecular mapping of genomic regions is our program to "saturate," with presumed point mutations, specific regions of the mouse genome associated with the same long, radiation-induced deletion mutations that are the targets of our molecular-mapping analyses. These germline mutagenesis experiments, which employ the supermutagen N-ethyl-N-nitrosourea (ENU), are designed: (1) to estimate the minimum number of genes within a region that are mutable to specific, biologically significant phenotypes; (2) to provide, for several regions of the genome, a fine-structure functional map based on a series of heritable intragenic mutations with characteristic phenotypes, which can subsequently be correlated with detailed molecular/physical maps; and (3) to provide fundamental genetical, logistical, and statistical information on which to base strategies for subsequent large-scale expansion of the functional maps of mammalian genomes.

Once again, the region of chromosome 7 surrounding the c locus is serving as a model to illustrate these "saturation-mutagenesis" strategies. The experimental protocol involves the 6- to 11-cM region defined by the $Df(c\ sh\text{-}1)^{Fp1}$ deletion of the c locus, which is probably the second-longest c deletion in our panel and may include up to 10% of the chromosome. Males carrying a standard, nonlethal albino (c) marker are treated with a highly mutagenic dose of ENU. Daughters ($+/c$) are crossed to tester $[c^{ch}\ +/Df(c\ sh\text{-}1)^{Fp1}]$ males, and albino progeny $[c/Df(c\ sh\text{-}1)^{Fp1}]$ are inspected for new phenotypes associated with the hemizygous expression of a newly induced, recessive mutation on the c-bearing chromosome that falls within the region deleted in $Df(c\ sh\text{-}1)^{Fp1}$. Absence of the albino class suggests the presence of a newly induced, lethal mutation (on the c-bearing chromosome) that likewise falls within the limits of the $Df(c\ sh\text{-}1)^{Fp1}$ deletion.

Such a "hemizygosity screen" of 900 $+$ /c F_1 females and, therefore, of 900 mutagenized gametes has detected three new confirmed lethal mutations; other presumed lethals are undergoing testing. We have also detected two repeat (i.e., noncomplementing, nonclustered) mutations of the neurological locus *shaker-1 (sh-1)* and two repeat mutations at a newly defined locus that result in a runting syndrome.

Preliminary deletion-mapping and time-of-death experiments have revealed several interesting characteristics of two of these presumably intragenic mutations. The first lethal mutation that was detected (*181SB*) appears to map to a distal subregion of the albino deletion complex (near *sh-1*) that has not yet been associated with a lethal phenotype. Moreover, the hemizygous *181SB* genotype [i.e., c *181SB*/$Df(c$ $sh-1)^{Fp1}$] appears to be always lethal before birth; however, some c *181SB*/c *181SB* homozygotes can survive past birth, but always die before weaning. The preliminary mapping data also suggest that *181SB* may map to the same deletion-defined subregion as the DNA-defined locus *D7OR1* mentioned previously. Hence, the potential exists for future molecular study of both this locus and this interesting ENU-induced lethal mutation.

Preliminary data also suggest that the "fitness" mutation (*494SB*), which gives rise to a runting syndrome in both hemizygotes and homozygotes, may map to subregions of the albino deletion complex heretofore associated with survival of the implantation embryo. It will be interesting to determine whether this particular mutation defines a later-acting locus whose effects are masked by the early-gestation death of animals homozygous for early-acting lethal deletions that also include this locus, or whether *494SB* represents a minor, more tolerable, intragenic mutation in one of the implantation lethals residing within this subregion.

FUTURE DIRECTIONS

The molecular-genetic analysis of the c region, as outlined here, will be facilitated by identifying additional DNA clones that map to $Df(c$ $sh-1)^{Fq1}$. The detection and cloning of the many deletion breakpoint/fusion fragments carried by the panel of mutant stocks will enable chromosomal "jumping" within the region, and, with the development of long-range restriction maps derived from the application of large-fragment DNA techniques, will contribute to a detailed molecular map of approximately 10% of chromosome 7. The continuing identification of ENU-induced single-gene mutations will likewise play an important role in defining the correlations between sequences of DNA and the location and function of specific genes.

Indeed, we anticipate that these new, (presumably) individual gene mutations, in addition to refining the functional maps of genomic regions associated with deletions, will also be important as function-deficient (or
function-altered) hosts for receiving segments of cloned, wild-type DNA via
transgenic mouse technology. These types of correction-of-phenotype
experiments, if technically feasible, will comprise the ultimate strategy of
gene identification for expressed DNA sequences derived from these regions
and will be a central component in a strategy for accomplishing in-depth
molecular and functional characterization of segments of the mouse
genome.

These functional- and physical-mapping strategies are also being actively
applied to two other regions of the mouse genome: one surrounding the p
(*pink-eyed dilution*) locus in chromosome 7, associated with 43 radiation-
induced lethal mutations; and one surrounding the b (*brown*) locus in
chromosome 4, associated with 28 lethal mutations. As with the c region,
many loci important for normal development can be accessed and studied
using the deletions as molecular and genetic "reagents." Experiments are
currently under way to screen 3000 mutagenized gametes for new ENU-
induced intragenic mutations in both the c and p regions.

Because of the many instances of linkage conservation and gene homology
between the mouse and human genomes (for review, see Searle et al.,
1987), we anticipate that such detailed physical and functional mapping of
chromosomal segments within such an experimentally malleable model
system will be directly applicable to the molecular-genetic study of the
human and other complex genomes. Molecular and mutational analysis of
mouse genomic regions, therefore, might not only define new developmental functions, but might also directly associate functions with human DNA
sequences that might otherwise be characterized only at a structural
(DNA sequence) level.

ACKNOWLEDGMENTS

Research was sponsored by the Office of Health and Environmental
Research, U.S. Department of Energy, under contract DE-AC05-84OR21400
with Martin Marietta Energy Systems, Inc. We thank Drs. L. B. Russell
and R. P. Woychik for their critical reading of the abstract.

This manuscript has been written by a contractor of the U.S. Government
under contract No. DE-AC05-84OR21400. Accordingly, the U.S. Government retains a nonexclusive, royalty-free license to publish or reproduce the
published form of this contribution, or allow others to do so, for U.S.
Government purposes.

REFERENCES

Deol, MS. 1956. The anatomy and development of the mutants pirouette, shaker-1, and waltzer in the mouse. Proc R Soc Lond (Biol) 145:206-213.

Gluecksohn-Waelsch, S. 1979. Genetic control of morphogenetic and biochemical differentiation: Lethal albino deletions in the mouse. Cell 16:225-237.

Lewis, SE. 1978. Developmental analysis of lethal effects of homozygosity for the c^{25H} deletion in the mouse. Dev Biol 65:553-557.

Lewis, SE, HA Turchin, and S Gluecksohn-Waelsch. 1976. The developmental analysis of an embryonic lethal (c^{6H}) in the mouse. J Embryol Exp Morphol 36: 363-371.

Lewis, SE, HA Turchin, and TE Wojtowicz. 1978. Fertility studies of complementing genotypes at the albino locus of the mouse. J Reprod Fertil 53:197-202.

Loose, DS, PA Shaw, KS Krauter, C Robinson, S England, RW Hanson, and S Gluecksohn-Waelsch. 1986. *Trans* regulation of the phospho*enol*pyruvate carboxykinase (GTP) gene, identified by deletions in chromosome 7 of the mouse. Proc Natl Acad Sci USA 83:5184-5188.

Mikaelian, DO and RJ Ruben. 1964. Hearing degeneration in the shaker-1 mouse. Arch Otolaryngol 80:418-430.

Niswander, L, D Yee, EM Rinchik, LB Russell, and T Magnuson. 1988. The albino deletion complex and early postimplantation survival in the mouse. Development (Camb) 102:45-53.

Rinchik, EM, LB Russell, NG Copeland, and NA Jenkins. 1985. The dilute-short ear (*d-se*) complex of the mouse: Lessons from a fancy mutation. Trends Genet 1:170-176.

Rinchik, EM, LB Russell, NG Copeland, and NA Jenkins. 1986. Molecular genetic analysis of the dilute-short ear (*d-se*) region of the mouse. Genetics 112:321-342.

Rinchik, EM, R Machanoff, CC Cummings, and DK Johnson. 1989. Molecular cloning and mapping of the ecotropic leukemia provirus *Emv-23* provides molecular access to the albino-deletion complex in mouse chromosome 7. Genomics 4:251-258.

Robert, B, P Barton, A Minty, P Daubas, A Weydert, F Bonhomme, J Catalan, D Chazottes, J-L Guenet, and M Buckingham. 1985. Investigation of genetic linkage between myosin and actin genes using an interspecific mouse back-cross. Nature 314:181-183.

Russell, LB. 1971. Definition of functional units in a small chromosomal segment of the mouse and its use in interpreting the nature of radiation-induced mutations. Mutat Res 11:107-123.

Russell, LB and GD Raymer. 1979. Analysis of the albino-locus region of the mouse. III. Time of death of prenatal lethals. Genetics 92:205-213.

Russell, LB and EM Rinchik. 1987. Genetic and molecular characterization of genomic regions surrounding specific loci of the mouse. Banbury Rep 28:109-121.

Russell, LB, CS Montgomery, and GD Raymer. 1982. Analysis of the albino-locus region of the mouse. IV. Characterization of 34 deficiencies. Genetics 100:427-453.

Russell, LB, WL Russell, and EM Kelly. 1979. Analysis of the albino-locus region of the mouse. I. Origin and viability. Genetics 91:127-139.

Russell, WL. 1951. X-ray-induced mutations in mice. Cold Spring Harbor Symp Quant Biol 16:327-336.

Schmid, W, G Müller, G Schütz, and S Gluecksohn-Waelsch. 1985. Deletions near the albino locus on chromosome 7 of the mouse affect the level of tyrosine amino-transferase mRNA. Proc Natl Acad Sci USA 82:2866-2869.

Searle, AG, J Peters, MF Lyon, EP Evans, JH Edwards, and VJ Buckle. 1987. Chromosome maps of man and mouse, III. Genomics 1:3-18.

Silver, J. 1985. A defective ecotropic provirus closely linked to the albino locus. J Virol 55:494-496.

REPETITIVE SEQUENCES IN THE HUMAN GENOME*

R. K. Moyzis

Genetics Group, Los Alamos National Laboratory, Los Alamos, NM 87545

Key words: *Genomic structure, repetitive DNA, chromosomes 17 and 18*

ABSTRACT ONLY

Twenty-five percent of human DNA consists of repetitive DNA sequences. A general outline of the chromosomal organization of these repetitive sequences is discussed. Our working hypothesis is that certain classes of human repetitive DNA sequences "encode" the information necessary for defining genomic structure.

Using a combination of biochemical, cytological, computational, and recombinant DNA approaches, the organization of interspersed, centromeric, and telomeric repetitive DNA in the human genome has been investigated. The distribution of interspersed repeats can be adequately described by models that assume a random spacing, with an average distance of 3 kb. This observed distribution for the "integration" of interspersed repetitive DNA is expected for sequences that transpose randomly throughout the genome. However, local regions of "preference" or "exclusion" for integrating certain classes of repetitive DNA are suggested by the data.

Centromeric repetitive sequences, on the other hand, can be highly chromosome specific. While certain classes of centromeric repetitive DNA, such as alphasatellite sequences, are found at the centromeres of all chromosomes, subfamilies of the classical satellites I, II, and III are localized to distinct chromosomes. Our laboratory has isolated three recombinant DNA clones of human repetitive DNA sequences that hybridize specifically to the heterochromatic positions 1qh, 9qh, and 16qh, respectively. These locations were determined by fluorescent *in situ* hybridization, and confirmed by DNA hybridizations to human chromosomes sorted by flow cytometry. *In situ* hybridizations to intact interphase nuclei showed a well-defined, localized organization for all three DNA sequences. In addition, targeted oligomer synthesis of discrete repetitive sequence domains has allowed the synthesis of chromosome-specific, *in situ* probes for chromosomes 17 and 18. The ability to localize defined human chromosome domains in both metaphase spreads and intact interphase nuclei allows novel approaches to the detection of chromosome abnormalities. It should allow the ultimate generation of a three-dimensional human genome map to complement the linear map.

*This work was supported by the U.S. DOE under Contract No. W-7405-ENG-36.

In related research, a highly conserved, repetitive DNA sequence has been isolated from a human repetitive DNA sequence library. Quantitative hybridizations to chromosomes sorted by flow cytometry indicate that comparable amounts of this sequence are present on each human chromosome. Fluorescent *in situ* hybridization experiments indicate that the major clusters of this sequence occur at the telomeres of all mammalian chromosomes. The evolutionary conservation of this sequence and its chromosomal location, and its similarity to telomeres isolated from lower eukaryotes, indicate that this sequence is a functional human telomere.

HUMAN CHROMOSOME-SPECIFIC PHYSICAL MAPPING: THEORETICAL AND EXPERIMENTAL APPROACHES AND APPLICATIONS

C. E. Hildebrand,[1] R. L. Stallings,[1] J. L. Longmire,[1] L. L. Deaven,[2] T. Beugelsdijk,[3] K. M. Sirotkin,[4] W. B. Goad,[4] T. G. Marr,[4] and R. K. Moyzis[1]

[1]Genetics Group, Life Sciences Division, Los Alamos National Laboratory, Los Alamos, NM 87545

[2]Cell Biology Group, Life Sciences Division, Los Alamos National Laboratory, Los Alamos, NM 87545

[3]Mechanical and Electronic Engineering Division, Los Alamos National Laboratory, Los Alamos, NM 87545

[4]Theoretical Biology Group, Theoretical Division, Los Alamos National Laboratory, Los Alamos, NM 87545

Key words: *Human genome, physical maps, chromosome-specific libraries, pulsed-field gel electrophoresis*

ABSTRACT

As part of the U.S. Department of Energy initiative to construct physical maps of the human genome, the physical mapping efforts of our laboratory are focused on two primary activities: (1) development of accelerated approaches to physical mapping and (2) demonstrating the applicability of multiple complementary mapping strategies in constructing a physical map of human chromosome 16. The goal of the physical mapping effort is to produce both a linear analytical map that provides the locations of identifiable landmarks (e.g., genes or anonymous restriction fragment-length polymorphisms) in molecular distances (i.e., kilobase pairs) as well as an overlapping set of cloned DNA fragments that span the length of chromosomes from telomere to telomere. Various approaches have been proposed for constructing both analytical ("top-down") and overlapping ("bottom-up") clone maps. Computer simulations based on a model human chromosome constructed from human DNA sequences in GenBank, interspersed with multiple classes of repetitive sequences, are being used to evaluate the relative efficiency and accuracy of each mapping strategy.

Analytical physical mapping approaches are based on macrorestriction analyses of long-range genome order using infrequently cutting restriction enzymes and pulsed-field gel electrophoresis. Initial studies are directed toward centromeric and telomeric regions and the cytogenetic region 16q22, which contains five gene loci (including two multigene families) and a total of more than 20 markers. The analytical map will be needed to span large regions of the genome that are either "unclonable" or contain extensive clusters of repetitive sequences and to close gaps between islands of overlapping clones that arise from the clone-ordering procedures.

To develop an overlapping clone map of chromosome 16, chromosome-16-specific partial-digest phage and cosmid libraries are being constructed from both flow-sorted chromosomes 16 and from a mouse × human somatic cell hybrid containing one copy of chromosome 16. Identification of overlapping phage or cosmid clones is under evaluation, using several clone "finger-printing" approaches. Random-ordering strategies will produce islands of overlapping clones separated by gaps. The progress of ordering strategies for human chromosomal DNA can be monitored using results from the simulations described.

Integration of overlapping clone maps with analytical maps will be essential for closing the physical map. Furthermore, the connectivity of genetic linkage maps to the physical maps via polymorphic "anchor" loci will provide a valuable tool for rapid access to a specific gene or region of interest. Using the overlapping clones from the region of interest, it will be possible to proceed to the highest level of resolution—the DNA base sequence. Multiple applications of long-range physical maps and the overlapping clone repositories are envisioned in biomedical areas, in understanding the molecular bases of genetic alterations, and in unraveling the hierarchies of chromatin and chromosome organization.

As part of the U.S. Department of Energy initiative to undertake a multidisciplinary program to analyze and understand the human genome (Office of Energy Research, 1987), our laboratory has developed the Center for Human Genome Studies to facilitate both intra- and interinstitutional research relevant to the Human Genome Project. The Los Alamos program has been built on the laboratory's long-term research commitments to understanding the mechanisms of radiation and chemical damage to complex genomes and the mutagenic and carcinogenic consequences of such actions. The National Laboratory Gene Library Project (see Deaven and Van Dilla, this volume) and the capability to isolate human chromosomes by fluorescence-activated chromosome sorting have provided essential tools for starting the analysis of the human genome. Expertise in theory, computational sciences, and database management led to the development of the central DNA sequence data base, GenBank, at Los Alamos. Additional capabilities in the physical, chemical, and engineering sciences have become the focus for development of new technology to expedite the mapping and ultimate sequencing of the human genome and the genomes of other species.

The Center for Human Genome Studies has integrated research projects in several areas including: (1) human genome physical mapping; (2) theory and simulation of physical mapping and sequencing strategies; (3) informatics encompassing data acquisition and management for large-scale mapping and sequencing projects; (4) laboratory robotics and automation to expedite the preparation and management of the enormous number of samples that will be required to obtain chromosome maps; and (5) advanced DNA sequencing technology to accelerate acquisition of sequence information.

In this brief review, we focus on the physical mapping component of the Los Alamos program. The rationale for constructing physical maps of the human genome has been a subject of intense national and international discussion and debate for the past 2 yr as part of the larger issue of whether and when to commit to a focused program to sequence the human genome (Office of Technology Assessment, 1988; National Research Council, 1988). Very low resolution physical maps of the human genome (e.g., cytogenetic maps of the human karyotype) have been known for more than three decades, and higher resolution (G- or Q-banded) cytogenetic maps have been available for more than two decades. More recently, *in situ* hybridization of specific gene fragments, or anonymous DNA fragments, to metaphase chromosomes has been used to reveal low-resolution physical arrangement of these markers along the chromosome.

The development of recombinant DNA technology and its application to human genetics have played a fundamental role in tracing the inheritance of anonymous DNA markers in relation to specific phenotypes. Application of this technology, focused on disease phenotypes, has led to the development of genetic linkage maps that place genetic markers or loci in linear order along chromosomes relative to the frequencies with which they recombine with one another during the process of meiosis (White et al., 1986). The distance between markers established by genetic linkage analyses is measured in percent recombination; the standard unit is the centimorgan (cM), or 1% recombination. In terms of physical distance, 1 cM is highly variable, but on average equals approximately 1 million base pairs (megabase pairs, or Mb). The various levels of physical and genetic mapping are summarized in Figure 1 with two applications of physical maps and ordered contiguous clones ("contigs") for studying nuclear topography (i.e., the organization of chromosomes in the interphase nucleus) and long-range organization and hierarchies of chromosome structure.

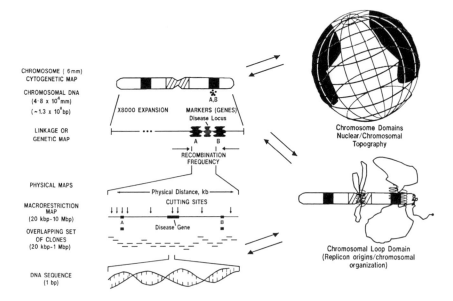

CHROMOSOME (6mm)
CYTOGENETIC MAP

CHROMOSOMAL DNA
(4·8 x 10⁴mm)
(~1.3 x 10⁸bp)

X8000 EXPANSION   MARKERS (GENES)
Disease Locus

LINKAGE OR
GENETIC MAP

A   B
RECOMBINATION
FREQUENCY

PHYSICAL MAPS

Physical Distance, kb
CUTTING SITES

MACRORESTRICTION
MAP
(20 kbp-10 Mbp)

A   Disease Gene   B

OVERLAPPING SET
OF CLONES
(20 kbp-1 Mbp)

DNA SEQUENCE
(1 bp)

Chromosome Domains
Nuclear/Chromosomal
Topography

Chromosomal Loop Domain
(Replicon origins/chromosomal
organization)

Figure 1. Multiple levels of mapping of human chromosomes. At lowest level of resolution, human genome is characterized by 22 pairs of autosomal chromosomes and two sex chromosomes, X and Y. Individual chromosomes can be distinguished by size, position of centromeric constriction relative to telomeres (centromeric index), and patterns of banding induced by staining with DNA-specific dyes after treatments to partially remove chromosomal proteins (G- and Q-banding). Locations of specific genes or markers (A and B in this diagram) along a chromosome can be determined by *in situ* hybridization using cloned DNA probes. Order of, and relative distances between, genes or markers along human chromosomes are established using polymorphic DNA markers or fragments of gene regions to follow inheritance of specific alleles in multigeneration families with large sibships. Distances in genetic linkage maps are given as percent recombination between markers; a distance of 1% recombination [1 centimorgan (cM)] is generally estimated to represent 1 million base pairs of DNA. Next level of resolution can be represented by analytical physical, or macrorestriction, map developed using rare-cutting restriction enzymes and pulsed-field gel electrophoresis to separate megabase-sized DNA fragments. Markers are located on macrorestriction maps relative to restriction sites, and distances can be measured in kilobase pairs. As an example of the value of long-range restriction maps, distances can be determined between markers flanking a disease locus. This information can then expedite identification of cloned large DNA fragments corresponding to the disease locus. Options from molecular genetics available for this purpose include using overlapping sets of cloned DNA from phage or cosmid vectors, or yeast chromosomes engineered to accept foreign DNA. A clone subset provides substrate for obtaining the DNA sequence, the ultimate physical map. Maps from cytological level to DNA sequence are retained in various data bases. Two applications of long-range physical maps: nuclear topography studies use *in situ* hybridization and confocal laser scanning microscopy for three-dimensional views of chromosome locations, chromosome subregions, or genes in interphase nucleus; probes explore hierarchies of chromosomal architecture.

The initial phase of physical mapping will be directed toward a single chromosome, and will employ several independent but complementary methods to produce (1) a set of overlapping, cloned DNA fragments spanning an entire chromosome, and (2) a large-scale restriction map that provides distances in terms of tens to hundreds of kilobase pairs between genes or DNA markers to span regions that are unclonable by current technology. Integration of the various types of physical maps with one another and with the other kinds of maps (see Figure 1) will be essential. Computational technology for automated mapping data acquisition, map integration, and large-scale database management and analysis is currently under development in our laboratory.

The Los Alamos physical mapping effort is directed toward human chromosome 16. This chromosome comprises approximately 3.5% of the human genome and is defined cytologically by 14 bands. More than 12 clinical disorders or syndromes are linked to chromosome 16 (McKusick, 1986); more than 24 loci, including three multigene families, have been assigned to this chromosome (Ropers et al., 1987). An extensive restriction fragment-length polymorphism (RFLP) map has been constructed by combined linkage studies from several laboratories (Donis-Keller et al., 1987). A panel of hybrid cell lines containing only human chromosome 16 or various deletions has been developed and facilitates the regional mapping of new probes (Callen et al., 1986).

Physical mapping of chromosome 16 is proceeding simultaneously along two complementary paths. These approaches are summarized in Figure 2. Analytical physical mapping approaches are based on macrorestriction analyses of long-range genomic order using infrequently cutting restriction enzymes and pulsed-field gel electrophoresis (PFGE) to resolve large DNA fragments ranging from less than 10 kb to several Mb (Cantor et al., 1987). Initial studies are directed toward centromeric and telomeric regions, as well as the cytogenetic band 16q22, which contains 5 gene loci (including two multigene families) and more than 20 markers (Ropers et al., 1987). The analytical map will be needed to span large regions of the genome that either are "unclonable" in existing vectors or contain extended regions of tandemly repeated sequences that present difficulties in mapping with overlapping clones. The analytical map will be essential for determining the order of sets of contiguous phage, cosmid, or yeast artificial chromosome (YAC) clones (Burke et al., 1987) and the sizes of gaps between contigs.

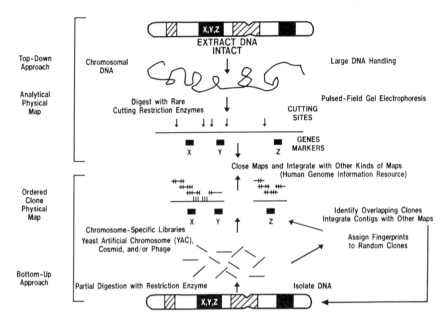

Figure 2. Schematic diagram of general complementary strategies for constructing long-range physical maps. Complementary strategies for generating physical maps of entire genomes or chromosomes are essential for achieving map closure. Various procedures have been developed or proposed for assigning fingerprints to individual random clones (Coulson et al., 1986; Livak et al., 1988; Poustka et al., 1980; Hildebrand et al., in preparation). Lander and Waterman (1988) have derived mathematical analyses for evaluating efficiency and accuracy of different mapping strategies and methods for monitoring progress of specific approaches.

To develop an overlapping clone map of chromosome 16, chromosome-16-specific libraries will be used as sources of contiguous clones. These contigs will be identified by efficient and accurate "fingerprinting" methods (Hildebrand et al., in preparation; Coulson et al., 1986; Livak et al., 1988), which are being compared computationally using a simulated human chromosome to uncover any potential unexpected pitfalls arising because of various classes of interspersed repetitive sequences. Chromosome-16-specific phage and cosmid libraries have been constructed from flow-sorted human chromosome 16 originating from a monochromosome hybrid cell line. These libraries are both well represented with respect to the expected frequency of multiple gene loci or anonymous single-copy markers, and are more than 92% free from contaminating rodent DNA fragments. Laboratory automation and robotic systems are being developed and integrated into sample preparation areas of the physical mapping problem to expedite and ensure reproducible quality in handling the massive number of samples required to construct a physical map of chromosome 16. Random clone-ordering strategies will produce islands of overlapping clones separated by "oceans" or gaps. Clearly, multiple libraries as well as analytical physical maps will be needed to close or bridge these gaps.

Integration of overlapping clone maps with analytical maps will be necessary to complete the low-resolution physical map. Further, the connectivity of genetic linkage maps to the physical maps via polymorphic "anchor" loci will provide a key resource for rapidly accessing any region of interest along the chromosome. Using overlapping clones from the region of interest, it will be possible to proceed efficiently to the highest level of resolution—the DNA sequence. Multiple applications of long-range physical maps and overlapping clone repositories can be envisioned in many areas of biomedical research, including understanding the molecular bases of a variety of genetic alterations and unraveling the hierarchies of chromatin and chromosome organization.

REFERENCES

Burke, DT, GF Carle, and MV Olson. 1987. Cloning of large segments of exogenous DNA in yeast. Science 236:806-812.

Callen, D, VJ Hyland, EG Baker, A Fratini, RN Simmers, JC Mulley, and GR Sutherland. 1986. Fine mapping of gene probes and anonymous DNA fragments to the long arm of chromosome 16. Genomics 2:144-153.

Cantor, C, CL Smith, and MK Matthew. 1987. Pulsed-field gel electrophoresis of very large DNA molecules. Annu Rev Biophys Biophys Chem 17:287-304.

Coulson, A, J Sulston, S Brenner, and J Karin. 1986. Toward a physical map of the genome of the nematode *Caenorhabditis elegans*. Proc Natl Acad Sci USA 83:7821-7825.

Donis-Keller, H, P Green, C Helms, et al. 1987. A genetic linkage map of the human genome. Cell 51:319-337.

Lander, ES and MS Waterman. 1988. Genomic mapping by fingerprinting random clones: A mathematical analysis. Genomics 2:231-239.

Livak, K, PN Korolkoff, and S Brenner. 1988. The use of fluorescent DNA terminators to map overlapping DNA fragments, pp. 12-13. In: *Genome Mapping and Sequencing*. Cold Spring Harbor Laboratory, Cold Spring Harbor, NY.

McKusick, V. 1986. *Mendelian Inheritance in Man*, 7th ed. Johns Hopkins University Press, Baltimore, MD.

National Research Council. 1988. *Mapping and Sequencing the Human Genome. Report of Committee on Mapping and Sequencing the Human Genome.* National Research Council, National Academy of Sciences, Washington, DC.

Office of Energy Research. 1967. *Subcommittee on Human Genome, Health and Environmental Research Advisory Committee, Report on Human Genome Initiative.* Prepared for the Office of Health and Environmental Research, Office of Energy Research, U.S. Department of Energy, Germantown, MD.

Office of Technology Assessment. 1988. *Mapping Our Genes—The Genome Projects: How Big, How Fast?* U.S. Congress, Office of Technology Assessment, Washington, DC.

Poustka, A, T Pohl, DP Barlow, G Zehetner, A Craig, F Michiels, E Ehrlich, A-M Frischauf, and H Lehrach. 1986. Molecular approaches to mammalian genetics. Cold Spring Harbor Symp Quant Biol 51:131-139.

Ropers, HH, T Gedde-Dahl, Jr., and DW Cox. 1987. Report of committee on the genetic constitution of chromosomes 13, 14, 15, and 16. Human Gene Mapping Workshop 5. Cytogenet Cell Genet 46:213-241.

White, R, M Leppert, P O'Connell, Y Nakamura, C Julier, S Woodward, A Silva, R Wolff, M Lathrop, and J-M Lalouel. 1986. Construction of human genetic linkage maps. I. Progress and perspectives. Cold Spring Harbor Symp Quant Biol 51:29-38.

Quantifying Molecular End Points in Differentiated Cells

OVERVIEW OF TECHNIQUES OF ANALYSIS OF CELL DAMAGE

P. Todd,[1] S. S. Hymer,[2] S. G. Delcourt,[3] and M. E. Kunze[4]

[1]Center for Chemical Engineering, National Institute of Standards and Technology, Boulder, CO 80303

[2]Pharmacia Diagnostics, San Diego, CA

[3]Department of Biochemistry, Hitchner Hall, University of Maine, Orono, ME 04469

[4]The Pennsylvania State University, 405 Althouse Laboratory, University Park, PA 16802

Key words: *Cell damage, flow cytometry, somatic mutagenesis*

ABSTRACT

Most physical and chemical methods for analyzing cell damage have been developed for cells damaged *in vitro*. In many cases, these methods can be transferred, with minor modifications, to the analysis of cell damage *in vivo*. Molecular end points for cell damage include: chemical modifications of DNA, chromosome aberrations, point mutations, gene deletions/translocations, malignant transformation, and reproductive death.

For each of these end points, *in vivo* methods of analysis have been developed, including centrifugation and electrophoresis of unlabeled DNA, use of probes to detect DNA damage, characterization of severe chromosome damage by flow cytometry, somatic mutant cell identification by image analysis and flow cytometry, electrophoresis of cellular proteins, and flow cytometry, image analysis, and electrophoresis for detecting cell population shifts. In most cases, problems of sensitivity, specificity, and analysis of large cell populations had to be solved to apply these methods *in vivo*. Affinity labeling and recombinant DNA technology have played an important role in nearly all cases.

Many of these methods are also useful in cell bioprocessing and biotechnology. Newer techniques, developed mainly for biotechnology applications but with potential for analysis of cell damage, include selective cell retrieval by laser scanning microscopy, single cell manipulation by optical trapping, and cell electroporation and electrofusion.

INTRODUCTION

The application of two-dimensional (2-D) gel electrophoresis to human proteins (searching for several needles in the entire haystack), the restriction

109

mapping of oncogenes, blot and *in situ* hybridization of nucleic acids (finding a brightly shining needle in the haystack), flow karyotyping, *in situ* hybridization in flow cytometry, and the analysis of blood cells for somatic mutants by flow cytometry (seeking a specific needle in a haystack), have all brought biochemical and molecular genetics directly to the whole organism. The advent of flow cytometry alone has made *in vivo* cells much more accessible. The need to administer large amounts of radioisotopes has been alleviated, and dividing cell populations can be distinguished from nondividing cells, etc. This short report introduces highlights and achievements of these methods and presents some original work designed to address issues of *in vivo* somatic mutagenesis.

OVERVIEW

Two-Dimensional Gel Electrophoresis

Two-dimensional protein gel electrophoresis, in which molecular weights and isoelectric points can be determined for some 200 proteins simultaneously, has been considered a likely method with which to address human mutagenesis. Questions to be answered include: Can statistically adequate evidence be found, in the relatively small populations of humans available, that ionizing radiation causes human heritable or somatic mutations? This method has the advantage of increasing the number of loci that can be examined, since the number of exposed individuals cannot be increased. It may also be able to distinguish between deletions/translocations and single-locus mutations. Molecular methods of direct genetic analysis have, for several applications, overtaken 2-D protein electrophoresis.

Oncogene Characterization *In Vivo*

By applying a combination of restriction mapping and sequencing to oncogenes in mouse tumors, Guerrero et al. (1984) were able to identify single-base-pair substitutions in the murine lymphoma *K-ras* oncogene as a consequence of activation by gamma radiation. This datum is evidence that gamma radiation does cause intragenic changes in mammalian cells. The sensitivity of this approach to genetic damage analysis is enhanced by using the "polymerase-chain-reaction" method. This method provides about 1 million repeats of a single-copy gene through repeated denaturation and enzymatic extension *in vitro*, and has been applied to the sequencing of mutant *K-ras* and *Ha-ras* oncogenes.

Sequence Changes *In Vivo*

Restriction fragment mapping with Southern blot analysis of electrophoresed fragments of specific genes is another route to the characterization of damage at specific loci. By applying these methods to cells grown *in vitro*, Stankowski and Hsie (1986) were able to show that ionizing radiation caused mixed mutagenic damage, including complete deletions, partial gene deletions, and damage undetectable by restriction mapping. This technology is extendable to cells *in vivo*.

The study of DNA synthesis and repair replication has been greatly aided by the use of bromodeoxyuridine (Brdu) and its antibody (Gratzner, 1982; Khochbin et al., 1988). Antibodies to other adducts have been developed, and Lesko et al. showed (this volume) that antibodies against thymine dimers in DNA can be used to detect less than 10^6 dimers per cell and that the number of damage sites can be estimated directly by using a fluorescence calibration method.

Somatic Cell Methods *In Vivo*

Most early flow cytometry experiments were confined to the study of cells grown *in vitro*, immunological and hematological cells, and certain tumor cells. Improved cell dispersal methods have broadened the applicability of flow cytometry to include even retrospective analysis of tissue cells embedded in paraffin (Kute et al., 1988). Flow karyotyping, the study of isolated metaphase chromosomes in suspension by flow cytometry, has advanced to a high level of sophistication, and the effects of genotoxic agents are detected in the form of modified fluorescence intensity distributions. If translocations have been replicated, for example, these will appear as new peaks in the flow karyogram. If extensive fragmentation has occurred, the "baseline" between chromosome peaks will rise.

Mutant gene products can also be sought by flow cytometry. By instrumenting the flow cytometer to detect "rare events" and using a highly specific fluorescent antibody stain, it is possible to detect one cell per few million circulating erythrocytes that have a mutated surface protein. This approach was applied by Bigbee et al. (this volume) to demonstrate that variant human erythrocytes expressing neither the M nor N glycophorin A gene occur more frequently in individuals bearing repair-defect genes or in those exposed to genotoxic agents.

Metabolic characterization of cells suspended from solid tissues can be performed using blue autofluorescence (an indicator of NADH/NADPH levels), rhodamine 123 staining (mitochondrial activity), and pyronin Y staining (RNA content). These markers have been exploited by Johnson et al. (this volume) in the characterization of airway epithelial cells isolated by centrifugation and noninvasive flow sorting. The combination of these techniques made it possible for them to follow differentiation pathways in heterotopic tracheal grafts of pure populations of basal and secretory cells.

Cytometry and *In Situ* Hybridization

The characterization of mRNA being made by cells *in vivo* is possible through *in situ* hybridization using cloned probes of cDNA synthesized with known mRNA as template. Highly radioactive probes, either synthesized or nick-translated using ^{32}P-labeled nucleotides, can be used in Northern blots and cell autoradiography. DNA can also be tagged with fluorescent or immunoenzymatic labels or with biotin, and methods have been developed for applying such labeled probes to whole cells in suspension. These cells can then be evaluated by flow or image cytometry.

Image cytometry was used by Lucas et al. (this volume) to detect translocations involving human chromosome 1 by using two fluorescent cDNA repeat-sequence probes specific for two regions on chromosome 1. Similarly, a whole chromosome 4 cDNA library was used to detect translocations involving that chromosome. Although these techniques were demonstrated on proliferating human lymphocytes, they should be applicable to any cell in metaphase. The same principle was applied by Eastmond et al. (this volume) to detect multiple copies per cell of a specific chromosome and hence aneuploidy.

A sensitive method was developed in which oncogene amplification can be detected on the basis of quantitative *in situ* hybridization experiments involving biotinylated cDNA probes stained with avidin coupled to a fluorescent coumarin derivative (AMCA). The method requires cell fixation, *in situ* hybridization in suspension, and a dual laser flow cytometer. By using Brdu and its fluorescent antibody, it is also possible to ask whether cells with amplified genes were synthesizing DNA at the time of fixation.

NOVEL APPROACHES

Interactive Microscopy

The use of a laser beam as a microsurgical instrument is a sophisticated extension of the UV microbeam concept introduced by Zirkle and Bloom (1953) and exploited by Perry to discover the nucleolus as the site of rRNA production. Trosko et al. (1988) reported that, using an interactive laser microscope, it was possible to demonstrate that certain toxic agents interfere with intercellular communication.

New questions about cell damage and repair are reopening the door to individual-cell experimentation, and Braby and Reece (this volume) have developed a system for charged-particle irradiation of single cells that also facilitates multiple treatments of individual cells and the study of end points other than colony formation.

Optical Trapping

Focused light beams from diode lasers, which emit light at wavelengths exceeding 900 nm, are capable of "trapping" and of being used to manipulate single cells, apparently with minimal damage (Buican et al., 1987; Ashkin et al., 1987). Thus a potential exists for maneuvering, exposing, "parking," and examining single cells automatically, possibly eliminating the need to study multiplying cells, and introducing a method for studying, *in vitro*, individual differentiated cells while they remain alive. No genotoxicological studies using this method have been published, except for the observation that yeast cells held in an optical trap in nutrient medium retained their ability to divide while held in a dual-beam optical trap (Ashkin et al., 1987).

Early-Passage Diploid Human Cells

Human diploid skin fibroblasts have been a significant study material for genotoxicology research since their introduction by Puck et al. (1957) in early *in vitro* cellular radiation studies. Extensive mutagenesis studies have been performed using human foreskin fibroblasts in primary or early-passage culture (Maher et al., 1979). There is still very little documentation of somatic mutagenesis study in diploid human differentiated or epithelioid cells, especially at very early passage *in vitro* when cultures should most closely resemble *in vivo* cell behavior. It is possible that early-passage fibroblast cultures are a reasonable genotoxicological model for differentiated human cells.

AN EXPERIMENTAL APPROACH TO SINGLE-LOCUS SOMATIC MUTAGENESIS

A series of experiments was conducted using first an established line of cultured Chinese hamster cells and subsequently low-passage-number human embryonic kidney cells to test the hypothesis that somatic cell mutants at the Na^+, K^+-ATPase locus could be detected by flow cytometry.

Materials and Methods

Test-of-principle experiments were performed using Chinese hamster lung cells (V79-171B) cultivated in F-12 medium with 10% fetal bovine serum (see Delcourt, 1985, for details). Cultured diploid human embryonic kidney cells at the third passage in culture were obtained from Microbiological Associates (Rockville, MD) and cultivated in epithelioid growth medium "MM1" (see Sheble, 1986). The indocarbocyanine dye $DilC_1(3)$ was used as a flow cytometric test (Shapiro, 1981; Shapiro et al., 1979) for resistance to the membrane-depolarizing effect of the cardiac glycoside ouabain. In both cases, colony formation survival curves in ouabain and after exposure to UV light and x rays were determined.

Results and Discussion

Wild-type Chinese hamster cells were resistant to ouabain below 0.001 M, and wild-type human cells were resistant to ouabain below 1.0 μM. Cells derived from mutant clones of Chinese hamster cells were shown to resist the membrane-depolarizing effect of ouabain (Figure 1) (Delcourt, 1985). Cultured human embryonic kidney cells were found to have a maximum plating efficiency in conditioned medium of 10%. These cells were responsive to the membrane-depolarizing effect of ouabain (Figure 2). Exposure to 6.2 J/m^2 of UV light at 256 nm (a 15% survival dose) resulted in a mutation frequency of 3.0 ± 0.7 × 10^{-6} mutants per surviving cell (Sheble, 1986). This datum compares favorably with the frequency of 1.0 × 10^{-6} found in human fibroblastic cells exposed to a 40% survival dose (Buchwald, 1977).

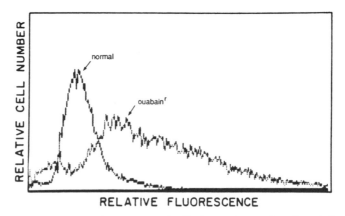

Figure 1. Flow cytometric fluorescence distributions of normal and ouabain-resistant Chinese hamster V79 cells incubated 2 hr in 1 mM ouabain in serum-free medium before staining with 2 μM DilC$_1$(3). Ouabain-resistant cells were not depolarized and had the same fluorescence distribution as untreated controls.

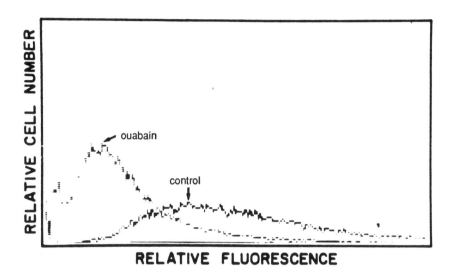

Figure 2. Flow cytometric fluorescence distributions of normal and ouabain-treated human embryonic kidney cells incubated 30 min in 0.1 mM ouabain in serum-free medium before staining with 2 μM DilC$_1$(3).

Conclusions

Differentiated human embryonic kidney cells capable of forming colonies *in vitro* possess a sensitivity to UV mutagenesis at the ouabain locus similar to that of cultured fibroblasts, ensuring that such studies on fibroblasts are potentially meaningful. The fluorescence distributions of Figure 2 overlap too heavily to allow the use of DilC$_1$(3) uptake in the presence of ouabain as a means of detecting low-frequency mutants at this locus.

ACKNOWLEDGMENTS

This research was supported by National Cancer Institute Grant RO1 CA35370 from the U.S. Public Health Service.

The U.S. Government does not endorse any particular brand name of products or manufacturer. Brand names are used in this article only for adequate specification of experimental procedures. This contribution, from the National Institute of Standards and Technology, an agency of the U.S. Government, is not subject to copyright.

REFERENCES

Ashkin, A, JM Dziedzic, and T Yamane. 1987. Optical trapping and manipulation of single cells using infrared laser beams. Nature 330:769-771.

Buchwald, M. 1977. Mutagenesis at the ouabain-resistance locus in human diploid fibroblasts. Mutat Res 44:401-412.

Buican, TN, MJ Smyth, HA Crissman, GC Salzman, CC Stewart, and JC Martin. 1987. Automated single-cell manipulation and sorting by light trapping. Appl Optics 26:5311-5316.

Delcourt, SG. 1985. *An Estimate of the Intragenic Mutation Induction Frequency by ^{60}Co Gamma Radiation in Chinese Hamster Cells.* M.S. Thesis. The Pennsylvania State University, University Park, PA.

Gratzner, HG. 1982. Monoclonal antibody to 5-bromo- and 5-iododeoxyuridine. A new reagent for detection of DNA replication. Science 218:474-475.

Guerrero, I, A Villasante, V Corces, and A Pellicer. 1984. Activation of a *c-K-ras* oncogene by somatic mutation in mouse lymphomas induced by gamma radiation. Science 225:1159-1162.

Khochbin, S, A Chabanas, P Albert, J Albert, and J-J Lawrence. 1988. Application of bromodeoxyuridine incorporation measurements to the determination of cell distribution within the S phase of the cell cycle. Cytometry 9:499-503.

Kute, TE, B Gregory, J Galleshaw, M Hopkins, D Buss, and D Case. 1988. How reproducible are flow cytometry data from paraffin-embedded blocks? Cytometry 9:494-498.

Maher, VM, DJ Dorney, AL Mendiala, B Konze-Thomas, and JJ McCormick. 1979. DNA excision-repair processes in human cells can eliminate the cytotoxic consequences of ultraviolet radiation. Mutat Res 62:311-323.

Puck, TT, SJ Cieciura, and HW Fisher. 1957. Clonal growth *in vitro* of human cells with fibroblastic morphology. Comparison of growth and genetic characteristics of single epithelioid and fibroblast-like cells from a variety of human organs. J Exp Med 106:145.

Shapiro, HM. 1981. Flow cytometric probes of early events in cell activation. Cytometry 1:301.

Shapiro, HM, PJ Natale, and LA Kamentsky. 1979. Estimation of membrane potentials of individual lymphocytes by flow cytometry. Proc Natl Acad Sci USA 76:5728.

Sheble, SK. 1986. *A Study of Colony Formation, Transmembrane Potential, and UV-Induced Ouabain Resistance in Human Fetal Kidney Cells.* M.S. Thesis. The Pennsylvania State University, University Park, PA.

Stankowski, LF, Jr., and AW Hsie. 1986. Quantitative and molecular analyses of radiation-induced mutation in AS52 cells. Radiat Res 105:37-48.

Trosko, JE, BV Madhukar, B Bombick, and CC Chang. 1988. Mechanisms and consequences of chemical modulators of intercellular communication studied by interactive laser cytometry. Cytometry (Suppl) 2:17.

Zirkle, RE and W Bloom. 1953. Irradiation of parts of individual cells. Science 117:487-493.

QUESTIONS AND COMMENTS

Q: Park, PNL, Richland, WA
    Is there information on the effects of "optical traps" on the cells?

A: Yes, Arthur Ashkin of Bell Laboratories has held yeast cells in a laser optical trap and observed a few cycles of budding, implying little or no genotoxic effect (**Ashkin** et al., **1987**).

Q: Gantt, NCl, Rockville, MD
    Do cells lose much of their asymmetry when suspended for flow cytometry?

A: Most animal cells suspended by the most common techniques (chelators and/or proteolytic enzyme) from solid tissues or monolayers become very round in shape (with a few exceptions) but may retain some functional asymmetry.

MOLECULAR ANALYSIS OF SPECIFIC DNA SEQUENCES USING THE POLYMERASE CHAIN-REACTION METHOD*

G. L. Stiegler and M. E. Frazier

Pacific Northwest Laboratory, P. O. Box 999, Richland, WA 99352

Key words: DNA, sequencing, polymerase, chain reaction method

ABSTRACT

We are using the polymerase-chain-reaction (PCR) method to enzymatically amplify specific genomic sequences. The end result of the enzymatic amplification is the synthesis of many copies (amplification of $>10^6$) of a defined targeted genomic sequence. The process involves priming, followed by extension of two specific oligonucleotide probes that flank the DNA sequences of interest, so that the end products of the polymerase reaction overlap across the DNA sequence. The method consists of repetitive cycles of denaturing, rehybridization of the oligonucleotide probes, and polymerase extension. The PC reaction results in an exponential increase in the amount of fragment defined by the positions of the 5' ends of the two primers on the template DNA.

The PCR method provides a powerful tool for obtaining direct DNA-sequence data from single-copy genes in mammalian genomes. As an application, we are currently developing a PCR method to analyze gene activations that occur in the Ha-*ras* and Ki-*ras* oncogenes. Missense mutations at amino acid 12 (first exon) or 61 (second exon), which can result in cell transformation in culture, are observed in many types of tumors. The PCR method will be used for amplification and subsequent DNA-sequence analysis of Ha-*ras* and Ki-*ras* exons 1 and 2.

INTRODUCTION

The polymerase chain reaction (PCR) overcomes the limitation of minimal available amounts of nucleic acid for molecular analysis. The PCR method, by enriching for specific DNA sequences, can amplify a particular DNA sequence by a factor of 10^6. The PCR technique has been used to characterize β-thalassemia mutations (Wong et al., 1987) and length variations in human mitochondrial DNA (Wrischnik et al., 1987) by direct DNA sequencing of amplified product. A description of the molecular analysis of the murine c-H-*ras* first exon is used here as an example of the analytical potential of the PCR method.

---

*This work was supported by the U.S. DOE under Contract No. DE-AC06-76RLO 1830.

The PCR amplification uses two oligonucleotide primers that are complementary to the mouse c-H-*ras* sequences flanking the *ras* 1st exon. This
sequence (Figure 1) was amplified (Figure 2) by repeating cycles of enzymatic extension of the two primers. During the first cyclic stage, the DNA is
heat denatured at 94°C. Immediately after denaturation the temperature
is decreased, and the primers are annealed at 37°C. The primers are
extended enzymatically in the final stage using DNA polymerase and designed so that they hybridize to opposite strands of the target sequence.
Their orientation (5'- to 3'-) directs polymerase extension to proceed across
the region bound by the two primers. With each completion of a cycle of
synthesis, a doubling in effect occurs in the amount of the DNA segment
defined by the two primer boundaries.

5'-ATGACAGAATACAAGC-3'
ATG ACA GAA TAC AAG CTT GTG GTG GTG GGC GCT GGA GGC GTG

GGA AAG AGT GCC CTG ACC ATC CAG CTG ATC CAG AAC CAC TTT

GTG GAC GAG TAT GAT CCC ACT ATA GAG
3'- CATACTAGGGTGATATCTC-5'

Figure 1. Mouse c-H-*ras* 1st exon. Primers used for PCR amplification are underlined.

In the early stages of PCR development, enzymatic amplification was
carried out using the polymerase activities of the Klenow fragment of
Escherichia coli DNA polymerase 1. Use of the Klenow fragment made the
PCR method more tedious because the heat denaturation destroyed its
enzymatic activity, requiring fresh enzyme at the beginning of each amplification cycle. This step, in addition to being tedious, was also a major
obstacle to automating the PCR method. Fortunately, a new heat-resistant
polymerase, purified from the thermophilic bacterium, *Thermus aquaticus*
(Taq), has replaced the Klenow fragment. The Taq enzyme survives extended incubation of 94°C and does not need to be replenished at each
cycle, allowing automation of the procedure and eliminating much of the
laborious and error-prone process of the manual PCR method.

We are developing the PCR method for amplification and DNA sequence
analysis of the first and second exons of the mouse c-H-*ras* and c-K-*ras*
oncogenes. The *ras* (H-, K-, and N-*ras*) family of oncogenes was chosen
because they appear to be those most frequently activated in primary
human and rodent tumors (Der et al., 1982; Guerrero et al., 1984 a). H- and

K-*ras* were first identified in rat retroviruses (Tsuchida et al., 1982; Dhar et al., 1982). N-*ras* was first found in a human tumor cell line (Taparowsky et al., 1983) and has been associated with carcinogen-induced mouse lymphoma (Guerrero et al., 1984b). All three genes encode nearly homologous proteins with a molecular weight of about 21,000 (p21); the most significant differences between the proteins are the C-terminal 40 amino acids. The *ras* genes are expressed in most, if not all, cells, and have been shown to have GTP/GDP binding (Gibbs et al., 1984) and GTPase activity (McGrath et al., 1984). The p21 proteins are proposed to be regulatory proteins involved in the normal growth control of cells.

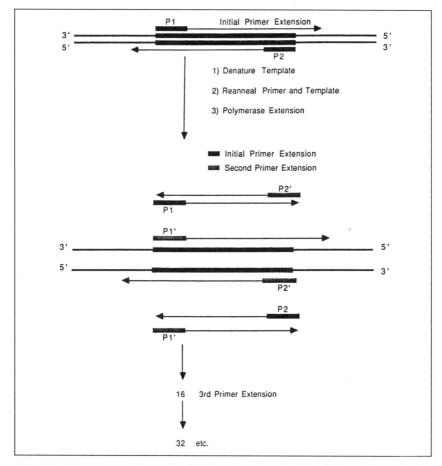

Figure 2. Polymerase chain reaction (PCR) cycle is repeated 20 to 30 times. Theoretically, doubling of yield occurs at each step.

In general, the activated *ras* genes differ from their normal cellular complements by a single point mutation that alters either the 12th or the 61st amino acid (located in the first and second exons, respectively; see Figures 1 and 2) of the protein (Tabin et al., 1982). Alterations in the *ras* coding regions (12th and/or 61st codon) have previously been experimentally detected by differential hybridization of oligonucleotide probes, changes in restriction enzyme cleavage sites brought about by point-mutation base alteration or by molecular cloning and DNA sequence analysis of the coding regions encompassing the 12th or 61st codon. The first two approaches are preferred for detecting point mutations in a population of molecules. Molecular cloning and DNA sequence analysis yield a more complete examination of the coding region and point mutation changes, but are restrictive in use because the techniques are laborious and more difficult. Also, the results may be more artifactual because of the manipulations involved in cloning and selective analysis of only one molecule from a population of molecules. Examination of the 1st and 2nd exon of the c-H-*ras* gene by the PCR method combines a rapid procedure such as restriction enzyme or oligonucleotide analysis with the comprehensive analysis of direct nucleotide sequencing while examining a whole population of molecules.

We are currently pursuing more than one approach to DNA sequence analysis of amplified PCR products. The first method, shown schematically in Figure 3A, uses the chemical degradation sequencing procedure of Maxam and Gilbert (Maxam and Gilbert, 1980). We amplify PCR products that are selectively ^{32}P-labeled at either 5' end by radiolabeling one of the extension primers before PCR amplification. The products, selectively labeled at one 5' end, are separated by polyacrylamide gel electrophoresis, and excised and purified from the gel matrix. The purified products are then sequenced by the chemical degradation method. The second sequencing procedure uses the dideoxy chain termination method developed by Sanger (Sanger et al., 1977) (Figure 3B). The amplified PCR products are again separated and purified by polyacrylamide gel electrophoresis. The purified fragments are then sequenced by PCR primer extension in the presence of dideoxy chain terminators using either Sequenase or the Taq enzyme.

The PCR method allows us to examine archived tumor tissue from previous in-house studies and will be the basis of new research efforts. Because we can readily amplify DNA and RNA sequences, rapid sequence analysis of mutants and variants at a known gene locus is facilitated. The ability to amplify and manipulate a target sequence present in only one copy per cell in a sample of 10^6 cells has great value in analysis of gene expression or gene rearrangement in single cells. The PCR procedure also has clinical application in diagnostic development for infectious disease and chromosomal rearrangements.

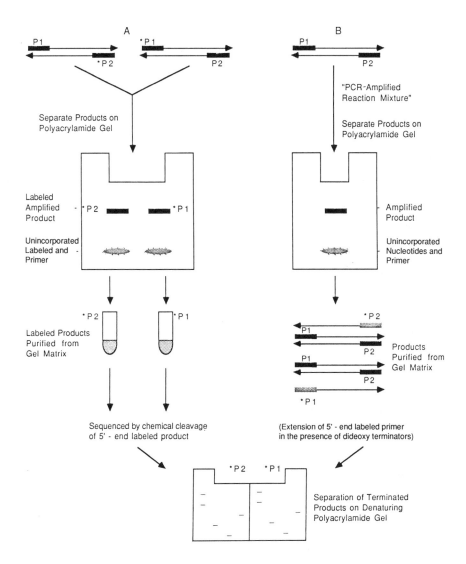

Figure 3. A and B. DNA sequencing strategy.

ACKNOWLEDGMENT

Work was supported by the U.S. Department of Energy under Contract No. DE-AC06-76RLO 1830.

REFERENCES

Der, CJ, TG Krontiris, and GM Cooper. 1982. Transforming genes of human bladder and lung carcinoma cell lines are homologous to the ras genes of Harvey and Kirsten sarcoma viruses. Proc Natl Acad Sci USA 79:3637-3640.

Dhar, R, RW Ellis, TY Shih, S Oroszlan, B Shapiro, J Maizel, D Lowy, and E Scolnick. 1982. Nucleotide sequence of the p21 transforming protein of Harvey sarcoma virus. Science 217:934-936.

Gibbs, JB, IS Sigal, M Poe, and EM Scolnick. 1984. Intrinsic GTPase activity distinguishes normal and oncogenic ras p21 molecules. Proc Natl Acad Sci USA 81: 5704-5708.

Guerrero, I, P Calzada, A Mayer, and A Pellicer. 1984a. A molecular approach to leukemogenesis: Mouse lymphomas contain an activated c-ras oncogene. Proc Natl Acad Sci USA 81:202-205.

Guerrero, I, A Villasante, V Corces, and A Pellicer. 1984b. Activation of a c-K-ras oncogene by somatic mutation in mouse lymphomas induced by gamma radiation. Science 225:1159-1162.

Maxam, A and W Gilbert. 1980. Sequencing end-labeled DNA with base-specific cleavages. Methods Enzymol 64:499-580.

McGrath, JP, DJ Capon, DV Goeddel, and AD Levison. 1984. Comparative biochemical properties of normal and activated human ras p21 protein. Nature 310: 644-649.

Sanger, F, S Nicklen, and AR Coulson. 1977. DNA sequencing with chain terminating inhibitors. Proc Natl Acad Sci USA 74:5463-5467.

Tabin, C, S Bradley, C Bargmann, R Weinberg, A Papageorge, E Scolnick, R Dhar, D Lowy, and E Chang. 1982. Mechanism of activation of a human oncogene. Nature 300:143-148.

Taparowsky, E, K Shimizu, M Goldfarb, and M Wigler. 1983. Structure and activation of the human N-ras gene. Cell 34:581-586.

Tsuchida, N, T Ryder, and E Ohtsubo. 1982. Nucleotide sequence of the oncogene encoding the p21 transforming protein of Kirsten murine sarcoma virus. Science 217:937-938.

Wong, C, CE Dowling, RK Saiki, RG Higuchi, HA Erlich, and HH Kazazin Jr. **1987.** Characterization of β-thalassaemia mutations using direct genomic sequencing of amplified single copy DNA. Nature 330:384-386.

Wrischnik, LA, RG Higuchi, M Stoneking, HA Erlich, N Arnheim, and AC Willson. **1987.** Length mutations in human mitochondrial DNA: Direct sequencing of enzymatically amplified DNA. Nucleic Acids Res 15:529-542.

THREE-COLOR FLOW CYTOMETRIC *IN SITU* HYBRIDIZATION ASSAY TO DETERMINE IF SPECIFIC GENE AMPLIFICATION GIVES CELLS A PROLIFERATIVE ADVANTAGE*

F. A. Dolbeare and J. W. Gray

Biomedical Sciences Division, Lawrence Livermore National Laboratory, Livermore, CA 94550

Key words: *Flow cytometric assay, CHO, c-myc, carcinogenesis, gene amplification*

ABSTRACT ONLY

During carcinogenesis, a number of genes that control growth and cell differentiation are genetically altered, in particular by gene amplification. We are interested in knowing whether these genetic changes also give a proliferative advantage to host cells over populations that do not contain amplified genetic sequences.

To attack this problem, we are using high- and low-copy *c-myc*-containing Chinese hamster ovary cells, which are pulsed with bromodeoxyuridine (Brdu) at specific intervals before the cells are fixed for flow cytometric analysis. The cells are then processed for *in situ* hybridization, using specific *c-myc* biotinylated probes, then treated with monoclonal *anti*-Brdu-fluorescein-isothiocyanate (FITC). A 7-amino-4-methylcoumarin acetic acid (AMCA) conjugated avidin is used to detect the biotinylated probe, and propidium iodide fluorescence is used to measure total cellular DNA. A dual laser-flow cytometer is used to analyze the cells. Populations with faster cell-doubling times are revealed by differences in the Brdu/DNA bivariate distributions. The AMCA/FITC distributions indicate the relationship between *c-myc* copy number and cell proliferation.

The technique can be applied to the analysis of cells containing other proto-oncogenes and to screen for specific DNA amplifications that cause increased cell proliferation.

---

*This work was performed under the auspices of the U.S. DOE by the Lawrence Livermore National Laboratory under Contract W-7405-ENG-48.

127

CONTROLLING RADIATION DOSE TO INDIVIDUAL CELLS

L. A. Braby and W. D. Reece

Pacific Northwest Laboratory, P.O. Box 999, Richland, WA 99352

Key words: *Collimator, microbeam irradiation, low dose, charged particle, cell damage*

ABSTRACT

One factor that contributes to the uncertainty in our understanding of the relationships between the initial deposition of energy by high-linear-energy-transfer ionizing radiation and the final effect is the random nature of energy deposition events in cell nuclei. Since the specific energy per event is large (20 rad for a 1-MeV proton crossing a 5-μm-diameter nucleus), the probability of the event in any specific nucleus is small at low doses. As a result, those processes that depend on the interaction of products, or on the time between events, happen very rarely, and their effects are mixed with the response of cells that received either no energy or only a single event.

To make it easier to relate the effects of specific energy deposition patterns to the consequences at the cellular level, we are developing a system for irradiating single cells with specified numbers of charged-particle tracks. The critical components of this system are (1) a positive ion accelerator that delivers about 100 particles per μm^2 per second, (2) a collimator that limits the beam to a diameter of about 0.5 μm, (3) a scintillator and photomultiplier that detect each particle as it leaves the accelerator vacuum system, (4) a shutter in the beam line that controls the number of particles (usually, a single particle), and (5) a microscope and stage to position cells over the collimator.

To avoid the difficulty of aligning very small holes, the 0.5-μm collimator will be made by positioning knife edges to define the beam and block edge-scattered particles. The edges will be positioned using special micrometer screws with 0.15-μm resolution. Preliminary tests with a 5-μm-diameter collimator indicate that the thin materials needed to minimize slit edge-scattering in the collimator can withstand the high particle fluence needed to detect the beam during alignment. Plastic scintillator films that are a few micrometers thick have been tested and can be used, with a microscope, to detect passage of single alpha particles. The microbeam irradiation system currently being assembled will be used to study the interaction of damage produced by charged-particle events that are separated in time. We will also use the system to study the relative importance of damage to different subcellular structures in producing different end effects.

THE PROBLEM

The biological effects of irradiation begin with the production of ionized or
excited molecules by passage of charged particles through the cell. These
ionizations are concentrated along the path of the charged particle, and the
density of ionization varies dramatically with the type and velocity of the
particle. Because the stochastic effects of irradiation, such as cancer induction, begin with damage to the DNA of a single cell, it is generally assumed
that the dose delivered to an individual cell nucleus will correlate with the
probability of damage to that cell and to the risk of adverse health effects.
The dose to a cell nucleus that has been traversed by a single proton, the
most common charged particle produced by neutron irradiation, is a random variable which depends on the actual number of ions produced, the
mass of the nucleus, and other factors, but is typically of the order of 0.2 Gy.
When an animal or a collection of cultured cells in an experimental dish is
exposed to a lower dose of neutrons, for example, 0.02 Gy, some of the
nuclei are traversed by recoil protons and others are not. The average dose
to those hit by a proton is 0.2 Gy, but the average, including 9 of 10
undamaged cells, is 0.02 Gy. Furthermore, the probability of being hit is a
Poisson random variable, so there is always the possibility that a cell will be
hit by two or three or more particles. For overall doses equal to the average
dose for a single charged particle crossing the cell nucleus, approximately
one-third of the cells receive a single track through the nucleus, one-third
receive no damage, and one-third receive two or more tracks. Thus, the
interpretation of the results of experiments done at low doses is complicated
by the presence of a wide range of doses in the irradiated population,
including a large fraction that receive no dose at all. If the dose is given at
low dose rates, further complications arise from the random timing of the
individual energy deposition events. If exactly two events occur in a cell or
nucleus, the time between the events will range from zero to the full length
of the irradiation.

THE SOLUTION

The effects of irradiation as a function of the dose and dose rate can be
evaluated with much greater confidence when individual cells are irradiated with known numbers of charged particle tracks. If we want to concentrate our research on damage to specific parts of the cell, for example, the
nucleus, this is most efficiently done by collimating a charged particle beam
to a few micrometers in diameter and placing the structure to be irradiated
over the collimator. Figure 1 is a schematic of the beam line components
needed to accomplish this with particles from an electrostatic accelerator.

This system is being assembled using the 2-MV tandem accelerator at Pacific Northwest Laboratory (PNL). A 90° bending magnet provides a vertical beam to irradiate dishes of cells without disturbing their culture medium. Cells to be irradiated will be placed on thin polyethylene terephthalate film stretched over a stainless steel ring, forming a dish that can be precisely positioned. The charged particle beam exits the accelerator vacuum system through a thin film of plastic scintillator. This scintillator is in contact with the dish bottom to minimize the effect of scattering in the scintillator. The light produced by the scintillator is collected by the microscope, which is also used to position the cell to be irradiated. During irradiation, the microscope illumination path is blocked by a shutter, and the shutter leading to a photomultiplier tube is opened. The exact number of particles passing through the target can be counted, and the irradiation is automatically terminated by closing a beam shutter at the specified dose.

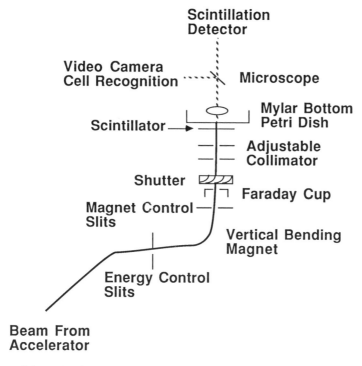

Figure 1. Schematic of the major components of the microbeam irradiation system. The microscope uses epi-illumination; thus, there are no optical components below the plane of the objects being irradiated.

Practical considerations in delivering low doses to living cells make it necessary to keep the particle fluence rate down to about 10 particles per second. This dictates use of a collimator rather than the lens that is typical of microbeam analytical systems. Scattering of particles by interaction with the edges of a collimator aperture can limit the resolution of a single aperture to a few micrometers. This limit can be reduced to a few tenths of a micrometer by using a second aperture, slightly larger than the first, to stop the edge-scattered particles. To align apertures of the order of 1 μm in diameter with the axis of the window and the Faraday cup used to monitor the beam, the apertures are formed by positioning four knife edges for each aperture. These edges are positioned by compound micrometer screws acting through pretensioned metal links with a final resolution of 0.2 μm per division.

This irradiation system can be used to irradiate single cells, or specific cells within small organisms, with a specific number of charged particles of known energy. Irradiation can be limited to specific cells in a tissue or to a specific portion of a cell, and the conditions of irradiation including the time between charged particle interactions can be made the same for the entire cell population. This eliminates much of the stochastic variation in dose and time between interactions that is inherent in populations exposed at low doses or low dose rates.

Table 1 summarizes the irradiation characteristics that are possible with the PNL system. The limitations are that the beam penetrates only a short distance, the range of the particular particle being used; as it penetrates the sample, multiple scattering causes it to diverge from the original path prescribed by the collimator.

Table 1. Characteristics of microbeam irradiation.

Particle type and energy:	Protons and deuterons, 1-4 MeV ^{3}He and ^{4}He, 2-6 MeV
Stopping power:	10-100 keV/μm
Collimator diameter:	Adjustable, 0.2-10 μm
Particle rate:	~10 per second
Shutter response time:	10 msec

ACKNOWLEDGMENT

Work was supported by the Office of Health and Environmental Research (OHER), U.S. Department of Energy, under Contract DE-AC06-76RLO 1830.

QUESTIONS AND COMMENTS

Q: Todd, NIST

Do you perceive that there are applications of the single-cell irradiation technique to differentiated cell systems and end points not related to proliferation?

A: Braby

Yes, there are a number of possible experiments dealing with cell function, such as cell-cell communication and the function of membranes, which can be devised. However, no specific experiments of this type have been planned yet. Experiments dealing with the regulation of cell growth in organized systems such as preimplantation embryos are planned. The only limitations on these experiments have to do with the limited range of the particles and the need to be able to recognize the intended target.

Q: Gantt, NCI

How long would it take to irradiate 500 cells with ~2 particles (average) to the nucleus?

A: The time needed to irradiate 500 cells depends almost entirely on the time it takes to find them under the microscope. The actual irradiation time is less than 0.5 sec each, or about 4 min. We are developing image-processing software to automatically identify 10T1/2 cell nuclei and position them for irradiation. Using real-time video processing electronics and motor-controlled optics positioning equipment, we expect to be able to find a target, position it, and irradiate it in 3 sec. This would be 25 min for the 500 cells. If a split dose is used, the second exposure could be faster because the positions of the cells are recorded by the computer. However, to keep a constant interval between doses, you have to use the same total irradiation time.

CHARACTERIZATION OF AIRWAY CELLS AND THEIR DIFFERENTIATION PATHWAYS*

N. F. Johnson, A. F. Hubbs, and D. G. Thomassen

Lovelace Inhalation Toxicology Research Institute, P.O. Box 5890, Albuquerque, NM 87185

Key words: *Epithelial cells, airways, cell differentiation*

ABSTRACT

The epithelium of conducting airways is the primary site for the development of neoplasms. These neoplasms can express a wide range and mixtures of phenotypes that are not seen in normal epithelial cells. The differentiation pathways of normal and aberrant epithelial cells are poorly understood. In this study, the differentiation pathways of normal epithelial cells from rat airways are investigated to identify morphological and cellular parameters associated with differentiation of particular cell types. Basal, secretory, and Clara cells have been isolated by flow cytometry, using bivariate analysis of forward and 90°C light-scatter signals, and by density gradient sedimentation. The cells have been characterized by flow cytometry and electron microscopy. The secretory cells have a well-developed synthetic apparatus and a pronounced, blue, autofluorescent signal (related to inherent NADPH levels). In contrast, basal cells have a poorly developed synthetic apparatus and low, blue, autofluorescent response. Similar differences occur with mitochondrial staining (rhodamine 123) and RNA staining (pyronin Y), where secretory cells have a more marked response than basal cells.

The expression of cell-surface sugar moieties has been studied as a means of identifying specific cell types. These moieties are thought to be modulated during the progression toward neoplasia. Analysis of the DNA content of viable basal and secretory cells has shown that the major proliferative cell in the trachea is the secretory cell. The separation of basal and secretory cells in high purity has allowed the differentiation pathways of individual cell types to be followed. Inoculation of denuded heterotopic tracheal grafts with pure populations of basal and secretory cells has shown that secretory cell progeny can give rise to a complete epithelium, while basal cells have only a limited progenitorial capacity. The combination of flow cytometry with pathology provides a powerful approach to defining cell phenotypes. Flow cytometry also allows separation of defined viable cell populations, the biological significance of which can be determined using heterotopic tracheal grafts.

---

*Research sponsored by the U.S. DOE Office of Health and Environmental Research under Contract No. DE-AC04-76VO1O13.

The lining epithelium of the lung is capable of neoplastic transformation. Lung tumors frequently coexpress many phenotypes, suggesting a common cellular ancestry. A common ancestry is also suggested by the pattern of embryonic development of the airway lining. Initially, the presumptive airways are lined by a single columnar cell type. During neonatal development, this single cell type ("prototype" cell) differentiates into all the major cell types present in normal adult epithelium: basal, secretory, and ciliated cells. Increasing our understanding of differentiation pathways will provide a basis to better delineate aberrant differentiation leading to neoplasia.

In the upper airways, basal and secretory cells are considered potential progenitor cells involved in the repair and maintenance of the normal epithelial lining. However, much of this information has come from histological investigations in which it is difficult to trace the lineage of specific cell types. This difficulty is compounded by the many cell types present in the lung. Our approach to determining the lineage of airway epithelial cells has been to dissociate the lining epithelium from the upper airways and to isolate and characterize purified cell subpopulations. Because most human lung cancers occur in the upper airway, these cells are the ones most likely to become neoplastic. We have used the rat trachea as a source of epithelial cells; the cells that line this tissue are morphologically similar to those found in human upper airways.

Lining epithelium from F344/N rat trachea was dissociated by enzymic methods and the cells used in flow cytometric analysis and sorting. Cells were stained with Hoechst 33342 alone or in combination with fluorescein-labeled lectins, pyronin Y, and propidium iodide (Sigma, St. Louis, MO) to determine DNA and RNA content and cell-surface sugar moieties. The cell suspension was analyzed using a dual laser flow cytometer (Los Alamos National Flow Cytometry Resource and Becton Dickinson FACTStar PLUS, Mountain View, CA). Cell populations were sorted on the basis of the inherent light-scatter characteristics ($2°$ and $90°$) of the cells. Two distinct populations of small agranular cells and larger granular cells were identified. Ultrastructural analysis showed these cells to be basal and secretory cells, respectively. The stored cell populations were 92% secretory cells and 95% basal cells, with a viability in excess of 98% as determined by trypan blue dye exclusion and propidium iodide fluorescence.

The ultrastructural appearance of the cells equated to their flow cytometric profile (Table 1). Ultrastructurally, the basal cells were small with scant cytoplasm containing few organelles but possessing prominent cytokeratin bundles. In contrast, the secretory cells were larger and contained prominent secretory granules and numerous organelles indicative of a metabolically active cell. Flow cytometry profiles showed that the secretory cells had high light-scatter signals, reflecting large size and granularity compared to the lower signals of the basal cells. The secretory cells also possessed high blue autofluorescence, indicative of high inherent NADPH levels, and high RNA content compared to the basal cells.

Table 1. Comparison of the flow cytometric and ultrastructural characteristics of basal and secretary cells from the rat trachea.

	Basal Cell	Secretory Cell
Flow Cytometric Characteristics		
Size	Small	Large
Granularity	Low	High
Redox potential	Low	High
RNA	Low	High
DNA	G/G	G/G, S, G, M
Ultrastructural and Growth Characteristics		
Size	Small	Large
Secretory granules	Absent	Present
Synthetic apparatus	Little	Ample
Growth in culture	Poor	Moderate

The lectin specificity of the cell surface was also determined. Basal cells stained intensely with *Wisteria floribunda* agglutinin and weakly with wheat-germ agglutinin, while secretory cells stained intensely with the latter lectin and with soya bean and *Banderiae simplifolia* agglutinin. These results show that differentiated secretory and basal cells have distinctive sugar moieties on their cell surfaces.

Flow cytometric analysis of the entire trachea cell suspension showed that there were few dividing cells in the tracheal epithelium but that most of those that were dividing were secretory cells. Less than 1% of cells were in the S, G_2, and M phases of the cell cycle. Of these dividing cells, the ratio of secretory to basal cells was 9:1. The increased proliferative capacity of secretory cells was also seen when sorted populations of basal and secretory cells were six times that of basal cells. These results show that secretory cells have a greater proliferative capacity than do basal cells, and that under normal circumstances in the upper airways, where the secretory cells are more numerous (45% secretory cells compared to 15% basal cells), secretory cells play the major role in repair and maintenance of the epithelial lining.

The progenitorial capacity of basal and secretory cells has been determined by inoculating denuded heterotopic grafts with sorted, highly purified populations of either cell type. Both cell types were capable of reestablishing an epithelial lining; however, the nature of the lining was markedly different. Inoculation of secretory cells resulted in a hypertrophic epithelium composed of all major cell types (basal, secretory, and ciliated cells). In contrast, basal cells gave rise to an epithelium composed only of basal and ciliated cells. These results suggest that the secretory cells have greater capacity to differentiate, are the main progenitor cells in the upper airways, and give rise to all the other main cell types (Figure 1).

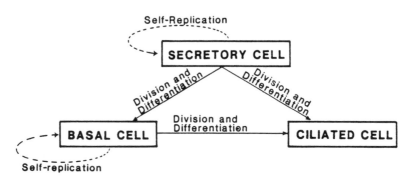

Figure 1. Schematic diagram showing the possible differentiation pathways of the three major tracheal epithelial cell types.

The approach used in this study to determine the lineage of airway epithelial cells, that is, isolation of pure cell populations used to repopulate denuded tracheal grafts, has shown that the secretory cell is the major proliferative and progenitorial cell type in the upper airways of the rat.

ACKNOWLEDGMENTS

Research was sponsored by U.S. Department of Energy's Office of Health and Environmental Research under Contract No. DE-AC04-76EV01013 in facilities fully accredited by the American Association for Accreditation of Laboratory Animal Care.

HUMAN MUTATION MONITORING USING THE GLYCOPHORIN A-BASED SOMATIC CELL ASSAY

W. L. Bigbee, R. G. Langlois, and R. H. Jensen

Biomedical Sciences Division, University of California, Lawrence Livermore National Laboratory, P.O. Box 5507, Livermore, CA 94550

Key words: *Glycophorin A, somatic mutation, cancer-prone syndromes*

ABSTRACT

A newly developed somatic cell mutation assay quantitates the level of *in vivo* genetic damage that occurs at the autosomal glycophorin A locus in humans. The glycophorin A gene occurs as two common alleles, M and N, which are codominantly expressed in MN heterozygotes. The assay uses monoclonal antibodies and flow-sorting to detect and quantify variant erythrocytes. The latter lack expression of a single allelic form of this cell-surface sialoglycoprotein in the peripheral blood of MN heterozygotes. The frequency of these null variant erythrocytes presumably reflects the level of genetic damage that results in gene expression loss mutations at this locus in erythroid progenitor cells.

The assay has been validated by analyzing blood samples from normal donors, from cancer patients receiving chemotherapy with mutagenic agents, from Hiroshima atomic-bomb survivors and Chernobyl nuclear-reactor-accident victims exposed to whole-body radiation, and from cancer-prone individuals with DNA repair/metabolism abnormalities. In individuals with no apparent exposure to mutagens, the frequency of null variant erythrocytes is ~10 per million cells, with small elevations apparent with smoking or increasing age. Patients who received chemotherapy with mutagenic agents showed elevations of two- to sevenfold over pretherapy controls, suggesting that the assay is sensitive to mutations induced by chemical mutagens. However, these increases persisted for only 3 mo after chemotherapy. A radiation-dose-dependent increase was observed in atomic-bomb survivors and in Chernobyl victims, indicating that radiation induces mutational lesions in long-lived erythroid stem cells that are capable of producing variant cells 40 yr after exposure. In studies of cancer-prone individuals with chromosome instability syndromes, elevations in the spontaneous variant cell frequency of ~10 fold were seen in ataxia-telangiectasia homozygotes; elevations of ~60 fold were observed in Bloom's syndrome homozygotes. These elevations demonstrate, for the first time, a correlation between increased spontaneous somatic mutation, cytogenetic instability, and cancer susceptibility in these individuals.

The results of all these studies demonstrate the utility of the assay in estimating somatic genotoxicity in cases of acute high-dose exposure. The usefulness of the assay for monitoring prospective cancer risk in situations of low-dose environmental and occupational exposures remains to be tested.

We have developed a new method for determining the frequency of specific locus mutations in human somatic cells *in vivo*. The assay estimates the level of genetic alterations at the autosomal glycophorin A (GPA) locus in erythroid cells by enumerating erythrocytes of variant GPA phenotype.

Glycophorin A is an erythroid-specific cell-surface sialoglycoprotein of 131 amino acids (see Anstee, 1980, for review), first expressed on erythroblasts (Yurchenco and Furthmayer, 1980; Ekblom et al., 1985; Loken et al., 1987; Kitano et al., 1988). Glycophorin A occurs in two common forms, GPA(M) and GPA(N), giving rise to the MN blood group (Race and Sanger, 1975). The two forms of GPA differ by two amino acids at positions 1 and 5 of the sequence (Furthmayer, 1978; Prohaska et al., 1981) and are the products of single-copy, codominantly expressed alleles mapped to chromosome 4, q28-q31 (Furthmayer, 1978; HGM7, 1984; Siebert and Fukuda, 1986; Rahuel et al., 1988). Thus, individuals of heterozygous MN blood type possess single copies of each allele, which produce approximately 5×10^5 molecules each of GPA(M) and GPA(N) on each erythrocyte (Langlois et al., 1985; Merry et al., 1986).

We have isolated and characterized a set of GPA(M)- and GPA(N)-specific monoclonal antibodies (Bigbee et al., 1983, 1984; Langlois et al., 1985). Our GPA assay (Langlois et al., 1986) uses pairs of these antibodies coupled to the distinguishable fluorophores fluorescein and Texas Red to label erythrocytes in peripheral blood samples from MN heterozygotes. Normal erythrocytes, expressing both GPA(M) and GPA(N), bind both the allele-specific antibodies and fluoresce both green and red. Rare variant cells, which lack expression of one allele, fail to bind one of the antibodies, and fluoresce only green or red. Flow-sorting is used to quantitatively enumerate these variant erythrocytes by rapidly screening (∼1500 cells per second) the erythrocyte population, detecting the single-color cells, and sorting them onto microscope slides for visual verification.

The frequency of null variant erythrocytes in the peripheral blood presumably reflects the level of fixed genetic alterations resulting in gene expression loss mutations at this locus in erythroid progenitor cells. Mutations that lead to variant erythrocytes of GPA allele-loss phenotype are likely to be selectively neutral, because individuals who heritably lack GPA are hematologically normal, and their erythrocytes have a normal lifetime (Furthmayer, 1978; Anstee, 1980).

We have developed several versions of the GPA assay using different pairs of monoclonal antibodies to permit the independent enumeration of hemizygous variant erythrocytes of NØ or MØ phenotype in the peripheral blood of MN heterozygotes. Mutational events that can give rise to variant cells of this phenotype include amino acid substitutions, deletions/insertions, and chromosome aneuploidy or nonhomologous somatic recombination. The assay can also detect, in MN individuals, homozygous variant erythrocytes of NN or MM phenotype that can result from homologous mitotic recombination, chromosome missegregation, or gene conversion (Langlois et al., 1986).

The assay has been validated by analyzing blood samples from normal donors, cancer patients receiving chemotherapy with mutagenic agents, Hiroshima A-bomb survivors, victims from the Chernobyl nuclear reactor and Goiana, Brazil, accidents exposed to whole-body radiation, and cancer-prone individuals with DNA repair/metabolism abnormalities. A summary of null variant cell frequencies in blood samples from healthy individuals, cancer patients, and A-bomb survivors is shown in Figure 1.

In normal persons with no apparent exposure to high levels of mutagens, the frequency of hemizygous (Figure 1, group 1) and homozygous variant erythrocytes is ~10 per million cells, with small elevations apparent with smoking or increasing age (Langlois et al., 1986; Jensen et al., 1988).

Cancer patients assayed before therapy showed hemizygous variant cell frequencies within the range observed for healthy controls (Figure 1, group 2); chemotherapy with mutagenic agents (notably cyclophosphamide and adriamycin) generally but not always resulted in elevations of hemizygous variant cell frequencies (Figure 1, group 3), suggesting that the assay is sensitive to mutations induced by chemical mutagens (Bigbee et al., in press). The observed variability in the response to chemotherapy is caused by differences in the chemotherapy agents used as well as differences in individual patient responses to similar therapy. Longitudinal sampling during and after therapy revealed a delay in the appearance of chemotherapy-induced variant cells after the beginning of therapy, with a maximum occurring at or shortly after the end of therapy. The elevated level then declined to near pretherapy levels within 6 mo. This time response suggests that the cells most susceptible to mutation by these agents are the rapidly proliferating erythroid precursor population.

We have observed increases in the frequency of variant cells in individuals exposed to whole-body ionizing radiation (Figure 1, groups 4 and 5). In Hiroshima A-bomb survivors, we observed a dose-dependent increase in hemizygous and homozygous variant cells (Langlois et al., 1987). The induced hemizygous cell frequency of $\sim0.2 \times 10^{-6}$/cGy falls within the range observed *in vitro* and *in vivo* for radiation-induced mutations at other loci. This finding and the fact that these results were obtained 40 yr after exposure support a mutational origin of the GPA variant cells and suggest that the radiation-induced mutational lesions must be fixed in long-lived hemopoietic stem cells. We have confirmed these results with observations of similar dose reponses in Chernobyl and Goiana victims sampled 1 to 2 yr after exposure (Bigbee et al., unpublished data).

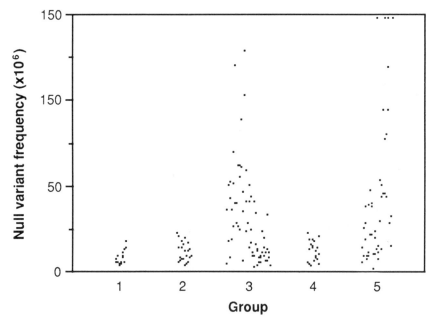

Figure 1. Glycophorin A hemizygous null variant cell frequencies in normal individuals, cancer chemotherapy patients, and A-bomb survivors. Data in group 1 are variant cell frequencies observed in blood samples from 16 healthy normal donors (range, 4 to 18 per million; mean, 8.4 per million). Group 2 data are from 22 cancer patients sampled before therapy (range, 4 to 23 per million; mean, 11.9 per million). Group 3 data are from 67 blood samples from cancer chemotherapy patients obtained after at least 120 days of therapy or within 120 days after completion of therapy (range, 3 to 129 per million; mean, 31.4 per million). Group 4 data are from 20 residents of Hiroshima in 1945 who received less than 1 cGy of radiation (range, 4 to 23 per million; mean, 12.4 per million). Group 5 data are from 47 Hiroshima A-bomb survivors (range, 2 to 668 per million; mean, 64.0 per million). The radiation doses estimated for this group (T65DR) range from 14 to 884 cGy (mean dose, 227 cGy). Samples from 4 of these individuals showed very high variant cell frequencies (244, 330, 366, and 668 per million) and are plotted at top of panel.

Finally, we determined spontaneous variant cell frequencies in cancer-prone individuals with chromosome instability syndromes. In persons with ataxia-telangiectasia we observed an ~10-fold elevation in the mean hemizygous variant cell frequency and an ~4-fold elevation in the mean homozygous frequency (Bigbee et al., 1989). These findings are the first evidence for an increased rate of somatic mutation in such individuals. Even higher elevations are found in Bloom's syndrome individuals: we observed a mean increase of ~70 fold for hemizygous variants and ~90 fold for homozygous variants (Langlois et al., 1989). This very high frequency of spontaneous hemizygous variants confirms previous reports of high *in vivo* specific locus mutations in these individuals (Gupta and Goldstein, 1980; Warren et al., 1981; Vijayalaxmi et al., 1983; Ben-Sasson et al., 1985). Our finding of a high frequency of homozygous variants is new evidence supporting the proposed elevated rate of *in vivo* somatic recombination in Bloom's syndrome individuals (German, 1964, 1982; German et al., 1974; Therman and Kuhn, 1976). Together, these findings demonstrate a correlation between increased spontaneous somatic mutation, cytogenetic instability, and cancer susceptibility in these individuals.

The results summarized here demonstrate that the GPA assay reveals an elevated level of spontaneous somatic mutation in cancer-prone individuals and that the assay responds in cases of acute high-dose exposures to chemical mutagens and radiation. The relationship between somatic genotoxicity at the GPA locus and cancer risk is unknown. However, the spectrum of genetic alterations detectable in the assay have been shown to be critical events in human carcinogenesis. These include activation of onocogenes by point mutation (Brodeur, 1986) and loss of functional alleles of tumor suppressor genes by gene deletion or inactivation, recombination, or chromosome loss (Friend et al., 1988). Further studies are required to determine the utility of the assay for estimating cancer risk in situations of low-dose environmental and/or occupational exposures.

ACKNOWLEDGMENTS

This work was performed under the auspices of the U.S. Department of Energy by the Lawrence Livermore National Laboratory under contract number W-7405-ENG-48 with support by grants R-808642-01 and R-811819-02-0 from the U.S. Environmental Protection Agency, and Interagency Agreements YO-1-ES-3-0114 from the U.S. National Institute of Environmental Health Sciences and 88-822 from the U.S. Department of Defense/Defense Nuclear Agency.

REFERENCES

Anstee, DJ. 1980. Blood group MNSs-active sialoglycoproteins of the human erythrocyte membrane, pp. 67-98. In: *Immunobiology of the Erythrocyte*, Sandler SG, J Nusbacher, MS Schanfield (eds.). Alan R Liss, New York.

Ben-Sasson, SA, T Cohen, and R Voss. 1985. Background allelic variant in normal hemopoietic cells and Bloom's syndrome erythrocytes and the possible implication of somatic crossingover. Cancer Genet Cytogenet 15:237-242.

Bigbee, WL, AW Wyrobek, RG Langlois, RH Jensen, and RB Everson. The effect of chemotherapy on the *in vivo* frequency of glycophorin A "null" variant erythrocytes. Mutat Res (in press).

Bigbee, WL, RG Langlois, M Swift, and RH Jensen. 1989. Evidence for an elevated frequency of *in vivo* somatic cell mutations in ataxia telangiectasia. Am J Hum Genet 44:402-408.

Bigbee, WL, RG Langlois, M Vanderlaan, and RH Jensen. 1984. Binding specificities of eight monoclonal antibodies to human glycophorin A studies using M^cM, and $M^kEn(UK)$ variant human erythrocytes and M- and MN^v-type chimpanzee erythrocytes. J Immunol 133:3149-3155.

Bigbee, WL, M Vanderlaan, SSN Fong, and RH Jensen. 1983. Monoclonal antibodies specific for the M- and N-forms of human glycophorin A. Mol Immunol 20:1353-1362.

Brodeur, GM. 1986. Molecular correlates of cytogenic abnormalities in human cancer cells: Implications for oncogene activation, pp. 229-256. In: *Progress in Hematology XIV*. Grune and Stratton, New York.

Ekblom, M, CG Gahmberg, and LC Anderson. 1985. Late expression of M and N antigens on glycophorin A during erythroid differentiation. Blood 66:233-236.

Friend, SH, TP Dryja, and RA Weinberg. 1988. Oncogenes and tumor-suppressing genes. N Engl J Med 318:618-622.

Furthmayer, H. 1978. Structural comparison of glycophorins and immunochemical analysis of genetic variants. Nature 271:519-524.

German, J. 1964. Cytological evidence for crossing-over *in vitro* in human lymphoid cells. Science 144:298-301.

German, J. 1982. Biological role of chromatid exchange in mammalian somatic cells, pp. 307-312. In: *Gene Amplification*, RT Schmike (ed.). Cold Spring Harbor Laboratory, Cold Spring Harbor, New York.

German, J, LP Crippa, and D Bloom. 1974. Bloom's syndrome. III. Analysis of the chromosome aberration characteristic of this disorder. Chromosoma (Berlin) 48:361-366.

Gupta, RS and S Goldstein. 1980. Diphtheria toxin resistance in human fibroblast cell strains from normal and cancer-prone individuals. Mutat Res 73:331-338.

HGM7 (Human Gene Mapping 7). 1984. Los Angeles Conference 1983. Seventh international workshop on human gene mapping, RS Sparkes, K Berg, HJ Evans, and HP Klinger (eds.). Cytogenet Cell Genet 37:1-666.

Jensen, RH, WL Bigbee, and RG Langlois. 1988. *In vivo* somatic mutations in the glycophorin A locus of human erythroid cells, pp. 149-159. In: *Banbury Report 28, Mammalian Cell Mutagenesis*, MM Moore, DM DeMarini, KR Tindall (eds.). Cold Spring Harbor Laboratory Press, Cold Spring Harbor, New York.

Kitano, K, E Kajii, S Ikemoto, Y Amemiya, N Komatsu, T Suda, and Y Miura. 1988. Confirmation of bone marrow engraftment by detection of M/N blood group antigens on erythroblasts in erythroid bursts. Br J Haematol 69:329-333.

Langlois, RG, WL Bigbee, and RH Jensen. 1985. Flow cytometric characterization of normal and variant cells with monoclonal antibodies specific for glycophorin A. J Immunol 134:4009-4017.

Langlois, RG, WL Bigbee, and RH Jensen. 1986. Measurements of the frequency of human erythrocytes with gene expression loss phenotypes at the glycophorin A locus. Hum Genet 74:353-362.

Langlois, RG, WL Bigbee, RH Jensen, and J German. 1989. Evidence for elevated *in vivo* mutation and somatic recombination in Bloom's syndrome. Proc Natl Acad Sci USA 86:670-674.

Langlois, RG, WL Bigbee, S Kyoizumi, N Nakamura, MA Bean, M Akiyama, and RH Jensen. 1987. Evidence for increased somatic cell mutations at the glycophorin A locus in atomic bomb survivors. Science 236:445-448.

Loken, MR, VO Shah, KL Dattilio, and CI Civin. 1987. Flow cytometric analysis of human bone marrow: I. Normal erythroid development. Blood 69:255-263.

Merry, AH, C Hodson, E Thompson, G Mallinson, and DJ Anstee. 1986. The use of monoclonal antibodies to quantitate the levels of sialoglycoproteins alpha, delta, and variant sialoglycoproteins in human erythrocyte membranes. Biochem J 233:93-98.

Prohaska, R, TAW Koerner, Jr., IM Armitage, and H Furthmayer. 1981. Chemical and carbon-13 nuclear magnetic resonance studies of the blood group M and N active sialoglycopeptides from human glycophorin A. J Biol Chem 256:5781-5791.

Race, RR and R Sanger. 1975. *Blood Groups in Man*, 6th Ed., pp. 92-138. Blackwell, Oxford.

Rahuel, C, J London, L d'Auriol, M-G Mattei, C Tournamille, C Skrzynia, Y Lebouc, F Falibert, and J-P Cartron. 1988. Characterization of cDNA clones for human glycophorin A. Use for gene localization and for analysis of normal and glycophorin-A-deficient (Finnish type) genomic DNA. Eur J Biochem 172:147-153.

Siebert, PD and M Fukuda. 1986. Human glycophorin A and B are encoded by separate, single copy genes coordinately regulated by a tumor-promoting phorbol ester. J Biol Chem 261:12433-12436.

Therman, E and EM Kuhn. 1976. Cytological demonstration of mitotic crossing-over in man. Cytogenet Cell Genet 17:254-267.

Vijayalaxmi, HJ Evans, JH Ray, and J German. 1983. Bloom's syndrome: Evidence for an increased mutation frequency *in vivo*. Science 221:851-853.

Warren, ST, RA Schultz, C-C Chang, MH Wade, and JE Trosko. 1981. Elevated spontaneous mutation rate in Bloom syndrome fibroblasts. Proc Natl Acad Sci USA 78:3133-3137.

Yurchenco, PD and H Furthmayer. 1980. Expression of red cell membrane proteins in erythroid precursor cells. J Supramol Struct 13:255-268.

QUESTIONS AND COMMENTS

Q: Gantt, NCI
   Were AT carriers normal for both normal and induced mutation?

A: Bigbee
   The purpose of the study of the ataxia-telangiectasia families was to determine background levels of glycophorin A variant cells, so only individuals with no known exposures to high levels of mutagens were included. Therefore the data presented for the obligate heterozygotes refer only to background variant cell frequencies; we have no data on induced levels in these individuals.

Q: Generoso, Oak Ridge National Laboratory, Oak Ridge, TN
   Do you have some measure of the magnitude of variant expressions not due to mutational events?

A: Bigbee
   We have no direct measure of the fraction of glycophorin A variant cells that may arise by nongenetic mechanisms because the assay can score only variant phenotypes. However, the assay has been designed to minimize such epigenetic events by requiring that null variant cells at one glycophorin A allele retain normal expression of the sister allele. Thus mutational and nonmutational mechanisms outside the glycophorin A locus that result in loss of expression of both alleles are excluded. We have made an indirect estimate of the frequency of nonmutational variants by examining blood samples from homozygous MM and NN individuals (Langlois et al., 1986). The frequency of

M-null or N-null cells in these samples arising by mutational mechanisms should be extremely low. We observed that the frequency of null variant cells in homozygous bloods is $< 10^{-6}$.

RAPID DETECTION OF HUMAN CHROMOSOME ABERRATIONS USING FLUORESCENCE *IN SITU* HYBRIDIZATION

J. N. Lucas, T. Tenjin, T. Straume, D. Pinkel, and J. Gray

University of California, Lawrence Livermore National Laboratory, Livermore, CA 94550

Key words: *Chromosome, aberrations, hybridization*

ABSTRACT

We present two methods for the rapid detection of translocations and dicentrics in human chromosomes. The first uses *in situ* hybridization with a pair of repeat-sequence DNA probes specific to the paracentric locus *1q12* and the telomeric locus *1p36* to fluorescently stain regions that flank human chromosome 1p. Translocations involving chromosome 1p are visualized by the presence of telomeric and paracentric hybridization regions on different chromosomes.

Human lymphocytes were irradiated with 0, 0.1, 0.25, 1.0, 2.0, or 4.0 Gy of gamma rays, and the frequencies of translocations and dicentrics per cell that involved 1p were determined. Both frequencies increased with dose, D, in a linear-quadratic manner. The δ, α, and β coefficients that resulted from a fit of the equation f(D) = $\delta + \alpha D + \beta D^2$ to the translocation frequency dose-response data were 0.0025, 0.0027, and 0.0037, respectively. The δ, α, and β coefficients that resulted from a fit to the dicentric frequency dose-response data were 0.0005, 0.0010, and 0.0028, respectively. Approximately 29,000 metaphase spreads were scored in this study; more than 20,000 of them were below 0.25 Gy. The average analysis rate was greater than 2 metaphase spreads per minute; however, an experienced analyst was able to find and score 1 metaphase spread every 10 sec.

The second method uses an entire chromosome-specific library as a probe. Hybridization of repetitive sequences in the probe to other chromosomes is suppressed by unlabeled human genomic DNA. This procedure allows the entire chromosome to be fluorescently stained. Using this procedure with chromosome 4 has permitted rapid identification of chromosome aberrations involving chromosome 4 in metaphase spreads. Extension of this technique to other chromosomes is being aggressively pursued. By applying it to other chromosomes, we expect to increase the aberration detection target size from the 1p arm of chromosome 1 to several chromosomes (e.g., chromosomes 1 to 4). The high contrast of the staining may eventually permit automated analysis of these structural aberrations at a much higher rate than currently possible. We believe that this new approach to

cytogenetic analysis will lead to better understanding of the induction of chromosome aberrations *in vitro* at low doses, and will permit meaningful screening of
individuals inadvertently exposed to genotoxins.

We have developed two methods for the rapid detection of translocations and
dicentrics in human chromosomes. The first uses fluorescence *in situ* hybridization with a pair of repeat-sequence DNA probes (Pinkel et al., 1986) specific to
the paracentric locus *1q12* (Cook and Hindley, 1979) and the telomeric locus
1p36 (Buroker et al., 1987) to fluorescently stain regions that flank human
chromosome 1p. Translocations involving chromosome 1p are visualized by the
presence of telomeric and paracentric hybridization regions on different chromosomes (Figure 1). A normal metaphase spread with the telomeric and centromeric fluorescent domains present on each of two large chromosomes is
shown in Figure 1A. Two kinds of chromosome rearrangements involving
chromosome 1p are shown in Figures 1B and 1C. (1) Translocations: Figure 1B
shows a pair of derivative chromosomes in which the paracentromeric locus is
present on one chromosome, and the telomeric locus is present on another
chromosome. Centromeric constrictions are evident on the two derivative chromosomes. (2) Dicentrics: Figure 1C shows one chromosome containing the
paracentromeric locus of chromosome 1 and one other centromere, and a
chromosome fragment containing the telomeric locus of chromosome 1.

Human lymphocytes were exposed *in vitro* to 0, 0.09, 0.18, 1.0, 2.0, 3.1, and
4.1 Gy of ^{60}Co irradiation, and the frequencies of translocations and dicentrics
per cell involving 1p were determined (Lucas et al., 1989). The frequencies
were fitted using the function $Y = \delta + \alpha D + \beta D^2$, where D was the radiation
dose. Figure 2 shows the data and computer fits for the translocation (A) and
dicentric (B) chromosome frequencies. These frequencies both increased with
dose, D, in a linear-quadratic manner. The low-dose portion of the ^{60}Co translocation dose-response curve is shown in the insert of Figure 2A. The δ, α, and β
coefficients were 0.0025, 0.0027, and 0.0037, respectively, for translocations
and 0.0005, 0.0010, and 0.0028, respectively, for dicentrics. Approximately
29,000 metaphase spreads were scored in this study; more than 20,000 were less
than 0.25 Gy. The average analysis rate was more than 2 metaphase spreads per
minute. However, an experienced analyst was able to find and score 1 metaphase spread every 10 sec.

The second method (chromosome painting) uses an entire chromosome-specific
library as a probe. Hybridization of repetitive sequences in the probe to other
chromosomes is suppressed by unlabeled human genomic DNA (Pinkel et al.,
1989). This procedure allows the entire chromosome to be fluorescently
stained; chromosomal rearrangements result in bicolor chromosomes. Using
this procedure with a chromosome 4-specific library has permitted rapid identification of chromosome aberrations involving chromosome 4 in metaphase
spreads (Figure 3). In the left panel, a normal metaphase spread is shown;

both number 4 chromosomes are light and background chromosomes are dark. A dicentric is shown in the top panel, while the bottom right panel illustrates a translocation involving one of the number 4 chromosomes.

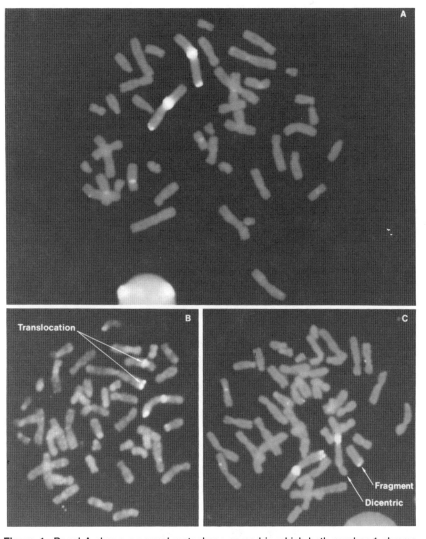

Figure 1. Panel A shows a normal metaphase spread in which both number 1 chromosomes are clearly labeled at the centromere and at the distal end of the short arm. Panel B shows a metaphase spread containing a translocation involving chromosome 1p. Panel C shows a metaphase spread containing a dicentric chromosome involving chromosome 1p.

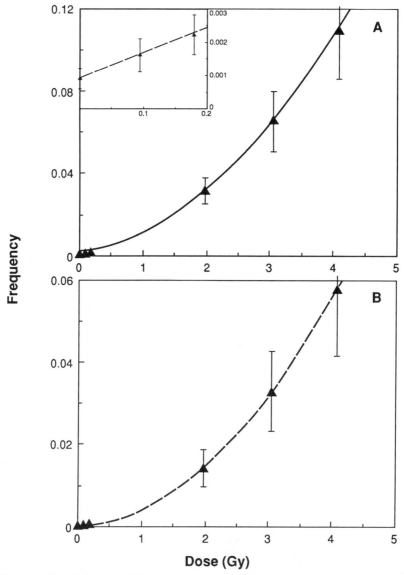

Figure 2. Aberration frequency dose-response curves for human chromosome 1p. Panel A shows translocation frequency dose-response data. Insert shows low-dose region of ^{60}Co study. Error bars indicate standard errors of measurements. *Solid line* shows fit of function $Y = \delta + \alpha D + \beta D^2$ to ^{60}Co-induced translocation frequencies. Panel B shows dicentric frequency dose-reponse data. Error bars indicate standard errors of measurements. *Long-dashed line* shows fit of function $Y = \delta + \alpha D + \beta D^2$ to ^{60}Co-induced dicentric frequencies.

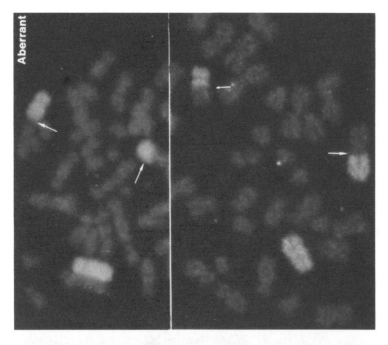

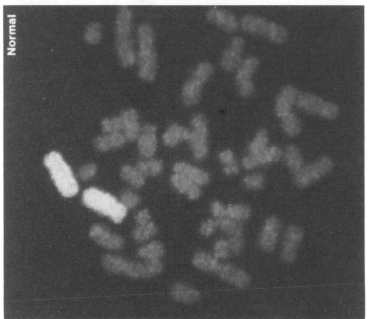

Figure 3. Detection of chromosome aberrations using chromosome painting. Shown on left, labeled normal, is normal metaphase with the four chromosomes painted. Right top panel shows dicentric involving chromosome 4. Right bottom panel shows translocation involving chromosome 4.

Extension of this technique to other chromosomes is being aggressively pursued. By staining multiple chromosomes simultaneously, we expect to substantially increase the target size for aberration detection. For example, the data of Figure 2 were obtained with pairs of probes for chromosome 1 (see Figure 1) that allowed detection of aberration with an efficiency of $\sim$8% of the genome. Use of whole-library probes for chromosomes 1, 2, 3, and 4 will increase this to more than 40%. Thus results reported here using repetitive probes could presumably be obtained by analysis of one-seventh of the metaphase using chromosome painting. The high contrast of the staining may eventually permit automated analysis of these structural aberrations at a much higher rate than is now possible visually. We believe that this new approach to cytogenetic analysis will lead to better understanding of induction of chromosome aberrations *in vitro* at low doses and will permit meaningful screening of exposed individuals.

ACKNOWLEDGMENT

Work performed under the auspices of the U.S. Department of Energy by the Lawrence Livermore National Laboratory under contract number W-7405-ENG-48.

REFERENCES

Buroker, N, R Bestwick, G Haight, RE Magenis, and M Litt. 1987. A hypervariable repeated sequence on human chromosome 1p36. Hum Genet 77:175-181.

Cooke, HJ and J Hindley. 1979. Cloning of human satellite III DNA: Different components are on different chromosomes. Nucleic Acids Res 10:3177-3197.

Lucas, JN, T Straume, D Pinkel, M Litt, and JW Gray. 1989. Rapid human chromosome aberration analysis using fluorescence in situ hybridization. Int J Radiat Biol (in press).

Pinkel, D, T Straume, and JW Gray. 1986. Cytogenetic analysis using quantitative high-sensitivity fluorescence hybridization. Proc Natl Acad Sci USA 83:2934-2938.

Pinkel, D, J Landegent, C Collins, J Fuscoe, R Segraves, J Lucas, and J Gray. 1989. Fluorescence *in situ* hybridization with human chromosome-specific libraries: Detection of trisomy 21 and translocations of chromosome 4. Proc Natl Acad Sci USA 85:9138-9142.

QUESTIONS AND COMMENTS

Q: Blazek, Argonne National Laboratory

What is the best current understanding of D^2 reponse for chromosomal translocation? I ask because our laboratory and others have recently observed evidence for D^2 reponse, or at least nonlinear response, for individual

DSB. Thus we would predict translocations proportional to D^4, or at least D_n^p, $n > 2$. (That evidence will be described in my presentation.)

A: Lucas
Our translocation results fit well a D^2 function, similar to results for dicentrics using conventional cytogenetic methods. Our data using chromosome painting are not consistent with a D^4 dose-response relationship.

Q: Brooks, Lovelace ITRI
What is the relationship between the translocations served in the Y-12 accident victims you scored and the frequency of rings and dicentrics scored at the time of the accident? This suggests little repair with time.

What is the lowest dose you have evaluated in these people?

A: Lucas
It should be pointed out that cytogenetic evaluation was not performed on the Y-12 accident victims until about 2 yr after the accident (**Bender** and Gooch, Radiat. Res. 16:44, **1962**). Due to loss of dicentrics and rings during this period and because they scored aberrations in 72-hr cultures (rather than the present convention of 48 hr), the early information from these accident victims cannot reliably be used for intercomparison.

The lowest dose evaluated for the Y-12 accident victims is 22.8 rad tissue kerma in air. We estimate this to be roughly 10 rad of absorbed marrow dose (about 8 rad of gamma rays and 2 rad of neutrons).

Q: Generoso, Oak Ridge National Laboratory
So far, what I have seen are chromosome-type radiation-induced aberrations. Have you tried your chromosome painting techniques to score for chemically induced chromatin-type rearrangements and deletions—those that result from alkylation of chromosomal DNA?

A: Lucas
We have not yet applied chromosome painting techniques to detect chemically induced chromatid-type rearrangements.

USE OF AN ANTIKINETOCHORE ANTIBODY AND DNA PROBES TO MEASURE ANEUPLOIDY INDUCTION IN INTERPHASE HUMAN LYMPHOCYTES AND CHINESE HAMSTER OVARY CELLS

D. A. Eastmond, J. D. Tucker, and D. Pinkel

Lawrence Livermore National Laboratory, Biomedical Sciences Division, University of California, P.O. Box 5507, Livermore, CA 94550

Key words: *Micronucleus, aneuploidy, antikinetochore antibody, DNA probes, in situ hybridization*

ABSTRACT

The rapid detection of aneuploidy-inducing chemicals is an important research priority in the fields of genetic toxicology and teratology. We have developed two new assays for identifying aneuploidy-inducing agents using new molecular and immunological techniques. The first approach utilizes the chemical induction of micronuclei in cytokinesis-blocked cells and an antikinetochore antibody to determine whether micronuclei contain kinetochores, a condition indicating potential aneuploidy. Using both human lymphocytes and Chinese hamster ovary cells, this approach was shown to be efficient in distinguishing a series of aneuploidy-inducing chemicals from clastogenic agents.

The second approach involves the use of *in situ* hybridization with fluorescently labeled chromosome-specific DNA probes. This permits the number of copies of a specific chromosome present in interphase nuclei to be determined rapidly. Initial studies using selected DNA probes and human lymphocytes indicate that this assay should be capable of measuring the frequency of nuclei hyperdiploid for a specific chromosome at a frequency as low as 0.013 when 1000-2000 cells are scored. These two new assays should facilitate more rapid identification of environmental agents with aneuploidy-inducing properties.

INTRODUCTION

Aneuploidy in germ cells is associated with birth defects, spontaneous abortions, and infertility, and in somatic cells aneuploidy may lead to cell death and carcinogenesis (Yunis, 1983; Hook, 1985). The nonrandom numerical chromosomal changes that are often observed in tumors or transformed cells suggest that aneuploidy induction by chemicals may be involved in carcinogenesis (Oshimura and Barrett, 1986). The identification of aneuploidy-inducing agents (aneuploidogens) and studies into the mechanisms by which aneuploidy may be involved in carcinogenesis are currently limited in that standard cytogenetic techniques are time consuming, require highly skilled personnel, and are prone to technical artifacts. Recent developments in immunology and molecular biology have produced new techniques that may allow simple and rapid identification of aneuploidogens. We report the development of two such new approaches. The first is the induction of micronuclei in human lymphocytes and Chinese hamster ovary (CHO) cells and the use of an antikinetochore antibody to determine whether micronuclei contain centromeres—a condition indicating potential aneuploidy. The second approach uses in situ hybridization with fluorescently labeled chromosome-specific DNA probes and the subsequent counting of the number of copies of that chromosome in the interphase nuclei of human lymphocytes.

Antikinetochore Assay

The antikinetochore assay is based on a modification of a micronucleus assay using cytokinesis-blocked human lymphocytes (Fenech and Morley, 1985). Micronuclei are formed when chromosomal fragments or whole chromosomes do not segregate properly during cell division. Cells with micronuclei containing a whole chromosome will result in aneuploid daughter cells if the micronucleus fails to segregate with the nucleus that is monosomic for that chromosome. Cells with a micronucleus containing a whole chromosome will therefore have a high probability of generating aneuploid daughter cells. In contrast, cells with a micronucleus containing an acentric fragment will not generate aneuploid daughter cells. Distinguishing between these two types of micronucleated cells is accomplished by using an antibody to the kinetochore that is obtained from individuals with the autoimmune disease CREST scleroderma. The kinetochore, a structure composed of centromere-associated proteins and nucleic acids, is the attachment site for the mitotic spindle apparatus.

Detailed procedures for performing the antikinetochore assay as well as a complete description of the basis for the assay can be found in Eastmond and Tucker (1989). Briefly, freshly isolated phytohemagglutinin-stimulated human peripheral lymphocytes are exposed to aneuploidogenic or clastogenic agents in vitro. Cytochalasin B is added at 44 hr to block cytokinesis, resulting in binucleated cells. At 72 hr, cells are centrifuged onto slides and fixed for 15 min in 100% methanol. The slides are either used immediately or are stored, desiccated, at -20°C under 100% nitrogen. An antikinetochore antibody (Antibodies Inc., Davis, CA) is applied in phosphate-buffered saline (PBS) containing 0.05% Tween 20. A fluoresceinated rabbit antihuman antibody in PBS containing 0.5% Tween 20 is then applied. 4'-6-Diamidino-2-phenylindole (DAPI; 0.25 μg/ml) is used to counterstain the nucleus. One thousand binucleated cells (approximately 500 from each of two duplicate cultures) were scored for micronuclei from coded slides using simultaneous phase contrast and DAPI fluorescence (maximal excitation at 355 nm, emission at 450 nm). After a micronucleated cell was located, the presence of a kinetochore in the micronucleus was determined using fluorescein filter settings (maximal excitation, 488 nm; emission, 520 nm). Chinese hamster ovary cells can also be used in this assay with minor modifications of culturing and treatment conditions.

The use of an antikinetochore antibody for determining the location of kinetochores within the nuclei and micronuclei of human lymphocytes is efficient. Rigorous attempts to enumerate individual kinetochores identified 35 to 46 fluorescein spots per interphase nucleus in untreated binucleated lymphocytes and 46 spots in virtually all metaphase spreads from Colcemid-arrested lymphocytes. In CHO cells, approximately 20 fluorescein spots were observed in each nucleus. The number of kinetochores visible within a cell varied, depending on the stage of the cell cycle, the microscopic plane of focus, the overlap of individual spots, and the efficiency of antibody penetration. Micronucleated cells were considered scorable for kinetochores only if the kinetochores in the main nuclei were numerous and distinctly visible. The frequency of scorable micronucleated cells ranged from 85% to 99.9%.

To determine the ability of this assay to distinguish aneuploidy-inducing compounds from clastogenic agents, a series of aneuploidogens and clastogens were tested for their ability to induce kinetochore-positive micronucleated cells (Figure 1). Colchicine and vincristine sulfate produced dose-related increases in kinetochore-positive micronucleated cells at concentrations ranging from 0.050 to 0.1 μM for colchicine and from 0.026 to 0.065 μM for vincristine. Diethylstilbestrol (DES) produced an unambiguous increase in kinetochore-positive micronucleated cells only at 30 μM, the highest dose tested. The potent clastogens sodium arsenite and ionizing radiation (from a ^{137}Cs source) induced dose-related increases of micronucleated cells at doses of 3-9 μM for arsenite and 100-400 rad for radiation.

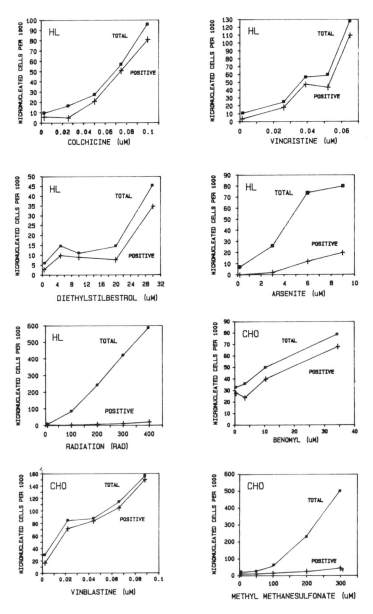

Figure 1. Induction of micronucleated human lymphocytes (HL) or Chinese hamster ovary cells (CHO) by various agents. Total number of binucleated cells with micronuclei (■) and number of binucleated cells containing one or more kinetochore-positive micronuclei (+) are shown for each instance. Zero dose has been slightly offset for clarity.

Most micronucleated cells induced by these two agents, however, lacked a kinetochore. Interestingly, both arsenite and radiation induced minor but statistically significant dose-related increases in kinetochore-positive micronucleated cells. This suggests that these agents might also be weak aneuploidogens in addition to their potent clastogenicity. A summary of the frequencies of kinetochore-positive and -negative micronucleated cells induced by these agents is shown in Table 1. For the aneuploidogens colchicine, vincristine, and DES, 92%, 87%, and 76%, respectively, of the induced micronucleated lymphocytes contained at least 1 kinetochore-positive micronucleus, whereas the frequencies of kinetochore-positive micronucleated lymphocytes produced by the potent clastogens sodium arsenite and ionizing radiation were only 19% and 3%, respectively.

Table 1. Frequencies of kinetochore-positive micronucleated cells induced by various agents.

	Kinetochore-positive (%)	Kinetochore-negative (%)
Human Lymphocytes		
Aneuploidogens		
Colchicine	92	8
Vincristine	87	13
Diethylstilbestrol	76	24
Clastogens		
Arsenite	19	81
Radiation	3	97
Chinese Hamster Ovary Cells		
Aneuploidogens		
Benomyl	92	8
Vinblastine	94	6
Clastogens		
Methyl methanesulfonate	11	89

Similar experiments were also performed using CHO cells (see Figure 1). The fungicide and aneuploidogen Benomyl (Du Pont de Nemours, Wilmington, DE) induced a significant increase in kinetochore-positive micronucleated cells at 34.4 μM, the highest concentration tested. Vinblastine sulfate, a potent chemotherapeutic and aneuploidy-inducing agent, induced significant dose-related increases in kinetochore-positive micronucleated cells at all test concentrations. The frequencies of kinetochore-positive micronucleated cells induced by Benomyl and vin-blastine sulfate were 92% and 94%, respectively (see Table 1). Experiments with the potent methylating and clastogenic agent methyl methanesul-fonate resulted in significant dose-related increases in micronucleated cells at test concentrations greater than 100 μM (see Figure 1). In this case, however, the micronucleated cells induced by methyl methanesulfonate contained a kinetochore-positive micronucleus only 11% of the time (see Table 1). These studies, using both human lymphocytes and CHO cells, indicate that this antikinetochore assay can readily distinguish between aneuploidy-inducing and clastogenic agents.

DNA Probe Assay

A second molecular approach for studying aneuploidy and identifying aneuploidy-inducing agents uses fluorescent *in situ* hybridization with DNA probes for specific human chromosomes. The assay involves simply counting the number of copies of a specific chromosome of interest in interphase nuclei. Detailed procedures for performing fluorescent *in situ* hybridization with DNA probes are described in Pinkel et al. (1986). The procedure for identifying aneuploidy-inducing agents is as follows. Freshly isolated phytohemagglutinin-stimulated human lymphocytes were treated with an aneuploidy-inducing agent *in vitro*. After 72 hr of culture, the cells were subjected to hypotonic treatment (0.075 M KCl) for 30 min and were fixed three times with methanol:acetic acid (3:1). The fixed cells were dropped on slides using a Pasteur pipet, allowed to dry, and stored at -20°C under 100% nitrogen. For hybridization, the slides are immersed in 70% formamide: 2 × SSC (1 × SSC is 0.15 M NaCl plus 0.015 M sodium citrate) at 70°C for 2 min to denature the DNA. Five nanograms of biotinylated probe DNA and 500 ng of sonicated herring carrier DNA are mixed with the hybridization mix (55% formamide: 1 × SSC/10% dextran sulfate), heated to 70°C to denature the probe, applied to the slide, and incubated overnight at 37°C. The slides are then washed in 50% for-mamide: 2 × SSC at 43° to 45°C. The biotinylated probe is detected with fluoresceinated avidin, and the hybridization signal is amplified using a biotinylated goat anti-avidin antibody followed by another layer of avidin. Propidium iodide was used to counterstain the nuclei, and the cells were scored using a fluorescein filter setting. For experiments with chemical treatments, the slides were coded, and 1000 cells (500 from each of two duplicate flasks) were scored at each dose point.

DNA probes for chromosome-specific repetitive sequences (mostly cen-tromeric) on about two-thirds of the human chromosomes are known

(Willard and Waye, 1987; Trask et al., 1988, and references therein). *In situ* hybridization with these probes results in the staining of discrete regions of the interphase nucleus; 8000 interphase nuclei from untreated 72-hr lymphocyte cultures were examined after hybridization with repetitive probes for chromosomes 1, 7, 9, or 17. The frequencies of nuclei containing zero, one, two, three, and four spots were 0.0024, 0.079, 0.9153, 0.0024, and 0.001, respectively. Based on these baseline frequencies, scoring 1000-2000 cells should allow detection of aneuploid cells with a 0.013 frequency of hyperdiploidy or a 0.11 frequency of hypodiploidy (α = 0.05; β = 0.80) for a specific chromosome in interphase nuclei. The higher apparent frequency of hypodiploid as compared to hyperdiploid nuclei (0.08 versus 0.003) in normal lymphocyte populations is consistent with calculations of the probability of overlap of the two spots on the basis of measurements of the spot and nuclear diameters.

The *in vitro* treatment of human lymphocytes with aneuploidy-inducing agents indicates that induction of aneuploidy can be readily detected by scoring the frequency of hyperdiploid interphase cells. The frequencies of cells hyperdiploid for chromosome 9 following colchicine, vincristine sulfate, and DES treatments were determined using a chromosome 9-specific repetitive probe. Colchicine treatment of lymphocytes at concentrations ranging from 0.025 to 0.1 μM resulted in a linear dose-related increase in hyperdiploid cells. All doses were significantly higher than the controls; frequencies of 50 hyperdiploid cells per 1000 were observed at the highest dose. In addition, significant increases in hyperploidy were also detected in colchicine-treated lymphocytes using repetitive probes for chromosomes 1, 7, 17, X, and Y. Cells treated with vincristine sulfate at 0.024- to 0.06-μM concentrations demonstrated a significant increase of hyperdiploid cells only at the highest dose. At this concentration, 20 hyperdiploid cells per 1000 were observed. Cells treated with DES at concentrations from 5 to 30 μM exhibited significant dose-related increases of hyperdiploid cells at concentrations greater than 5 μM. Frequencies of 37 and 36 hyperdiploid cells per 1000 were observed with DES concentrations of 20 and 30 μM, respectively.

CONCLUDING COMMENTS

These initial results indicate that both antikinetochore and DNA probe assays permit detection of aneuploidy-inducing agents. Both assays are much more rapid than standard cytogenetic techniques, and both require considerably less training to perform and score. Also, both approaches appear to be readily adaptable for *in vivo* biomonitoring studies. Although additional studies with a wider variety of aneuploidogenic and clastogenic agents are required to properly validate these approaches, the application of these assays should greatly facilitate identifying aneuploidy-inducing environmental agents and investigating the role of aneuploidy induction in carcinogenesis.

ACKNOWLEDGMENTS

We thank R. Moyzis, H. Willard, H. Cooke, and K. Smith for generously providing the chromosome-specific DNA probes. This work was performed under the auspices of the U.S. Department of Energy by the Lawrence Livermore National Laboratory under contract number W-7405-ENG-48, with additional support from the National Cancer Institute grant CA 45919. This research was conducted, in part, by an appointment to the Alexander Hollaender Distinguished Postdoctoral Fellowship Program supported by the U.S. Department of Energy, Office of Health and Environmental Research, and administered by Oak Ridge Associated Universities.

REFERENCES

Eastmond, DA and JD Tucker. 1989. Identification of aneuploidy-inducing agents using cytokinesis blocked human lymphocytes and an antikinetochore antibody. Environ Mol Mutagen 13:34-43.

Fenech, M and AA Morley. 1985. Measurement of micronuclei in lymphocytes. Mutat Res 147:29-36.

Hook, EB. 1985. The impact of aneuploidy upon public health: Mortality and morbidity associated with human chromosome abnormalities, pp. 7-33. In: *Aneuploidy, Etiology and Mechanisms*, VL Dellarco, PE Voytek, and A Hollaender (eds.). Plenum Press, New York.

Oshimura, M and JC Barrett. 1986. Chemically induced aneuploidy in mammalian cells: Mechanisms and biological significance in cancer. Environ Mutagen 8:129-159.

Pinkel, D, T Straume, and JW Gray. 1986. Cytogenetic analysis using quantitative, high-sensitivity, fluorescence hybridization. Proc Natl Acad Sci USA 83:2934-2938.

Trask, B, G van den Engh, D Pinkel, J Mulliken, F Waldman, H van Dekken, and JW Gray. 1988. Fluorescence *in situ* hybridization to interphase cell nuclei in suspension allows flow cytometric analysis of chromosome content and microscopic analysis of nuclear organization. Hum Genet 78:251-259.

Willard, H and JS Waye. 1987. Hierarchical order in chromosome-specific human alpha satellite DNA. Trends Genet 3:192-198.

Yunis, JJ. 1983. The chromosomal basis of human neoplasia. Science 221:227-236.

QUESTIONS AND COMMENTS

Q: Generoso, Oak Ridge National Laboratory, Oak Ridge, TN
Have you tried your methods on human sperm samples?

A: Personally, I have not used either of these techniques with human sperm. There are, however, two research groups at LLNL that are using chromosome-specific DNA probes on human sperm samples. One group headed by Andy Wyrobek has been using these probes to determine the number of copies of specific chromosomes in sperm. The other group headed by Brigitte Brandriff is getting some very interesting information using chromosome-specific DNA probes to study the sequence of events that occur following fertilization of hamster eggs with human sperm.

Although I don't know of anyone who has used the antikinetochore antibody on human sperm, del Mazo's group in Spain has used the antikinetochore antibody in studies of mouse spermatids and spermatozoa.

Q: Todd, NIST
What are the prospects for automation of this procedure through flow cytometry?

A: I think the prospects for automation are excellent. For the modified micronucleus assay, automation using an image analysis system is probably more likely than automation using a flow system. For the assay using DNA probes, automation using image analysis as well as flow cytometry will probably be feasible. There is currently a major effort at LLNL to automate scoring using the DNA probes for a number of types of cytogenetic analyses.

QUANTITATIVE *IN SITU* ASSAY FOR CYCLOBUTYLDITHYMIDINE DIMERS IN MAMMALIAN CELLS

S. A. Lesko, W. Li, G. Zheng, D. S. Kaplan, D. E. Callahan, W. R. Midden, N. Ni, and P. T. Strickland

Division of Biophysics, Division of Occupational Medicine and Division of Environmental Chemistry, The Johns Hopkins University, School of Hygiene and Public Health, Baltimore, MD 21205

Key words: *Thymidine dimer, immunofluorescence, enzyme-linked immunosorbent assay (ELISA), computer-assisted microfluorometry (CAM)*

ABSTRACT

An indirect immunofluorescence procedure was developed for measuring cyclobutyldithymidine dimers in DNA of individual Syrian hamster embryo cells, using a specific monoclonal antibody. A fluorescein-labeled secondary antibody and a fluorochrome that binds to DNA were used to measure the photoproduct and total DNA in the same nucleus. Fluorescence intensity was quantitated with a computer-assisted microfluorometric system, which was calibrated with a uranyl-oxide-impregnated glass slide. Similar dose-response curves, that is, normalized fluorescence intensity plotted as a function of dose of germicidal irradiation, were obtained with two different cell types.

Normalized fluorescence intensity per nucleus was related to thymidine dimer content with a competitive enzyme-linked immunosorbent assay, using DNA isolated from cells given doses of germicidal irradiation identical to those used in the immunofluorescence assay. We can readily detect thymidine dimer levels produced by 10 J/m^2 of germicidal irradiation ($\sim$8 $\times$ 10^5/nucleus) that allow for 15% to 30% cell survival.

A tritiated antibody that recognizes denatured DNA was used to relate fluorescence intensity to the number of antibody molecules bound per nucleus. When 3.6 $\times$ 10^5 molecules of tritiated antibody were bound to the nuclear DNA, the nuclei emitted a fluorescence signal that was 1.6% of that emitted by the uranyl oxide slide at a standard condition of high voltage and gain. From these data we calculated that about 45% of thymidine dimers in cells exposed to germicidal irradiation were being detected in the indirect immunofluorescence assay.

This technique can provide a sensitive means for measuring various types of DNA damage in individual cells if the appropriate probes are available. It can be

167

especially useful for monitoring occupational or environmentally exposed populations, where only small samples of cells or tissues are usually available.

Photochemical damage to DNA is generally thought to be an important factor in the development of skin cancer (Epstein, 1970; Gramstein and Sober, 1982). The availability of sensitive and specific methods for the direct measurement of individual DNA adducts at the single-cell level would greatly facilitate the study of the biological significance of these lesions.

In this investigation, we used Syrian hamster embryo cells treated with germicidal irradiation to optimize a quantitative immunostaining procedure. With appropriate processing of the cells, cyclobutyldithymidine dimers (T< >T) were rendered accessible to binding by a specific antibody, thereby generating a fluorescence signal whose intensity accurately described the T< >T dimer content per cell. Quantitation of T< >T dimers in single immunostained hamster cells was accomplished by means of computer-assisted microfluorometry (CAM) in conjunction with a competitive enzyme-linked immunosorbent assay (ELISA). A relationship was established between normalized fluorescence intensity and the number of T< >T dimers per cell. This method can be extended to other DNA adducts when the appropriate antibodies are available, and will be especially useful when only a small sample of cells or tissue is available, thus precluding the necessity for isolating DNA. Monitoring persons who are occupationally or environmentally exposed to genotoxic agents presents such a scenario. Immunofluorescence assays also allow for a direct study of the formation and persistence of adducts in the different cell types of a tissue, where a particular cell type may have enhanced proclivity to undergo neoplastic transformation.

CALIBRATION OF CAM SYSTEM

In conducting a quantitative immunofluorescence study, the first priority is a method to compare daily fluorescence measurements. Our microfluorometry system was calibrated using a uranyl-oxide-impregnated glass slide as the standard (Kaplan, 1985; Picciolo and Kaplan, 1984, 1986). Data were obtained with this standard using all combinations of high voltage and amplifier gain. The parameters were adjusted to prevent photomultiplier tube (PMT) saturation while maintaining distinguishable intensity levels. A standard curve was obtained that showed a linear relationship between log intensity and log high voltage. Fluorescence intensity data from any experiment can be compared by extrapolation to a standard condition (high voltage, 376; gain, 1) using regression line parameters (slope and intercept from standard curve). The fluorescence of the uranyl glass slide (0.43-0.54) measured at this standard condition was then used to normalize fluorescence intensity data obtained with cell nuclei.

IMMUNOCYTOCHEMICAL MEASUREMENT OF T< >T DIMERS

T< >T dimers and DNA fluorescence were measured in the same individual cell using fluorescein isothiocyanate (FITC) and propidium iodide, respectively. FITC fluorescence intensity per nucleus was determined as a percentage of the fluorescence intensity of the uranyl glass slide at the standard condition and normalized to propidium iodide fluorescence per nucleus. Measurements were made over a dose range of 0 to 120 J/m^2 for early passage, diploid fibroblasts (FC13), and a line of immortalized fibroblasts (21F). The data show that both cell types exhibited very similar responses with respect to T< >T dimer fluorescence per unit DNA fluorescence in relation to dose of germicidal irradiation.

Competitive ELISA for Quantitation of T< >T Dimers

To quantitate T< >T dimer formation in hamster cells with respect to ultraviolet (UV) dose, a competitive ELISA was performed with DNA isolated from FC13 and 21F fibroblasts that received identical doses of UV irradiation under the same conditions as cells used for immunocytochemical measurements. The ELISA was calibrated using serial dilutions of denatured UV-irradiated calf thymus DNA (one T< >T dimer per 20 and 2500 base pairs, high-performance liquid chromatography analysis) as standards. The T< >T dimer content of the various competitor DNA, which were isolated from UV-irradiated cells, was determined by comparing the amount of DNA required to reduce by 40% antibody binding to the immobilized DNA with the amount of standard DNA required to reduce antibody binding by 40%.

Quantitation of T< >T Dimers in Irradiated Syrian Hamster Embryo Cells

The relationship between T< >T dimer formation and fluorescence intensity measurements was compared, with respect to dose of germicidal irradiation, in early-passage FC13 cells and immortal 21F cells. Germicidal irradiation (10 J/m^2) produced about 9×10^5 T< >T dimers (1 per 7450 bases of DNA) in F13 cells with a normalized fluorescence intensity of 0.027%. The values for 21F cells at 10 J/m^2 were 7.5×10^5 T< >T per cell

(1 per 9750 bases) with a normalized fluorescence intensity of 0.021%. The limit of sensitivity of the immunofluoresence assay with the current anti-UV DNA antibody is about 5 J/m^2 (55%-75% survival). The antibody was tritiated by reductive alkylation and used to examine the relationship between the number of T< >T dimers per cell and the number of antibody molecules bound per cell. The data show that about 45% of the T< >T dimers in cells receiving 100 J/m^2 of germicidal irradiation were detected with the indirect immunofluorescence assay.

REFERENCES

Epstein, JH. 1970. Ultraviolet carcinogenesis, pp. 235-273. In: *Photophysiology, Current Topics in Photobiology and Photochemistry*, Vol. 5, AC Giese (ed.). Academic Press, New York, NY.

Gramstein, RD and AJ Sober. 1982. Current concepts in ultraviolet carcinogenesis. Proc Soc Exp Med 170:115-125.

Kaplan, DS. 1985. *Application of Quantitative Microfluorimetry to Clinical Serology*. Ph.D. Thesis, George Washington University, Washington, DC.

Picciolo, GL and DS Kaplan. 1984. Reducing in fading of fluorescent reaction product for microphotometric quantitation. Adv Appl Microbiol 30:197-234.

Picciolo, GL and DS Kaplan. 1986. Method and device for quantitative endpoint determination in immunofluorescence using microfluorophotometry. U.S. Patent Number 4, 622, 921, November 11, 1986.

QUESTIONS AND COMMENTS

Q: Todd, NIST
   What is the time between exposure and sampling? Is there any time for repair? Have you sought an effect of sampling delay?

A: The sample was obtained immediately after irradiation. Therefore, with the data presented here, there was no time for repair. We do however have tissue samples obtained at various times after exposure. These latter samples have not been analyzed as yet.

Q: Tenforde, PNL, Richland, WA
   Have you examined effects of repeated exposures of hamster skin? This might give information on inducible UV repair.

A: No, but we plan to do this.

Carcinogenesis and Developmental Studies with Multilevel Systems

DEVELOPMENT, REGENERATION, AND NEOPLASIA OF THE TRACHEOBRONCHIAL EPITHELIUM

E. M. McDowell

Department of Pathology, University of Maryland School of Medicine, Baltimore, MD 21201

Key words: *Tracheobronchial epithelium, development, regeneration, neoplasia*

ABSTRACT

Development, regeneration, and cell differentiation of mucociliary tracheo-bronchial epithelium (TBE) are quite similar in humans and hamsters, and similar events occur in both species during fetal development and regeneration of adult epithelium after injury *in vivo* and *in vitro*. Secretory cells and basal cells divide, but ciliated cells do not. Vitamin A is required for the division of secretory cells, but basal cells will continue to divide when vitamin A is deficient. Evidence is accumulating to suggest that secretory cells replicate to provide new secretory cells *and* ciliated cells, whereas basal cells divide only to replenish themselves. Following injury to the TBE, secretory cells divide and give rise to a transient epidermoid metaplasia that is normally reversible, and the mucociliary epithelium is rapidly restored (reversal of epidermoid metaplasia requires an adequate supply of vitamin A). However, if the TBE is injured repeatedly *and* exposed to carcinogens, the secretory cells replicate and give rise to a persistent state of epidermoid metaplasia, which may subsequently give rise to malignant tracheobronchial neoplasms.

Under normal conditions, the tracheobronchial epithelium (TBE) is pseu-dostratified and is composed of short basal cells and tall columnar secretory (mucous) and ciliated cells. All cell types rest on the basement membrane, but only the columnar cells reach to the airway lumen. For many years, the basal cell was considered to be the only stem cell for the TBE. Basal cells were thought to give rise to basal, secretory, and ciliated cells (reviewed by Otani, 1987). Moreover, basal cells were said to be the stem cell for pathological lesions such as epidermoid metaplasia, and the cell of origin of squamous cell carcinomas. However, this view was not held by all, and alternative hypotheses were presented by Bindreiter et al. (1968) and by Boren and Paradise (1978). These investigators suggested that basal cells gave rise to basal cells and secretory cells but not to ciliated cells. Moreover, they showed conclusively that differentiated secretory cells were capable of division, giving rise to new secretory cells *and* ciliated cells.

My colleagues and I have had the opportunity to examine a large number of human and hamster lung tumors and the closely associated TBE. A striking finding was that many of the keratinized cells in the foci of epidermoid metaplasia were producing mucus. Moreover, glandular differentiation and mucus production were commonplace in many of the lung tumors, including those with epidermoid (squamous) differentiation (Trump et al., 1978; Becci et al., 1978a,b; McDowell et al., 1978b). For these reasons, we have probed further into the normal and abnormal biology of the TBE during the last decade. Stages in the formation of the TBE during fetal and neonatal development share many similarities with regeneration of the adult TBE after diverse types of injury. Therefore, we studied epithelial cell differentiation and the progenitor roles of secretory cells and basal cells during normal development and after mechanical or nutritional injury (e.g., vitamin A deficiency) to the adult epithelium; the hamster trachea was our experimental model. Our results suggest that basal cells divide and give rise only to basal cells, whereas columnar secretory cells divide and give rise to secretory cells *and* ciliated cells; that is, the TBE has two populations of stem cells, each lineage giving rise to specific cell types.

The tracheal epithelium of adult hamsters consists of short basal cells (about 10%) with very scant cytoplasm, and columnar secretory (57%) and ciliated cells (33%) (Keenan et al., 1982a). When a focal mechanical injury is made such that the epithelial cells are scraped away, leaving the basement membrane intact, the viable cells adjacent to the wound edges flatten and migrate over the denuded basement membrane. Most of these flattened migrating cells are secretory cells. The mucous granules are expelled, but ultrastructural characteristics such as an expansive cytoplasm, a well-developed Golgi apparatus, and an abundant endoplasmic reticulum are retained. If the wound is not too large, the abraded area is covered by a layer of flattened secretory cells during the first 12 to 24 hr. Subsequently, cells within the wound site, as well as cells at the edges of the wound, undergo intense mitotic activity. Most (about 80%) of these dividing cells are secretory cells (Keenan et al., 1982b,c); a minority of dividing cells are basal cells (Figure 1). Within 48 hr, a stratified metaplastic epithelium is produced, composed, for the most part, of highly keratinized altered secretory cells. Shortly thereafter, mitotic activity subsides and large, pale-staining preciliated cells arise within the wound site. Preciliated cells often contain mucous granules in their apical cytoplasm that have been carried over from the progenitor secretory cell. However, the preciliated cells are not capable of synthesizing mucus and the mucous granules are rapidly expelled about the same time that cilia develop from the cell apices (Keenan et al., 1983). Labeling experiments with [^{3}H] thymidine ([^{3}H]TdR) showed that the preciliated cells and ciliated cells are end-stage cells that do not replicate (Boren and Paradise, 1978; Keenan et al., 1982c). The TBE returns to normal about 7 days after the injury.

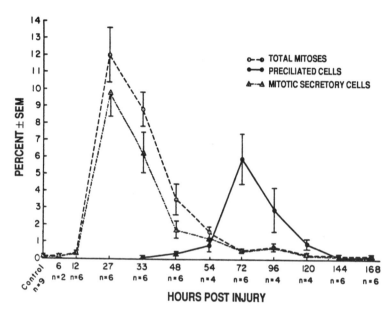

Figure 1. Comparison of total mitotic rates, secretory cell mitotic rates, and appearance of preciliated cells (mean percent ± 1 SEM) at different times after epithelial wounding in the hamster trachea (hamsters received colchicine 6 hr before sacrifice). Note that secretory cells contribute about 80% of all mitotic activity at 27 hr after wounding. (From Keenan et al., 1982c. Reprinted with permission from Springer-Verlag, Heidelberg.)

A similar sequence of events occurs in the human bronchial epithelium. The stratified keratinized cells within areas of epidermoid metaplasia are often mucus producing (Trump et al., 1978), and preciliated cells containing mucous granules are also seen (McDowell et al., 1978a).

Our most recent studies have shown that events associated with injury to the TBE are major determinants of the carcinogenic response. Acute studies on the effects of intratracheal cannulation (ITC) showed that tracheal cell proliferation increased significantly in ITC-induced mucosal wounds (Keenan et al., 1989a), and that the carcinogenic response induced in the respiratory tract of Syrian golden hamsters by repeated intratracheal instillations of benzo[a]pyrene (BaP) adsorbed to ferric oxide (Fe_2O_3) particles suspended in saline resulted from the interactions of these factors and the cannula-induced tracheal wounding (Keenan et al., 1989b). The study included the following variables: a single instillation by intralaryngeal cannulation (ILC) of N-methyl-N-nitrosourea (MNU) at 5 wk of age; and 15 weekly treatments (beginning at 7 wk of age) by ILC or ITC alone, or together with instillations of saline, or Fe_2O_3 saline, or BaP-Fe_2O_3 saline. Repeated ITC-induced tracheal wounds caused persistent tracheal epithelial hyperplasia, metaplasia, and/or atrophy, and submucosal fibroplasia during the observation period of 22 to 78 wk of age. Tracheal cancers (*in situ* or invasive carcinomas) were seen only in those hamsters receiving repeated ITC and one or both carcinogens. In the absence of mucosal injury, no malignant tumors were produced in the TBE. The cancer latency was shortest and the incidence of tracheal (50%) and main-stem bronchial (21%) cancers highest in hamsters given MNU and repeated ITC with BaP-Fe_2O_3 saline. Hamsters given carcinogens by ILC (which induced laryngeal but not tracheal wounds) developed proliferative lesions and cancers of the larynx but no tracheobronchial cancers. These data demonstrate the singular importance of repeated ITC-induced intratracheal wounding as an enhancing factor in respiratory carcinogenesis (Keenan et al., 1989b).

During fetal development, the airways are at first lined by simple, undifferentiated columnar cells. Ciliated cells and secretory cells are the first to differentiate, followed by basal cells (Plopper et al., 1986; Cutz, 1987). As soon as the basal cells are formed, the epithelium changes from simple columnar to pseudostratified, because the short basal cells do not reach the lumen. In fetal hamsters, small numbers of basal cells are first seen in the trachea on gestational day 13; however, throughout gestation and into the neonatal period, most mitotic activity is associated with columnar secretory cells, not basal cells (McDowell et al., 1985a,b; Otani et al., 1986). Preciliated cells that are formed during normal fetal development have the same characteristics as those formed in the adult epithelium regenerating after injury. Moreover, the timing of their appearance is similar in both situations: the preciliated cells appear about 1 to 2 days after the peak of mitotic activity when the rate of cell proliferation is beginning to approach baseline levels (Figure 2).

Methods are now available to culture dispersed hamster tracheal epithelial cells in serum-free medium on a collagen gel substrate (Wu et al., 1985). In the presence of defined growth factors and vitamin A, this technique supports the differentiation and maturation of the tracheal epithelial cells so that a functional mucociliary epithelium is restored within 7 days in culture, recapitulating many aspects of normal fetal development and regeneration after injury, as occurs *in vivo* (McDowell et al., 1987a,b). Using this technique, we demonstrated intense replication of secretory cells within 48 hr after seeding of the cells. By 4 and 5 days in culture, the rate of cell replication was waning. At this time, the secretory cells were differentiating, and secretory granules were accumulating at the cell apices. Pale-staining preciliated cells were present by 6 days in culture and, by 7 days, mature ciliated and secretory cells were well established.

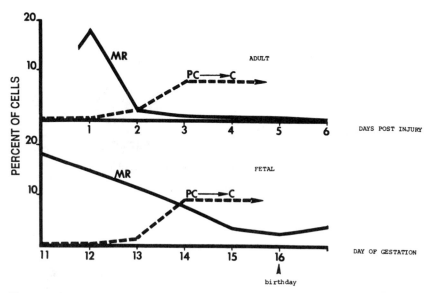

Figure 2. Similarities between normal fetal development (bottom) and regeneration after injury (top) in hamster tracheal epithelium. In normal adult epithelium, mitotic rate (MR) is very low, ~0.1%; 1 day after mechanical injury, MR peaks at wound site and is equivalent to rates of proliferation in fetus on 11th and 12th gestational days. Extent and timing of cell replication in relation to production of preciliated cells (PC) are very similar in both situations. Preciliated cells rapidly mature into ciliated cells (C). (From McDowell et al., 1987a. Reprinted with permission from Lippincott/Harper and Row, Philadelphia.)

Vitamin A was essential for this process. If retinoic acid was absent from the culture medium, a very different scenario occurred. After 24 hr, the secretory cells became extremely flattened, although at this time they were still capable of division. However, after 3 days of culture without vitamin A, the replication of secretory cells was greatly reduced, yet the small basal cells continued to divide. Consequently, the basal cells "outgrew" the quiescent flattened secretory cells, and islands of small, tightly packed basal cells became prominent (McDowell et al., 1987b). These *in vitro* experiments confirmed our previous *in vivo* analysis of the effect of vitamin A deficiency on the hamster tracheal epithelium. In normal hamsters, both secretory cells and basal cells replicate. As the animals become vitamin A deficient, subtle changes occur in the tracheal epithelium. Cell division of the secretory cells is greatly diminished, and their shape changes from columnar to cuboidal. Division of basal cells is far less affected, so that basal cells continue to divide and increase in number and density (McDowell et al., 1984a). When vitamin A is restored to the diet, the replication rate of secretory cells increases within 2 days and normal mitotic rates are restored after 3 to 4 days. Moreover, the number of preciliated cells (which approached zero in the vitamin-A-deficient epithelium) increases shortly after division of the secretory cells is reestablished. Normal mucociliary cell numbers and function are restored within 7 days of vitamin A repletion to the hamsters (McDowell et al., 1984b) (Figure 3).

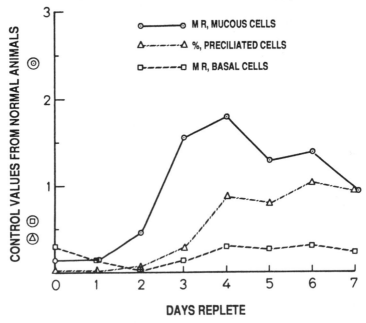

Figure 3. Relationship between proportion of preciliated cells and mitotic rates (MR) of mucous cells and basal cells in hamster trachea after vitamin A deprivation or repletion. All data are presented as mean percentages of total number of epithelial cells counted. Control values from normal animals are plotted and circled outside graph at left of y axis; vitamin-A-deprived (0 point on x axis) and days-replete data are plotted within graph. (From McDowell et al., 1984b. Reprinted with permission from Springer-Verlag, Heidelberg.)

In summary, development, regeneration, and cell differentiation of mucociliary TBE are quite similar in humans and hamsters, and similar events occur in both species during fetal development and regeneration of adult epithelium after injury *in vivo* and *in vitro*. Secretory cells and basal cells divide, but ciliated cells do not. Vitamin A is required for the division of secretory cells, but basal cells will continue to divide when vitamin A is deficient. Evidence is accumulating to suggest that secretory cells replicate to provide new secretory cells *and* ciliated cells, whereas basal cells divide only to replenish themselves. Following injury to the TBE, secretory cells divide and give rise to a transient epidermoid metaplasia that is normally reversible, and the mucociliary epithelium is rapidly restored (reversal of epidermoid metaplasia requires an adequate supply of vitamin A). However, if the TBE is injured repeatedly *and* exposed to carcinogens, the secretory cells replicate and give rise to a persistent state of epidermoid metaplasia, which may subsequently give rise to malignant tracheobronchial neoplasms (Figure 4).

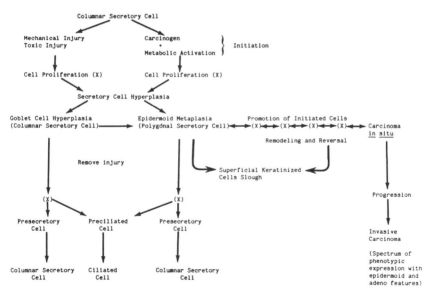

Figure 4. Probable interrelationships of secretory cells and their progeny in normal, hyperplastic, metaplastic, and neoplastic tracheobronchial epithelium. (From Keenan, 1987. Reprinted with permission from Churchill Livingstone, New York and London.)

REFERENCES

Becci, PJ, EM McDowell, and BF Trump. 1978a. The respiratory epithelium. IV. Histogenesis of epidermoid metaplasia and carcinoma *in situ* in the hamster. J Natl Cancer Inst 61:577-586.

Becci, PJ, EM McDowell, and BF Trump. **1978b.** The respiratory epithelium. VI. Histogenesis of hamster lung tumors induced by benzo(a)pyrene-ferric oxide. J Natl Cancer Inst 61:607-618.

Bindreiter, M, J Schuppler, and L Stockinger. **1968.** Zellproliferation und Differenzierung im Trachealepithel der Ratte. Exp Cell Res 50:377-382.

Boren, HG and LJ Paradise. **1978.** Cytokinetics of lung, pp. 369-418. In: *Pathogenesis and Therapy of Lung Cancer, Vol. 10, Lung Biology in Health and Disease,* CC Harris (ed.). Marcel Dekker, Amsterdam.

Cutz, E. **1987.** Cytomorphology and differentiation of airway epithelium in developing human lung, pp. 1-41. In: *Lung Carcinomas,* EM McDowell (ed.). Churchill Livingstone, New York & London.

Keenan, KP. **1987.** Cell injury and repair of the tracheobronchial epithelium, pp. 74-93. In: *Lung Carcinomas,* EM McDowell (ed.). Churchill Livingstone, New York & London.

Keenan, KP, JW Combs, and EM McDowell. **1982a.** Regeneration of hamster tracheal epithelium after mechanical injury. I. Focal lesions: Quantitative morphologic study of cell proliferation. Virchows Arch B Cell Pathol 41:193-214.

Keenan, KP, JW Combs, and EM McDowell. **1982b.** Regeneration of hamster tracheal epithelium after mechanical injury. II. Multifocal lesions: Stathmokinetic and autoradiographic studies of cell proliferation. Virchows Arch B Cell Pathol 41:215-229.

Keenan, KP, JW Combs, and EM McDowell. **1982c.** Regeneration of hamster tracheal epithelium after mechanical injury. III. Large and small lesions: Stathmokinetic and single pulse, and continuous thymidine labeling autoradiographic studies. Virchows Arch B Cell Pathol 41:231-252.

Keenan, KP, TS Wilson, and EM McDowell. **1983.** Regeneration of hamster tracheal epithelium after mechanical injury. IV. Histochemical, immunocytochemical and ultrastructural studies. Virchows Arch B Cell Pathol 43:213-240.

Keenan, KP, U Saffiotti, SF Stinson, CW Riggs, and EM McDowell. **1989a.** Morphological and cytokinetic responses of hamster airways to intralaryngeal and intratracheal cannulation with instillation of saline or ferric oxide particles in saline. Cancer Res 49:1521-1527.

Keenan, KP, U Saffiotti, SF Stinson, CW Riggs, and EM McDowell. **1989b.** Multifactorial hamster respiratory carcinogenesis with interdependent effects of cannula-induced mucosal wounding, saline, ferric oxide, benzo[a]pyrene and N-methyl-N-nitrosourea. Cancer Res 49:1528-1540.

McDowell, EM, KP Keenan, and M Huang. **1984a.** Effects of vitamin A-deprivation on hamster tracheal epithelium: A quantitative morphologic study. Virchows Arch B Cell Pathol 45:197-219.

McDowell, EM, KP Keenan, and M Huang. **1984b.** Restoration of mucociliary tracheal epithelium following deprivation of vitamin A: A quantitative morpho-logic study. Virchows Arch B Cell Pathol 45:221-240.

McDowell, EM, C Newkirk, and B Coleman. **1985a.** Development of hamster tracheal epithelium. I. A quantitative morphologic study in the fetus. Anat Rec 213:429-447.

McDowell, EM, C Newkirk, and B Coleman. **1985b.** Development of hamster tracheal epithelium. II. Cell proliferation in the fetus. Anat Rec 213:448-456.

McDowell, EM, LA Barrett, F Glavin, CC Harris, and BF Trump. **1978a.** The respiratory epithelium. I. Human bronchus. J Natl Cancer Inst 61:539-549.

McDowell, EM, JS McLaughlin, DK Merenyi, RF Kieffer, CC Harris, and BF Trump. **1978b.** The respiratory epithelium. V. Histogenesis of human lung car-cinomas. J Natl Cancer Inst 61:587-606.

McDowell, EM, T Ben, C Newkirk, S Chang, and LM De Luca. **1987a.** Differentia-tion of tracheal mucociliary epithelium in primary cell culture recapitulates normal fetal development and regeneration following injury in hamsters. Am J Pathol 129:511-522.

McDowell, EM, T Ben, B Coleman, S Chang, C Newkirk, and LM De Luca. **1987b.** Effects of retinoic acid on the growth and morphology of hamster tracheal epithelial cells in primary culture. Virchows Arch B Cell Pathol 54:38-51.

Otani, EM. **1987.** The basal cell progenitor of the tracheobronchial epithelium: Fact or folklore?, pp. 395-402. In: *Lung Carcinomas*, EM McDowell (ed.). Churchill Livingstone, New York & London.

Otani, EM, C Newkirk, and EM McDowell. **1986.** Development of hamster tra-cheal epithelium. IV. Cell proliferation and cytodifferentiation in the neonate. Anat Rec 214:183-192.

Plopper, CG, JL Alley, and AJ Weir. 1986. Differentiation of tracheal epithelium during fetal lung maturation in the rhesus monkey *Macaca mulatta*. Am J Anat 175:59-71.

Trump, BF, EM McDowell, F Glavin, LA Barrett, PJ Becci, W Schürch, HE Kaiser, and CC Harris. 1978. The respiratory epithelium. III. Histogenesis of epider-moid metaplasia and carcinoma in situ in humans. J Natl Cancer Inst 61:563-575.

Wu, R, E Nolan, and C Turner. 1985. Expression of tracheal differentiated func-tions in serum-free hormone-supplemented medium. J Cell Physiol 125:167-181.

QUESTIONS AND COMMENTS

Q: (Speaker did not identify himself)

John Little at Harvard has also described a pronounced effect of airway trauma on lung cancer induction in the hamster. Tracheal instillation of saline appears to be necessary to induce cancer following α-irradiation by polonium. Is this marked response peculiar to the hamster?

A: McDowell

No, I don't believe this response is peculiar to hamsters, nor is it likely to be peculiar to the lung. An association between wound healing and cancer production has been known for many years in different organs, in many species (**Haddow**, Adv. Cancer Res. 16:181-234, **1972**).

RECEPTORS FOR GROWTH FACTORS ARE EXPRESSED IN RADIATION-INDUCED LUNG TUMORS

G. Kelly,[1] P. R. Kerkof,[1,2] and P. J. Haley[1]

[1]Inhalation Toxicology Research Institute, P.O. Box 5890, Albuquerque, NM 87185

[2]Department of Biology, University of New Mexico, Albuquerque, NM 87131

Key words: *Oncogene expression, radiation, lung tumors, insulin receptor*

ABSTRACT

Improvement of human health risk estimates requires an understanding of the fundamental molecular processes involved in radiation-induced carcinogenesis. We are examining the radiation-induced activation of oncogenes in carcinomas of the respiratory tract, induced in beagle dogs exposed by inhalation to $^{239}PuO_2$, as a possible model for humans. In this work, we have examined a set of radiation-induced canine lung tumors for the aberrant expression of oncogenes by probing a battery of known oncogenes with labeled cDNA transcripts from primary tumor tissues. Six of 11 lung carcinomas examined expressed sequences that hybridize with one or more of the following oncogenes: met H, erb-B, ros, src, or neu at elevated levels. The protein products of each of these oncogenes have been characterized as growth-factor receptors containing conserved tyrosine kinase domains. The range of signals observed in these experiments may be the result of cross-hybridization between homologous sequences within each tyrosine kinase domain. These results suggest that an autocrine stimulative mechanism may play an important role in the proliferative potential of these tumors.

Lung cancer is a major cause of cancer-related deaths in the United States (Brown and Kessler, 1988). Concern is mounting that radon and radon daughters from naturally occurring geological outcrops may pose a significant lung-cancer risk to large segments of the population (Fleischer, 1986; BEIR, 1988). This concern has contributed to a heightened interest in the carcinogenic effects associated with inhalation of alpha-emitting radionuclides. Improved health risk estimates require an understanding of the fundamental molecular processes involved in radiation-induced carcinogenesis. The objective of our research is to develop a comprehensive understanding of the molecular mechanisms responsible for radiation-induced neoplasia.

181

Ongoing lifespan radiation carcinogenesis studies in the beagle dog at this Institute have produced a variety of alpha-radiation-induced lung neoplasms (McClellan et al., 1986). We have obtained a set of 10 primary lung tumors from beagle dogs exposed by inhalation to ^{239}PuO$_2$ and 2 primary lung tumors of spontaneous origin from control dogs in the Inhalation Toxicology Research Institute (ITRI) colony (Table 1).

Table 1. Histological diagnosis of lung tumors in dogs exposed to ^{239}Pu.

Dog Number	Total Alpha Dose (Gy) to Lung	Diagnoses
With ^{239}Pu-Induced tumors:		
1121S	1.0	Papillary adenocarcinoma
1320A	1.8	Papillary adenocarcinoma
1070B	3.3	Bronchioloalveolar carcinoma
1222T	3.5	Anaplastic, large cell adenocarcinoma
1057S	5.0	Bronchioloalveolar carcinoma
1220B	5.3	Adenosquamous carcinoma
1100B	6.0	Adenosquamous carcinoma
1145T	9.8	Papillary adenocarcinoma
1134B	11	Papillary adenocarcinoma
1364S	13	Papillary adenocarcinoma
With spontaneous tumors:		
770S	—	Papillary adenocarcinoma
859C	—	Papillary adenocarcinoma

One phenomenon occurring in the development of some neoplasms is the aberrant expression of normal c-onc genes in tumor tissue. The over-expression of proto-oncogenes has been implicated in the genesis of a variety of tumors (Slamon et al., 1984). We examined the 10 radiation-induced and 2 spontaneous tumors for aberrant expression of a variety of known oncogenes. Briefly, oncogene expression was examined by probing a battery of as many as 20 known oncogenes on a slot blot with labeled cDNA transcripts from the primary tumor tissues (Table 2 and Figure 1). Densito-metric scans of the resulting autoradiographs were used to identify those oncogenes expressed at elevated levels. This method should provide an accurate representation of the levels of expression of the genes included in the blot.

Table 2. Oncogenes used to examine expression in radiation-induced lung tumors.

Ras	Receptor Tyrosine Kinases	Cytoplasmic Protein Kinases	Others
c-H-ras	v-erb-B	v-raf	c-myc
c-Ki-ras	c-neu	v-mos	v-myb
c-N-ras	v-fms	v-src	v-bas
	v-ros	v-fes/v-fps	v-sis
	c-met	v-abl	v-fos
	c-trk		v-erb-A

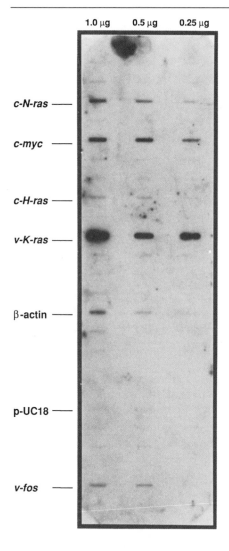

Figure 1. ^{32}P-labeled cDNA from papillary adenocarcinoma (1041B) taken from ^{239}PuO$_2$-exposed beagle dog was hybridized to a nylon filter containing clones of 19 different oncogenes. Oncogene transcripts expressed in this tumor (N-ras, c-myc, Ki-ras), are illustrated with β-actin, which served as positive control, and pUC18, which served as negative control.

Levels of oncogene cDNA were normalized to the level of β-actin gene expression in each tumor RNA preparation, enabling comparisons of relative levels of expression between tumors. Oncogene sequences hybridizing at levels 1.5-fold higher than sequences hybridizing to the β-actin clone were scored as positive for elevated expression. When RNA isolated from the lung of an unexposed beagle dog was examined in parallel experiments as a control, the oncogenes included in our battery were not expressed (Table 3).

Table 3. Oncogenes expressed in lung tumors induced by chronic alpha irradiation from $^{239}PuO_2$.[a]

Dog Number	c-myc	ras	v-ros	c-met	v-erb-B
1121S	+	+	+		
1320A	+	+			
1070B	+	+		+	
1222T	+	+		+	
1057S	+	+	+		
1220B	+	+			
1100B	+	+			
1145T		+	+	+	+
1134B	+	+			
1364S	+				
770S	+		+		+
859C					

[a]Oncogenes expressed at levels ≥ 1.5-fold level observed for β-actin gene were scored positive for expression. *Ras* column includes *c-N-ras, c-Ki-ras,* and *c-N-ras; v-ros, c-met,* and *v-erb-B* columns are oncogenes from receptor tyrosine kinase group (see Table 2) scoring positive in this assay.

Nine of 12 tumors examined expressed one or more members of the *ras* family of oncogenes: *N-ras* was expressed in 7 tumors, *H-ras* in 5 tumors, and *Ki-ras* in 4 tumors. Of 7 tumors expressing sequences similar to the *N-ras* oncogene, 6 tumors also expressed either *H-ras* or *Ki-ras;* 1 tumor, that from dog 1222T, expressed *H-, Ki-,* and *N-ras*-related sequences. Ten of 12 tumors examined expressed sequences that hybridized to the *c-myc* oncogene clone. One of the tumors negative for *c-myc* expression, that from dog 859C, expressed *c-myc*-like sequences at approximately the same level as β-actin. However, this level of expression was not scored as positive under the selection criteria employed.

We are not able to postulate a cause-and-effect relationship or definitive correlation between exposure, diagnosis and oncogene expression, and the high frequency of *ras*- and *myc*- related sequences expressed in the tumors we have examined to date. Enhanced expression of the *myc* oncogene has been correlated with the malignant progression of human neuroblastomas (Schwab et al., 1984) and colon carcinomas (Alitalo et al., 1983), and it has been found in a number of human lung-cancer cell lines (Little et al., 1983). The cellular *ras* oncogene is also expressed in a variety of malignant tumors; however, the association of *ras* expression with proliferation and malignancy has been inconsistent (Chesa et al., 1987). Interestingly, 3 of the 12 tumors we have examined do not express *ras*-related transcripts; 2 of the 3 *ras*-negative tumors are spontaneous tumors. The significance of this observation, if any, cannot be determined without additional experimentation with other spontaneous tumors.

We have been particularly interested in examining the expression of a number of oncogenes whose normal homologues are receptors for growth factors. Enhanced expression of the receptor for epidermal growth factor has been demonstrated in human lung carcinomas (Sobol et al., 1987) and human lung-tumor cell lines (Haeder et al., 1988), and in a variety of other human tumor cell lines of epithelial origin (Ullrich et al., 1984; Young-Hua et al., 1984; Filmus et al., 1987). The battery of known oncogenes used in these experiments included up to six clones encoding tyrosine kinase receptor-related oncogenes: *erb-B*, *c-neu*, *v-fms*, *v-ros*, *c-trk*, and *c-met* (Hanks et al., 1988). The *erb-B* oncogene, which encodes the cytoplasmic portion of the epidermal growth-factor receptor, was expressed in 1 of 11 tumors tested. *V-fms* and *c-neu* were not expressed in any of the tumors examined. Six of 12 tumors expressed sequences that hybridized with oncogene clones of *v-ros* or *c-met*. If we reduce the stringency of selection criteria to include those oncogenes expressed at a level equal to or greater than the level of β-actin, 9 of 12 tumors score positive for either *ros* and/or *met* expression. The *ros* and *met* clones both code for oncogenes whose normal homologues are transmembrane proteins related to the insulin receptor (Yarden and Ullrich, 1988).

The observation that a high proportion of the lung carcinomas included in these experiments express oncogenes related to the insulin receptor suggests that the alveolar type 2 cell may be the cell of origin for these tumors. Alveolar type 2 cells express receptors for insulin (Shapiro et al., 1986). The frequency with which the *ros* and *met* oncogenes are expressed in these lung tumors suggests that the autocrine stimulative mechanism, potentially involving one or more tyrosine kinase growth-factor receptors, may play an important role in the proliferative potential of these tumors. Elevated expression of growth-factor receptors could be involved in the cellular growth advantage underlying tumor progression (Filmus et al., 1987). Experiments to test this hypothesis are underway in our laboratory using a series of tumor cell lines derived from ^{239}Pu-induced canine lung tumors.

ACKNOWLEDGMENTS

The authors express their appreciation to Ms. Michelle Wood and Ms. Donna Klinge for their expert technical assistance. Research was sponsored by the U.S. Department of Energy's Office of Health and Environmental Research under Contract No. DE-AC04-76EV01013.

REFERENCES

Alitalo, K, M Schwab, CC Lin, HE Varmus, and JM Bishop. 1983. Homogeneously staining chromosomal regions contain amplified copies of an abundantly expressed cellular oncogene (c-myc) in malignant neuroendocrine cells from a human colon carcinoma. Proc Natl Acad Sci USA 80:1707-1711.

BEIR (National Research Council Committee on the Biological Effects of Ionizing Radiation). 1988. Health Risks of Radon and Other Internally Deposited Alpha-Emitters. BEIR Report IV. National Academy Press, Washington, DC.

Brown, CC and LG Kessler. 1988. Projections of lung cancer mortality in the United States: 1985-2025. J Natl Cancer Inst 80:43-51.

Chesa, PG, WJ Rettig, MR Melamed, LJ Old, and HL Niman. 1987. Expression of p21^{ras} in normal and malignant human tissues: Lack of association with proliferation and malignancy. Proc Natl Acad Sci USA 84:3234-3228.

Filmus, J, JM Trent, MN Pollack, and RN Buick. 1987. Epidermal growth factor receptor gene-amplified MDA-468 breast cancer cell line and its nonamplified variants. Mol Cell Biol 7:251-257.

Fleischer, RL. 1986. A possible association between lung cancer and a geological outcrop. Health Phys 50:832-827.

Haeder, M, M Rotsch, G Bepler, C Henning, K Haveman, B Heimann, and K Moelling. 1988. Epidermal growth factor receptor expression in human lung cancer cell lines. Cancer Res 48:1132-1136.

Hanks, SK, AM Quinn, and T Hunter. 1988. The protein kinase family: Conserved features and deduced phylogeny of the catalytic domains. Science 241:42-52.

Little, CD, MM Nau, DN Carney, AF Gazdar, and JD Minna. 1983. Amplification and expression of the c-myc oncogene in human lung cancer cell lines. Nature 306:194-196.

McClellan, RO, BB Boecker, FF Hahn, and BA Muggenburg. **1986**. Lovelace ITRI studies on the toxicity of inhaled radionuclides in beagle dogs, pp. 74-96. In: *Life-Span Radiation Effects Studies in Animals: What Can They Tell Us?*, RC Thompson and JA Mahaffey (eds.). CONF-830951. NTIS, Springfield, VA.

Schwab, M, J Ellison, M Busch, W Rosenau, HE Varmus, and JM Bishop. **1984**. Enhanced expression of the human *N-myc* consequent to amplification of DNA may contribute to malignant progression of neuroblastoma. Proc Natl Acad Sci USA 81:4940-4944.

Shapiro, DL, JN Livingston, WM Maniscalco, and JN Finkelstein. **1986**. Insulin receptors and insulin effects of type II alveolar epithelial cells. Biochim Biophys Acta 885:216-220.

Slamon, DJ, JB DeKernion, IM Verma, and MJ Cline. **1984**. Expression of cellular oncogenes in human malignancies. Science 224:256-262.

Sobol, RE, RW Astarita, C Hofedits, H Masui, R Fairshter, I Royston, and J Mendelsohn. **1987**. Epidermal growth factor receptor expression in human lung carcinomas defined by a monoclonal antibody. J Natl Cancer Inst 79:403-405.

Ullrich, A, L Coussen, JF Haylick, TJ Dull, A Gray, AW Tam, Y Yarden, TA Libermann, J Schlessinger, J Downward, ELV Mayes, N Whittle, MD Waterfield, and PH Seeburg. **1984**. Human epidermal growth factor receptor cDNA sequence and aberrant expression of the amplified gene in A431 epidermoid carcinoma cells. Nature 309:418-425.

Yarden, Y and A Ullrich. **1988**. Growth factor receptor tyrosine kinases. Annu Rev Biochem 57:443-478.

Young-Hua, X, N Richert, S Ito, GT Merlino, and I Pastan. **1984**. Characterization of epidermal growth factor expression in malignant and normal human cell lines. Proc Natl Acad Sci USA 81:7308-7312.

QUESTIONS AND COMMENTS

Q: Frazier, PNL, Richland, WA
   The normal lung contains as many as 70 different morphological cell types. How do you know that the levels of "oncogene" expression observed in the lung tumor are not normal levels of expression for the cell type from which the tumor arose? Or could the observed results reflect a cause/effect relationship?

A: At this time we have no way to answer this question. It is certainly a possibility that the oncogenes expressed in these tumors are not causally related to the formation of the tumor. If this is, in fact, the case, the description of the genes expressed at least provides a phenotype for the tumor and normal cells, which may allow us to identify the cells at risk in radiation-induced respiratory carcinogenesis.

One caveat to keep in mind is that these studies are preliminary in nature; as such, we have made no attempt to claim a cause/effect relationship for oncogene expression. We hope to establish such a relationship in future studies that will try to determine the molecular mechanisms responsive for the receptor protein kinase expression we have observed.

Q: Morgan, PNL, Richland, WA
Have you examined tissue adjacent and/or far removed from the tumor?

A: We generally have not looked at adjacent normal tissue from tumor-bearing dogs. In one case where we did look at "normal" lung tissue from an exposed/tumor-bearing dog, we did see low levels of *ras* and *myc*. When we went back to this dog's pathology records, we discovered that the primary tumor in this animal was extremely metastatic, suggesting that our ostensibly normal tissue actually contained tumor cells. We believe that by using normal lung tissue from a healthy, unexposed dog as a control, we can avoid complications such as that described above.

Q: Gantt, NCI
Were the spontaneous tumors relatively small? I have a vague recollection that there is a strong tendency for *ras* and/or *myc* to be strongly expressed at a later time in tumor growth.

A: I don't know the size of these tumors. We will shortly be reviewing the pathology of these tumors to attempt to establish correlations between clinical presentation, progression, and metastasis with the oncogenes that are expressed. I will certainly try and establish a size (age) for each tumor at that time.

USE OF ARCHIVED TISSUES FOR STUDIES OF PLUTONIUM-INDUCED LUNG TUMORS

C. L. Sanders, K. E. McDonald, K. E. Lauhala, and M. E. Frazier

Pacific Northwest Laboratory, Richland, WA 99352

Key words: *Archived tissues, lifespan studies, ^{239}Pu aerosols, rat lung tumors*

ABSTRACT

Nonciliated bronchiolar epithelium is the apparent target tissue for lung carcinomas induced by exposure to inhaled ^{239}PuO$_2$ in rats. The process of pulmonary carcinogenesis is being evaluated in archived tissues from lifespan and serial sacrifice studies in about 4000 rats.

Archived lung tissues are being examined for histopathological changes, by light microscopy, scanning electron microscopy, and transmission electron microscopy; cell proliferation, by nuclear labeling with tritiated thymidine; DNA aneuploidy, using flow cytometry of nuclei isolated from paraffin sections and microspectrometry of Feulgen-stained tissues; yield and fidelity of extracted DNA and sequencing of specific oncogenes; growth factor (bombesin, epidermal growth factor, transforming growth factors) binding; quantitative cellular changes, using morphometric techniques; and microdosimetric patterns, using quantitative light and scanning electron microscopy.

There is an association between plutonium particle aggregation near bronchioles and bronchiolization, which appears to lead to carcinoma formation. Formation of large plutonium aggregates, as well as bronchiolization and carcinoma formation, exhibit a threshold at about 1 Gy. Two waves of bronchiolar proliferation precede carcinoma formation. DNA aneuploidy in bronchiolar proliferative lesions may be suggestive of malignant potential.

Mutation of proto-oncogenes in nonciliated bronchiolar epithelium, followed by cell injury and proliferative repair of bronchiolar cells near plutonium aggregates, may lead to carcinoma formation.

INTRODUCTION

Previous lifespan studies in rats exposed to plutonium-239 aerosols indicated that lung tumor incidence might increase at radiation doses to the lung comparable to doses received by humans from a maximum permissible occupational lung deposition of 0.6 kBq ^{239}Pu (Sanders et al., 1976). A total of 3192 young adult, female, specific-pathogen-free (SPF), Wistar rats were used in the initial lifespan study: 2134 were exposed to ^{239}PuO$_2$ at initial lung burdens (ILB) ranging from 0.009 to 6.7 kBq, and 1058 were sham-exposed controls (Sanders et al., 1986). Histopathological analyses have been completed on 1707 of 3192 rats, including 554 sham-exposed controls and 1153 exposed animals. Cell kinetic, autoradiographic, and morphometric techniques are being used to evaluate the spatial-temporal dose-distribution patterns and the cellular events preceding lung-tumor formation in 140 serially sacrificed female Wistar rats given a single exposure to ^{239}PuO$_2$ (ILB, 3.9 kBq). Proto-oncogene activation, growth factors and growth-factor receptors, DNA cell content (by cell flow cytometry and microspectrophotometry), and cell proliferation [by ^{3}H-TdR (thymidine) nuclear labeling] are being examined in archival paraffin-block sections.

The percentages of all rats that had lung tumors (mean dose level in parentheses) were 0.7% (sham-exposed controls); 0.3% (6 rad); 0% (11 rad); 0.7% (23 rad); 2.1% (47 rad); 0% (83 rad); 12% (190 rad); 17% (350 rad); 66% (740 rad); and 81% (1500 rad). Four primary lung tumors, including 1 adenocarcinoma, were seen in 554 sham-exposed controls. A total of 116 lung tumors found in 1153 exposed rats included 60 squamous cell carcinomas, 29 adenocarcinomas, 10 hemangiosarcomas, 8 adenomas, 3 adenosquamous carcinomas, and 3 fibrosarcomas. To date, only 8 lung tumors have been found in 918 rats with lung doses ranging from >0 to <100 rad (malignant tumor incidence, 0.44%), while 108 lung tumors have been found in 235 rats with lung doses >100 rad (malignant tumor incidence, 44%). This indicates the presence of a "practical" threshold dose of about 100 rad for lung tumor formation from inhaled ^{239}PuO$_2$. The dose-response relationship is well fitted by a pure quadratic function. The lower dose range of the quadratic curve (>100 rad) appears to represent primarily initiation events; the much steeper, higher dose portion of the curve (>100 rad) appears to represent mostly promotion events caused by plutonium particle aggregation that result in the progressive expression of carcinogenesis (Sanders et al., 1988a).

The formation of promutagenic DNA damage is usually assumed to be linear; however, in the case of inhaled plutonium, the stimulation of cell proliferation in focal regions by plutonium particle aggregation is clearly dose dependent, exhibiting a threshold. In fact, the breaks in the tumor curve and in the curve showing plutonium particle aggregation are similar (Sanders et al., 1988a,b). At lung doses <1 Gy, we see no formation of large plutonium particle aggregates and little or no tumor response. A similar proliferative response has been seen with formaldehyde exposure and tumor formation of the respiratory tract (Anderson, 1987). A computer simulation study predicted a similar dose response for a very strong promotion effect. An independent promotion effect apparently results in models that are not low-dose linear but have a slope of zero at zero dose (Portier, 1987).

Primary lung carcinoma formation is preceded by a cellular evolution of focal inflammation, fibrosis and epithelial hyperplasia, and metaplasia associated with plutonium aggregates. In the serial sacrifice study, particle aggregation increased with time; well-defined focal inflammatory lesions appeared by 120 days and well-defined fibrotic lesions by 180 days after exposure. Alpha radiation doses averaging only 1.2 cGy/day were delivered to plutonium particle aggregate areas that were often adjacent to bronchioles (Sanders et al., 1988a). Nonciliated bronchiolar epithelial hypertrophy and hyperplasia were first seen at 15 days after exposure; bronchiolar tissue returned to normal a few months later. Alveolar bronchiolarization consisting of ciliated and nonciliated cells was first seen at 120 days and increased in severity and maximum incidence by 300 days after exposure. Adenocarcinoma was first seen at 600 days, squamous metaplasia at 270 days, and squamous carcinoma at 450 days after exposure.

A scanning electron microscope (SEM) autoradiographic technique gives a more nearly three-dimensional view of a comparatively large lung tissue mass than is possible with light or transmission electron microscope (TEM) autoradiography (Sanders et al., 1988b,c) (Figure 1). Plutonium particles were rapidly cleared from the surface of bronchioles during the first few weeks after exposure. Thereafter, about five times more alpha tracks intersected the bronchiolar epithelium from plutonium particles found in peribronchiolar alveoli than from plutonium found on the bronchiolar surface (Sanders et al., 1989). Plutonium lung clearance at an ILB of 3.9 kBq was considerably slower than clearance seen at an ILB of 0.4 kBq. Slower lung clearance at the higher ILB may have resulted from greater alveolar macrophage toxicity from plutonium particle concentration in macrophages during the early clearance phase and the formation of particle aggregates during the late clearance phase. Large plutonium particle aggregates are rarely seen at an ILB of 0.4 kBq but are proportionately more common with increasing ILB. Aggregated peribronchiolar plutonium particles appeared to be more often retained, whereas most alveolar particles were more rapidly cleared from the lung. Prolonged peribronchiolar particle retention appears to play a prominent role in the development of lung carcinomas.

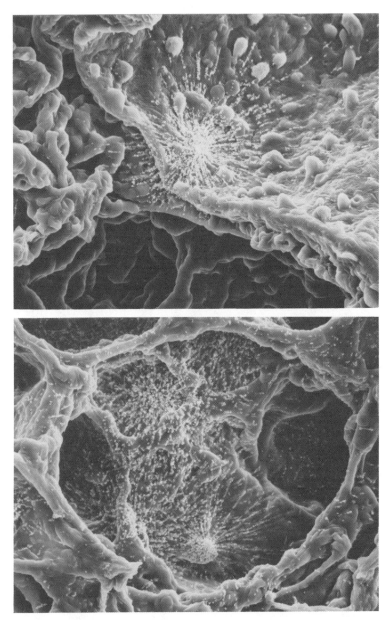

Figure 1. Scanning electron microscopic autoradiographs of rat lung after inhalation of $^{239}PuO_2$ particles. Top, alveoli; bottom, terminal bronchiole adjacent to alveoli.

Target cells for lung tumors in rats, nonciliated bronchiolar epithelium, and type 2 alveolar epithelium evidenced exposure to alpha particles (microdosimetry), proliferative response to injury, and capacity for neoplastic transformation after inhalation of $^{239}PuO_2$. Maximal increase in proliferation of alveolar cells (primarily type 2 cells) was seen by 60 days after exposure, decreasing gradually to control proliferation levels by 400 days. Excessive type 2 cell proliferation in response to continuing injury to type 1 cells may lead to cuboidal metaplasia (Adamson and Bowden, 1979). Death of type 2 cells and alveolar endothelial cells leads to fibroplasia and squamous metaplasia of alveoli (Adamson et al., 1977).

Bronchiolar epithelial proliferation appeared in two phases. The first proliferative phase, seen at 15 days after exposure, probably was associated with initial deposition on and clearance of plutonium particles from bronchiolar surfaces. The second phase, reaching maximum proliferation at about 250 days, appeared to be associated with peribronchiolar plutonium aggregate formation. Only nonciliated bronchiolar epithelial cells exhibited nuclear labeling. All epithelial dysplastic and neoplastic lesions in the lung exhibited labeling indices much greater than those of unexposed alveolar or bronchiolar epithelium (Rhoads et al., 1983). A temporal relationship was seen in labeling of cells associated with alveolar bronchiolarization; higher proliferative rates were seen in early lesions. Proliferative rates of adenocarcinomas were similar to those of alveolar bronchiolarization lesions; squamous metaplastic lesions and squamous carcinomas had similarly high proliferative rates, indicating an evolution of squamous metaplastic cells into squamous carcinoma. The association of cells involved with alveolar bronchiolarization and adenocarcinoma formation is less clear. Both type 2 alveolar epithelium and nonciliated bronchiolar epithelium in terminal bronchioles may participate in alveolar bronchiolarization and carcinoma formation.

Nuclear DNA flow cytometry of paraffin sections correlates well with analysis of fresh tissue samples from the same specimen (Hedley et al., 1983). DNA aneuploidy often correlates with increased proliferation and neoplasia. Aneuploid tumors have a more aggressive life history than diploid tumors of the same histopathology. More than 80% of human lung carcinomas are aneuploid; patients with DNA aneuploid tumors had a significantly shorter survival time than those with diploid tumors (Coon et al., 1987; Moran and Melamed, 1984). Replicate aneuploid DNA indices strongly suggest a common origin for multiple tumors within the lung. DNA aneuploidy in metaplastic or hyperplastic epithelial lesions may occur before histological evidence of invasive carcinoma.

Proto-oncogenes are among proposed cellular targets for physical and chemical carcinogens. Some proto-oncogenes affect cell proliferation and differentiation, and neoplastic expression, through the production of growth factors. Proto-onocogenes may mutate to cancer genes, amplifying growth-factor production (Cline, 1987). A deficiency in DNA repair during the G_2 phase of the cell cycle combined with a proliferative stimulus such as oncogene activation may be necessary for the evolution of a neoplastic population of squamous cells (Sanford et al., 1986). Bronchial epithelial cells show strong nuclear reactivity to *c-myc* oncoprotein (Loke et al., 1988). Squamous cell carcinomas of the lung have two to five times the number of epidermal growth factor (EGF) receptors as normal skin (Hendler and Ozanne, 1984). Amplification of the EGF receptor gene is seen in squamous cell carcinomas but not in adenocarcinomas (Berger et al., 1987). Peptides such as gastrin-releasing peptide and bombesin act as mitogens on normal bronchial epithelium and lung carcinomas (Wiley et al., 1984; Weber et al., 1985).

Promotion is the ability to induce cell proliferation, either as a direct primary mitogenic event or as a secondary regenerative effect after cell death. A strong association occurs between inflammation, proliferation, and carcinogenesis during the promotion phase of tumor development (Lewis and Adams, 1987). The dependence of tumor expression on a round of cell proliferation may indicate a need for DNA replication to effect the change in gene expression related to radiation-induced DNA alteration. Thus, if the initiated cells are to form tumors, they must be stimulated to proliferate without showing normal terminal differentiation (Farber, 1987; Nettesheim et al., 1987).

The end product of tumor promotion is generally a benign lesion or preneoplastic foci of cells. These cells must undergo one or more additional heritable changes during the progression to a malignant neoplasm. The progression of benign tumors to malignant cancers is a phase of carcinogenesis clearly distinct from promotion. Morphological evidence for multiple steps in the progression from dysplastic lesions to carcinoma *in situ* and ultimately to malignant carcinomas is well established. Oncogene amplification has been shown in some tumors to correlate with the degree of neoplastic progression (Slamon et al., 1987). When chronic exposure is involved, as seen with inhaled plutonium particles, few if any insults will affect only one stage in the multistep carcinogenic process.

ACKNOWLEDGMENT

This research was supported by the U.S. Department of Energy under Contract DE-AC06-76RLO 1830.

REFERENCES

Adamson, IYR and DH Bowden. 1979. Bleomycin-induced injury and metaplasia of alveolar type 2 cells. Am J Pathol 96:531-544.

Adamson, IYR, DH Bowden, MG Cote, and H Witschi. 1977. Lung injury induced by butylated hydroxytoluene: Cytodynamic and biochemical studies in mice. Lab Invest 36:26-32.

Anderson, MW. 1987. Issues in biochemical applications to risk assessment: How do we evaluate individual components of multistage models? Environ Health Perspect 76:175-179.

Berger, MS, WJ Gullick, C Greenfield, S Evans, BJ Addis, and MD Waterfield. 1987. Epidermal growth factor receptors in lung tumours. J Pathol 152:297-307.

Cline, MJ. 1987. Keynote Address: The role of proto-oncogenes in human cancer. Implications for diagnosis and treatment. Int J Radiat Oncol Biol Phys 13:1297-1301.

Coon, JS, AL Landay, and RS Weinstein. 1987. Biology of disease. Advances in flow cytometry for diagnostic pathology. Lab Invest 57:453-479.

Farber, E. 1987. Possible etiologic mechanisms in chemical carcinogenesis. Environ Health Perspect 75:65-70.

Hedley, DW, ML Friedlander, JW Taylor, CA Rugg, and EA Musgrove. 1983. Method for analysis of cellular DNA content of paraffin-embedded pathological material using flow cytometry. J Histochem Cytochem 31:1333-1335.

Hendler, F and B Ozanne. 1984. Human squamous cell lung cancers express increased epidermal growth factor receptors. J Clin Invest 74:647-651.

Lewis, JG and DO Adams. 1987. Inflammation, oxidative DNA damage, and carcinogenesis. Environ Health Perspect 76:19-27.

Loke, S-L, LM Neckers, G Schwab, and ES Jaffe. 1988. c-myc protein in normal tissue. J Pathol 131:29-37.

Moran, RE and MR Melamed. 1984. Flow cytometric analysis of human lung cancer. Anal Quant Cytol 6:99-104.

Nettesheim, P, DJ Fitzgerald, H Kitamura, CL Walker, TM Gilmer, JC Barrett, and TE Gray. 1987. In vitro analysis of multistage carcinogenesis. Environ Health Perspect 75:71-79.

Portier, CJ. 1987. Statistical properties of a two-stage model of carcinogenesis. Environ Health Perspect 76:125-131.

Rhoads, K, JA Mahaffey, and CL Sanders. 1983. Dosimetry and response in rat pulmonary epithelium following inhalation of $^{239}PuO_2$, pp. 59-65. In: Current Concepts in Lung Dosimetry, CONF-820492, Pt. 1. NTIS, Springfield, VA.

Sanders, CL, KE McDonald, and KE Lauhala. 1988a. Promotion of pulmonary carcinogenesis by plutonium particle aggregation following inhalation of $^{239}PuO_2$. Radiat Res 116:393-405.

Sanders, CL, KE McDonald, and JA Mahaffey. **1988b.** Lung tumor response to inhaled Pu and its implications to radiation protection. Health Phys 55:455-462.

Sanders, CL, KE McDonald, and KE Lauhala. **1988c.** SEM autoradiography: Aggregation of inhaled ^{239}PuO$_2$. Int J Radiat Biol 54:115-121.

Sanders, CL, KE McDonald, and KE Lauhala. **1989.** Quantitative scanning electron microscopic autoradiography of inhaled ^{239}PuO$_2$. Health Phys 56:321-325.

Sanders, CL, KE McDonald, BW Killand, JA Mahaffey, and WC Cannon. **1986.** Low-level lifespan studies with inhaled ^{239}PuO$_2$ in rats, pp. 429-449. In: *Life-Span Radiation Effects Studies in Animals: What Can They Tell Us?* CONF-830951. NTIS, Springfield, VA.

Sanders, CL, GE Dagle, WC Cannon, DK Craig, WJ Powers, and DM Meier. **1976.** Inhalation carcinogenesis of high-fired ^{239}PuO$_2$ in rats. Radiat Res 68:349-360.

Sanford, KK, R Gantt, JS Rhim, R Parshad, and FM Price. **1986.** Enhanced G2 chromatid radiosensitivity: An early stage in the neoplastic transformation of human epidermal keratinocytes in culture. Proc Annu Meet Am Assoc Cancer Res 27:104.

Slamon, DJ, GM Clark, SG Wong, WI Levin, A Ullrich, and WL McGuire. **1987.** Human breast cancer: Correlation of relapse and survival with amplification of the *HER-2/neu* oncogene. Science 235:177-182.

Weber, Z, JE Zuckerman, DG Bostwick, KG Bensch, BI Sikic, and TA Raffin. **1985.** Gastrin-releasing peptide is a selective mitogen for small cell lung carcinoma *in vitro*. J Clin Invest 75:306-309.

Wiley, JC, JF Lechner, and CC Harris. **1984.** Bombesin and the C-terminal tetradecapeptide of gastrin-releasing peptide are growth factors for normal human bronchial epithelial cells. Exp Cell Res 153:245-248.

QUESTIONS AND COMMENTS

Q: Thomassen, Lovelace Inhalation Toxicology Research Institute
    What fraction of the lung is irradiated by clusters of plutonium over the time course of the study?

A: Less than 10%.

Q: Is the distribution of tritium-labeled cells uniform in the lung or associated with clusters of plutonium?

A: Tritium-labeled cells are about 10 times more abundant in areas of plutonium particle aggregation than in other alveolar regions of the lung.

EVIDENCE FOR ONCOGENE ACTIVATION IN RADIATION-INDUCED CARCINOGENESIS

M. E. Frazier,[1] T. M. Seed,[2] L. L. (Scott) Whiting,[1] and G. L. Stiegler[1]

[1]Pacific Northwest Laboratory, P. O. Box 999, Richland, WA 99352
[2]Argonne National Laboratory, Chicago, IL 60439

Key words: *Oncogenes, lung cancer, plutonium, transfection, transcription*

ABSTRACT

Control and tumor tissue (from the same animals) are being examined to detect tumor-specific changes in oncogene sequences resulting from radiation-induced malignancies. The types of oncogenes that are activated and the molecular lesions which cause their activation are being identified.

High molecular weight (HMW) DNA from primary lung tumors or leukemic cells was added to NIH 3T3 cells in the transfection assay. Dominant-acting transforming genes were detected both in alpha-radiation-induced lung tumors and in gamma-radiation-induced leukemias. Further, when HMW DNA from tumor and normal tissues from the same animals were isolated and digested with the restriction endonucleases and probed with viral oncogene probes, a number of novel restriction fragments were detected in plutonium-induced lung tumors. Finally, we detected enhanced transcription of several oncogenes in the malignant cells.

The evidence from these studies suggests that the changes found in the oncogene sequences of cells from radiation-induced cancers are more extensive than the changes in single-base pairs that have been observed in oncogenes from chemically induced tumors. The radiation appears to cause amplification and/or rearrangement of the affected genes. The data also suggest that the lesions that caused the restriction fragment-length polymorphisms activated the oncogenes.

The isolated oncogenes are being sequenced to identify the activating lesions, an important first step in determining whether radiation causes distinctive patterns of genetic change.

INTRODUCTION

This research examines the role of known oncogenes in radiation-induced malignancies. The first model examines the lung tumors that develop in animals following the inhalation of $^{238}PuO_2$, $^{239}PuO_2$, or $^{239}Pu(NO_3)_4$. Radiation-related deaths were caused by radiation pneumonitis, lung tumors, or bone tumors (Dagle, 1987; Park, 1987). The second cancer model is myelogenous leukemia, which develops in dogs as the result of continuous, whole-body, low-daily-dose gamma radiation. These models provide a means for determining whether gamma irradiation caused the same kinds and frequencies of molecular damage as alpha irradiation.

Dominant-acting oncogenes present in the plutonium-induced lung tumors from beagle dogs are being detected, isolated, characterized, and compared with the proto-oncogene sequences present in normal canine DNA. In a second aspect of the research, DNA from these radiation-induced tumors and accompanying cohort cells are examined to determine whether tumor-specific changes in or adjacent to known proto-oncogene sequences can be detected as novel restriction fragments. RNA from tumor and cohort cells are being studied for evidence of altered or enhanced oncogene transcription. Finally, methods are being developed for detecting, isolating, and sequencing oncogenes from archived samples that have been formalin fixed and/or paraffin embedded.

METHODS

Eighteen-month-old beagles were administered single aerosol exposures of $^{238}PuO_2$, $^{239}PuO_2$, or $^{239}Pu(NO_3)_4$ (Dagle, 1987; Park, 1987). For each isotope, the animals were divided into six dose levels of $\sim$20 dogs per group. Exposure groups included dogs with initial lung burdens ranging from 74 to 215,000 Bq, corresponding to respective radiation doses that are approximately 1, 8, 40, 150, 700, and 2800 times, respectively, the current maximum permissible lung dose for a plutonium worker.

In the leukemia model, 13-month-old beagles were exposed daily (22 hr/day) to whole-body ^{60}Co gamma irradiation at dose rates ranging from 0.3 to 26.8 Gy (Seed et al., 1980). The dogs were monitored clinically and hematologically. The dogs that developed leukemia went through five clinical stages: radiotoxic suppression of hematopoietic cells, partial recovery, accommodation, preleukemia, and overt leukemia (Seed et al., 1985).

Tumors and normal cohort tissues were obtained at necropsy, immediately frozen, and stored in liquid nitrogen until processed for DNA or RNA extraction. Cellular DNA was extracted using proteinase K and phenol/chloroform (Maniatis et al., 1982). DNA was transfected onto NIH 3T3 mouse fibroblasts by the calcium phosphate precipitation technique of Wigler et al. (1978). The DNA to be examined for restriction fragment-length polymorphisms were digested with restriction endonuclease and probed with ^{32}P-labeled oncogene sequences, using the method of Southern (1975). RNA purification was performed by the method of Chirgwin et al. (1979).

To generate a canine DNA fragment library, DNA from a normal dog was partially digested with the restriction enzyme *Sau* 3A to generate DNA fragments between 9 and 22 kbp in size. These DNA fragments were ligated into the Lambda Dash phage cloning vector, which had been completely digested with *Bam* HI. The resultant concatameric DNA was then packaged into individual bacteriophage particles using a packaging mix obtained from Stratogene (La Jolla, CA). The bacteriophage were then used to infect *Escherichia coli* p2392 cells. The resulting plaques were screened by Southern analysis (Southern, 1975) for the presence of oncogene sequences, using a variety of cloned oncogene probes.

RESULTS

Plutonium-Induced Lung Tumors

Cellular DNA can be efficiently taken up and integrated into the chromosomal DNA of NIH 3T3 cells in a process called transfection. If the DNA contains an active oncogene, the recipient cells will convert to neoplastic phenotypes. Using high molecular weight DNA in the NIH 3T3 transfection assay, we detected dominant-acting transforming genes in nine of nine plutonium-induced lung tumors (Table 1). By contrast, only 10% -20% of naturally occurring human tumors have been found to contain an active oncogene by this assay. None of the cohort or control DNA from beagles consistently caused transformation.

Table 1. Transforming genes in DNA isolated from canine cells.

DNA Source	Number of Samples (Positive/Total)	Number of Samples Growing in Soft Agar (Positive/Total)	Efficiency of Transformation (Foci/μg DNA)[a]
Lung tumors (plutonium-induced)	9/9	7/7	0.02-0.05
Plutonium-exposed lung tissue (no tumor)	0/4	0	< 0.006
Myeloproliferative disorders (gamma-irradiation-induced)	3/3	3/3	0.01-0.06
Lymphoproliferative leukemia (spontaneous)	0/1	0	< 0.006
Plutonium-exposed spleen tissue (no tumor)	1/4[b]	0[b]	< 0.006
NIH 3T3 cells	0/11	0	< 0.006

[a] Number of transformants produced per microgram of DNA. Each DNA sample was examined in two or more transfection experiments.
[b] DNA from the spleen of dog 1033 transformed NIH 3T3 cells in two of five assays. Transformants grew in soft agar and produced 0.01 transformants/μg of DNA.

A malignant cell is assumed to contain more than one activated oncogene. Unfortunately, the standard transfection assay identifies only the subset of transforming genes that are dominant effectors (usually, *ras* oncogenes). Because it is well documented that radiation can cause deletion, translocation, and other gross chromosomal rearrangements and that proto-oncogenes can be activated by these same genetic mechanisms, we pursued a strategy for detecting activated oncogenes other than dominant effectors. This strategy involved examining the H-*ras*, K-*ras*, erb B, src, myc, and sis oncogene DNA restriction patterns in lung tumors and normal tissues from the same animals for tumor-specific restriction fragment-length polymorphisms. The most frequently observed were in K-*ras* (8/11) and erb B (6/11), and these were observed in a number of plutonium-induced tumors (Table 2). Because the changes were observed using more than one restriction enzyme, they are not caused by point mutations. Rather, these alterations in normal restriction patterns indicate the presence of deletions, translocations, or other gross rearrangements in the DNA of these tumor cells. In addition to altered banding patterns, gene amplification (as many as 60 copies per cell) of *ras*- or erb B-related sequences were detected in lung tumors from dogs 889 and 796, respectively (Figure 1). These data support our hypothesis that alpha radiation causes large lesions in DNA, resulting in oncogene activation.

Table 2. Summary of oncogene restriction fragment-length polymorphisms.

Dog Number	Exposure	Tentative Diagnosis	Tumor-Specific Restriction Fragment-Length Polymorphisms[a]				
			erb B	src	myc	Ha-ras	Ki-ras
727	$^{239}PuO_2$	Bronchiolar adenocarcinoma	-	-	-	-	+
777	$^{239}PuO_2$	Adenosquamous carcinoma	-	+	-	-	-
783	$^{239}PuO_2$	Adenosquamous carcinoma	+	-	-	-	+
796	$^{239}PuO_2$	Squamous cell carcinoma	+*	-	-	-	-
880	$^{239}PuO_2$	Adenosquamous carcinoma	+	-	-	+	+
889	$^{239}PuO_2$	Adenosquamous carcinoma	+	-	-	+*	+
1033	$^{238}PuO_2$	Papillary adenocarcinoma	-	-	-	-	+
1342	$^{239}Pu(NO_3)_4$	Adenosquamous carcinoma	+*	-	-	-	-
1391	$^{239}Pu(NO_3)_4$	Adenocarcinoma	-	-	+	+	+
1640	$^{239}Pu(NO_3)_4$	Adenosquamous carcinoma	-	-	-	-	+
1655	$^{239}Pu(NO_3)_4$	Adenosquamous carcinoma	+	-	-	-	-*

[a] Symbols: -, negative; +, positive; *, amplified gene.

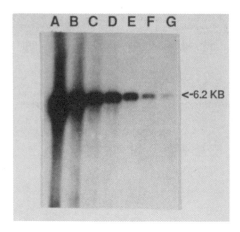

Figure 1. Detection of amplified Ki-*ras* sequences in a plutonium-induced lung tumor. Cellular DNA digested with *Eco*RI were electrophoretically separated on 1% agarose, transferred to nitrocellulose, and hybridized to a ^{32}P-labeled *Bam*HI fragment of v-Ki-*ras*. Ten micrograms of genomic DNA from animal 1655 lung tumor was added to lane A. Serial dilutions of DNA from lung tumor 1655 were added to lanes B through G: Lane B, 1:4 dilution; lane C, 1:8 dilution; lane D, 1:16 dilution; lane E, 1:32 dilution; lane F, 1:64 dilution. Lane G contains 10 μg of dog 1655 DNA extracted from lung tissue without a detectable tumor.

(In figure: A B C D E F G; <-6.2 KB)

Although observations of these RFLP do not, in themselves, prove that a specific oncogene is involved in the carcinogenic process, they do help us decide which genes may be the most important to study. We also think that analysis of the total data may provide some evidence for a specific pattern of oncogene activation. To determine whether there are any correlations between specific changes in oncogene restriction endonuclease patterns and gene expression, we measured oncogene transcription, using both Northern and quantitative dot blot hybridization. Tissues examined included those from normal lung and lung tumors from radiation-exposed animals. Steady-state levels of *ras* and *erb B* gene transcripts were higher in dogs with plutonium-induced lung cancer tissue than in normal tissues from the same animals (data not shown). These data are consistent with the observed tumor-specific changes in oncogene-related DNA sequences and indicate that those changes can cause increased transcription. Further, the evidence indicates that alpha radiation caused gross changes, for example, gene amplification and/or rearrangements in the affected proto-oncogenes.

Gamma Irradiation-Induced Myelogenous Leukemia

Transforming sequences were also detected in DNA from three dogs with myeloproliferative disorders (but not a lymphocytic leukemia) using the NIH 3T3 mouse transformation assay (see Table 1). Subsequent studies with these same leukemic dogs showed that their DNA contained leukemia-specific restriction fragment-length polymorphisms associated with N-*ras*, *abl*, and *fms* proto-oncogene sequences but not with *myc*, *erb B*, Ha-*ras*, or Ki-*ras* genes (Table 3). Finally, transcription levels of a number of oncogenes were examined using dot blot procedures. Enhanced expression of *myb*, *fms*, and *ras* as well as decreased expression of *sis* were associated with development of myelogenous leukemia (Table 4).

Table 3. Restriction fragment-length polymorphisms in γ-radiation-induced leukemias.

Dog Number	Leukemia	Restriction Fragment-Length Polymorphisms[a]					
		Ki-*ras*	*erb-B*	N-*ras*	*myc*	*abl*	*fms*
1688	Lymphocytic	-	-	-	-	-	-
2331	Myelomonocytic[b]	-	-	+*	-	+	+
2385	Myelomonocytic[b]	-	-	+	-	-	+
3863	Myelomonocytic[b]	-	-	+*	-	+	+

[a] γ-, negative; +, positive; *, amplified gene.
[b] Radiation-induced leukemia.

Table 4. Onocogene expression in γ-radiation-induced leukemias.

Dog Number	Leukemia	Expression of Oncogene[a]					
		ras	*sis*	*myb*	*abl*	*fms*	*src*
1688	Lymphocytic	±	0	±	0	0	0
2331	Myelomonocytic[b]	+	-	+	+	+	0
2385	Myelomonocytic[b]	+	-	+	±	+	0
3863	Myelomonocytic[b]	+	-	+	+	+	0

[a] Key: 0, no detectable change in expression relative to normal spleen;
          -, decreased expression relative to normal spleen;
          ±, slightly increased expression relative to normal spleen;
          +, increased expression relative to normal spleen (>fivefold).
[b] Radiation-induced leukemia.

DISCUSSION

Certain types of carcinogens cause unique or unusual types of cancer. For example, vinyl chloride causes hemangiosarcomas of the liver, and asbestos induces mesotheliomas in lungs of exposed individuals. Unfortunately, the causative agents responsible for most types of cancers cannot be identified in this manner.

A long-term goal of this research is to devise methods for detecting molecular differences in the DNA of tumor cells to help identify the agent (whether chemical or radiation) that initiated the carcinogenic process. To accomplish this, we first must know where in the DNA to look for these cancer-causing lesions. It is now known that not all DNA damage results in cancer. Rather, existing evidence implicates a subset of genes in carcinogenesis; these genes, which are called proto-oncogenes, have an important role in normal growth and development. However, exposure to either physical or chemical agents can cause mutations in their DNA sequences, causing these proto-oncogenes to become activated into oncogenes (cancer-causing genes) that transform the cell into a cancerous cell. The proto-oncogenes may be activated and contribute to neoplastic transformation of cells through point mutations, frame shifts, deletions, translocations, gene amplification, or other genetic mechanisms. This activation results in either an altered protein with a modified function, increased amounts of gene product, or some combination of these events. Any can contribute to the carcinogenic process.

Evidence is now accumulating that a number of carcinogens produce exactly the same change in DNA time after time. These changes can convert a proto-oncogene into an activated oncogene (cancer-causing gene). For example, nitrosomethylurea (Table 5) appears to cause a characteristic point mutation in the Ha-*ras* gene in 61 of 61 rat mammary tumors (Zarbl et al., 1985). Similar results have been reported by Balmain et. al. (1984) with a similar but different specific mutation in 33 of 37 dimethyl-benz[a]anthracene- (DMBA-) induced skin tumors.

Table 5. Specific mutagenesis of Ha-*ras*.

Species	Tumor	Insult[a]	Mutation[a]	Incidence
Rat[b]	Mammary carcinoma	NMU	G->A (codon 12)	61/61
		DMBA	A->N (codon 61)	5/5
Mouse[c]	Skin papilloma or carcinoma	DMBA	A->T (codon 61)	45/50

[a] NMU, nitrosomethylurea; DMBA, dimethylbenz[a]anthracene; G, guanine; A, adenosine; N, any nucleotide; T, thmidine. Sequence of codon 12, GCT; sequence of codon 61, CAA.
[b] Zarbl et al., 1985.
[c] Quintanilla et al., 1986.

Dominant-acting transforming oncogenes from the *ras* family have been detected both in plutonium-induced lung tumors and in gamma-radiation-induced leukemias. Furthermore, some of these animals have tumor-specific restriction fragment-length polymorphisms in *ras*-related DNA sequences, and Northern analyses show an increased expression of the *ras* gene. However, the radiation-caused changes from tumor cell DNA detected in *ras*-related oncogene sequences often appear to be extensive, resulting in gross chromosomal rearrangements. This is supported by the presence of cytogenetic alterations, in the q arm of the first chromosome, in a number of dogs having or developing gamma-radiation-induced chronic myeloproliferative disorders. In addition, gene amplification has been detected in two of three animals with myelomonocytic leukemia (Figure 2).

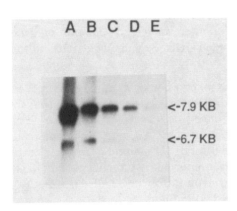

Figure 2. Detection of amplified N-*ras* sequences in a radiation-induced myelomonocytic leukemia. Cellular DNA digested with *Eco*RI were electrophoretically separated on 1% agarose, transferred to nitrocellulose, and hybridized to a ^{32}P-labeled fragment of c-N-*ras*. Ten micrograms of genomic DNA from animal 3863 (spleen) was added to lane A. Serial dilutions of DNA from spleen 3863 were added to lanes B through E: Lane B, 1:5 dilution; lane C, 1:15 dilution; lane D, 1:45 dilution. Lane E contains 10 μg of DNA extracted from a "normal" spleen.

ACKNOWLEDGMENT

Work was supported by the U.S. Department of Energy under Contract No. DE-AC06-76RLO 1830 and W-31-109-ENG-38.

REFERENCES

Chirgwin, JJ, AE MacDonald, and WJ Rutter. 1979. Isolation of biologically active ribonucleic acid from sources enriched in ribonuclease. Biochemistry 18:5294-5299.

Dagle, GE. 1987. Inhaled plutonium nitrate in dogs, pp. 21-25. In: *Pacific Northwest Annual Report for 1986 to the DOE Office of Energy Research*, PNL-6100, Pt. 1. NTIS, Springfield, VA.

Maniatis, T, EF Fritsch, and J Sambrook. 1982. *Molecular Cloning. A Laboratory Manual*. Cold Springs Harbor Laboratory, Cold Springs Harbor, NY.

Park, JF. 1987. Inhaled plutonium oxide in dogs, pp. 5-19. In: *Pacific Northwest Annual Report for 1986 to the DOE Office of Energy Research*, PNL-6100, Pt. 1. NTIS, Springfield, VA.

Quintanilla, M, K Brown, M Ramsden, and A Balmain. 1986. Carcinogen-specific mutation and amplification of Ha-*ras* during mouse skin carcinogenesis. Nature 322:78-80.

Seed, TM, LV Kaspar, TE Fritz, and DV Tolle. 1985. Cellular responses in chronic radiation leukemogenesis. In: *The Role of Chemicals and Radiation in the Etiology of Cancer*, E Huberman, SH Barr (eds.). Raven Press, NY.

Seed, TM, SM Cullen, LV Kaspar, DV Tolle, and TE Fritz. 1980. Hemopathological consequences of protracted gamma irradiation: Alterations in granulocyte reserves and granulocyte mobilization. Blood 56:42-51.

Southern, EM. 1975. Detection of specific sequences among DNA fragments separated by gel electrophoresis. J Mol Biol 98:503-517.

Wigler, M, S Silverstein, A Pellicer, and R Axel. 1978. Biochemical transfer of single-copy eucaryotic genes using total cellular DNA as donor. Cell 14:725-731.

Zarbl, H, S Sukumar, AV Arthur, D Martin-Zanca, and M Barbacid. 1985. Direct mutagenesis of Ha-*ras*-1 oncogenes by *N*-nitroso-*N*-methylurea during initiation of mammary carcinogenesis in rats. Nature 315:382-385.

INVOLVEMENT OF GROWTH FACTORS AND THEIR RECEPTORS IN RADIATION-INDUCED CARCINOGENESIS

F. C. Leung, J. R. Coleman, G. E. Dagle, and F. T. Cross

Pacific Northwest Laboratory, P. O. Box 999, Richland, WA 99352

Key words: *Carcinogenesis, growth-factor receptor, lung tumors*

ABSTRACT

In this presentation we examine the role of growth factors (GF) and growth-factor receptors (GFR) in radiation-induced lung tumors. We hypothesize that inappropriate activation or overexpression of GF and GFR plays a role in oncogenesis in the lung. In human lung tumors, for example, the abnormal expression of epidermal growth-factor receptor (EGFR) and bombesin has been reported to be associated primarily with non-small-cell carcinoma and small-cell carcinoma of the lung, respectively. Using the radioreceptor binding and immunocytochemical assays, we have examined the expression of EGFR in plutonium-induced lung tumors in beagle dogs. By both assays, EGFR levels were found to be significantly higher in plutonium-induced lung tumors than in normal lung tissue (from controls). Scatchard analysis revealed that the increase in EGFR resulted from increased receptor numbers rather than from greater binding affinity. In one plutonium-induced dog lung tumor that we examined, EGFR level increased but the expression of transforming growth factor-α (TGF-α), EGF, and bombesin was also abnormally elevated, as measured by immunocytochemical assays. Abnormally high expression of GF and GFR by immunocytochemical assays is mainly associated with epidermoid carcinoma of the lung. In radon-induced rat lung tumors, EGFR was also abnormally high, as measured by immunocytochemical assays.

In the substantial number of malignant lung tumors observed in lifespan experiments at the Pacific Northwest Laboratory (PNL), the abnormally high expression of GF/GFR in radiation-induced lung tumors suggests their involvement in radiation-induced oncogenesis in the lung.

INTRODUCTION

In humans, it is well established that all kinds of tumors produce polypeptide hormones and that lung tumors produce these hormones most frequently. With the aid of radioimmunoassays and immunocytochemistry, Abe et al. (1984) reported that various hormones are present in tumors from both patients presenting with ectopic hormone syndrome and those without this syndrome. Data collected so far suggest that production of hormones may be a universal phenomenon of neoplasia. The growth of normal cells is largely controlled by growth factors (GF) and their receptors (GFR). Circumstantial and direct evidence supports the hypothesis that abnormal expression of GF and/or GFR can lead to malignant transformation (Heldin and Westermark, 1984). Many types of tumor cells synthesize and secrete GF when cultured *in vitro*, and many types of tumor cells have abnormally high numbers of GFR, altered receptors, or altered postreceptor signaling pathways. It is hypothesized that the GF/GFR act via the autocrine and/or the paracrine pathways; therefore, abnormally expressed GF/GFR can be viewed as transforming proteins, a hypothesis supported by experimental observations. The phenotypic transformation of nonneoplastic rat kidney (NRK) fibroblasts by GF requires transforming growth factor-α (TGF-α) and platelet-derived growth factor (PDGF). Using the gene transfer technique, three independent groups of investigators (Di Fiore et al., 1987; Velu et al., 1987; Riedel et al., 1988) recently demonstrated the ligand-dependent transforming potential of NIH 3T3 mouse fibroblasts transfected with a human epidermal growth-factor receptor (EGFR) gene. Recent studies have also shown abnormally high levels of EGFR in human epidermoid carcinomas and of bombesin in small-cell carcinomas of the human lung. We hypothesized that radiation- and chemical-induced lung tumors, in both animals and humans, would have different, unique, and specific profiles of abnormally expressed GF and/or GFR. To test this hypothesis, we are using radioreceptor binding assays to examine EGFR from lung tumors obtained at necropsy from radiation-exposed and control animals. Using immunocytochemical assays, we are also examining archived, paraffin-block lung-tumor specimens obtained from previously exposed animals.

MATERIALS AND METHODS

Tissue Samples

For the radioreceptor binding assay, primary lung-tumor tissues were obtained from 5 dogs exposed to plutonium and from 1 control dog (Table 1). In addition, normal lung tissue was obtained from 2 dogs with lung tumors and from 13 additional dogs. These specimens were immediately frozen and stored at -70°C until assayed.

For the immunocytochemical assays, primary lung-tumor specimens from dogs and rats, embedded in paraffin blocks, were obtained from current and past lifespan studies at PNL that investigated radiation effects in animals.

Table 1. Radionuclide exposure and tumor classification for dogs exposed to inhaled plutonium.

Identification	Sex	Radionuclide	Initial Lung Burden (nCi)	Tumor Type
A	F	$^{238}PuO_2$	22	Bronchioloalveolar carcinoma
B	F	$^{239}Pu(NO_3)_4$	72	Papillary adenocarcinoma
C	F	$^{239}PuO_2$	140	Papillary adenocarcinoma
D	M	$^{239}Pu(NO_3)_4$	54	Papillary adenocarcinoma
E	M	$^{238}PuO_2$	17	Papillary adenocarcinoma
F	M	Control	0	Papillary adenocarcinoma

Radioreceptor Assay

The detailed methodology for the EGFR radioreceptor assay (RRA) is described in Leung et al. (submitted). Briefly, mouse EGF (Collaborative Research, Bedford, MA) was iodinated by a modified lactoperoxidase method as described by Leung (1980). Labeled EGF was separated from free EGF by gel filtration; specific activity of the ^{125}I-labeled EGF was usually between 80 and 100 $\mu Ci/\mu g$. For the binding assay, 300 μg of microsomal membrane protein preparation from normal and tumorous lung tissue was incubated with $[^{125}I]EGF$. Nonspecific binding was determined by incubation with excess unlabeled EGF. Competitive binding studies were performed with various concentrations of unlabeled EGF, and the binding affinity and binding capacity of the lung-tissue samples were obtained from Scatchard plot analyses.

Immunocytochemical Assays

Paraffin-block sections of the normal and tumorous lung tissue were taken from formalin-fixed and routinely processed histological specimens. The Vectastain® ABC (peroxidase) system was used to detect enzymes in 5-μm-thick paraffin sections. A monclonal anti-EGF receptor (clone no. 29.1, mouse IgG1) was obtained from Sigma (St. Louis, MO). This monoclonal antibody is produced from mice immunized with the A431 carcinoma cell line. Polyclonal rabbit antiserum generated against bombesin was obtained from ICN ImmunoBiologicals (Lisle, IL); a polyclonal rabbit antiserum against EGF was obtained from Collaborative Research Incorporated (Bedford, MA); and a polyclonal goat antiserum against TGF-α was obtained from Biotop (Seattle, WA). The appropriate Vectastain ABC kits were used, based on the species of the primary antibody, and appropriate (isotype) normal animal sera were used as a blocking reagent for both the specific and nonspecific sections. The nonspecific section (also 5 μm thick), taken from tissue adjacent to the specific section, was treated with exactly the same reagents as the specific section, except that normal serum was substituted for the primary antibody. The EGFR antibody (AB) AB-1 was diluted 1:50-500; bombesin AB-1, 1:500-2000; TGF-α AB-1, 1:500-2000; EGF AB-1, 1:500-1000. Positive tissue samples for immunocytochemistry were also examined in each assay: human placenta for EGFR and TGF-α; rat and dog salivary glands for EGF; and rat duodenum for bombesin. Normal rat lung and tumor-free dog lung tissues were also examined in each assay as negative controls. Immunohistochemistry slide samples were graded as positive or negative.

RESULTS

Specific EGFR binding in lung-tumor tissue was compared with that in normal lung tissue from tumor-free dogs. The percentage of specific EGFR binding in the lung tumors was almost 10 fold that in normal lung tissue: 32% compared to 4% (Figure 1). Scatchard analyses of tumors and normal lung tissue revealed a single class of EGFR, and the summary of the analysis indicated that the increase in EGFR binding in the lung tumors resulted from an increase in receptor capacity without significant change in receptor affinity.

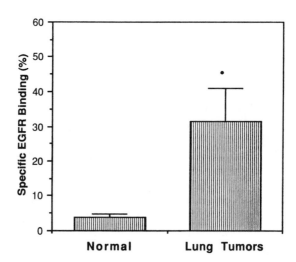

Figure 1. Specific epidermal growth-factor receptor (EGFR) binding in normal and tumorous lung tissue from dogs. Normal, N = 13; lung tumor, N = 8. The symbol • = p < 0.01 between normal and lung tumor by Student's t test.

The microsomal membrane preparations from the lung tumors had approximately 10 times more EGFR binding capacity than did normal lung tissue. Immunocytochemical analysis of the same tumor samples revealed positive EGFR staining, with varying intensity, in all tumors. Plutonium-induced dog lung serial sections stained positively with antibodies against EGFR, EGF, TGF-α, and bombesin are shown in Figures 2 and 3. When bronchial epithelium samples from a dog with tumors were examined microscopically, both "normal" and hyperplastic tissue stained positive for EGFR (Figure 4). When we examined serial sections of a radon-induced rat epidermoid carcinoma of the lung by immunocytochemical assays, the carcinoma stained positively with all four antibodies (Table 2).

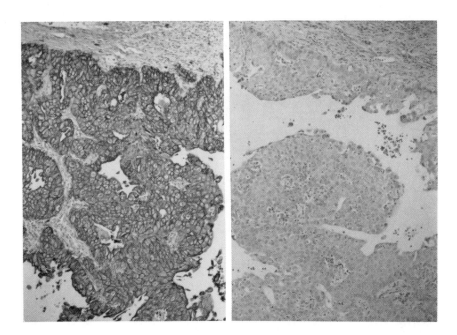

Figure 2. Plutonium-induced squamous carcinoma of dog lung, immunocytochemically stained for epidermal growth-factor receptor (EGFR). Left, specific staining with monoclonal antibody; right, nonspecific staining with normal serum.

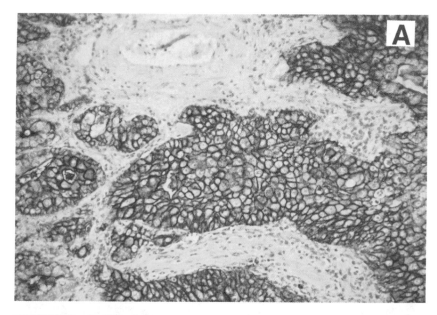

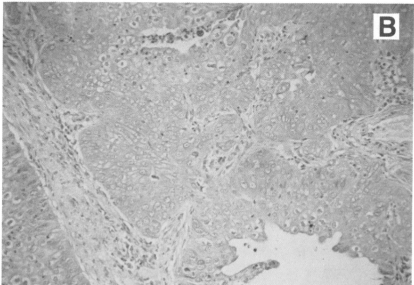

Figure 3. A and B. Serial sections of plutonium-induced squamous carcinoma of dog lung specifically immunocytochemically stained for (A) epidermal growth-factor receptor (EGFR) and (B) epidermal growth factor (EGF). (Continued on following page.)

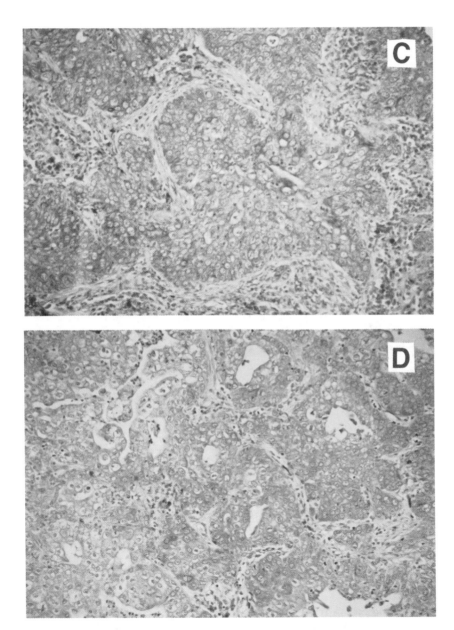

Figure 3 (continued). C and D. Serial sections of plutonium-induced squamous carcinoma of dog lung specifically immunocytochemically stained for (C) transforming growth factor-α (TGF-α) and (D) bombesin.

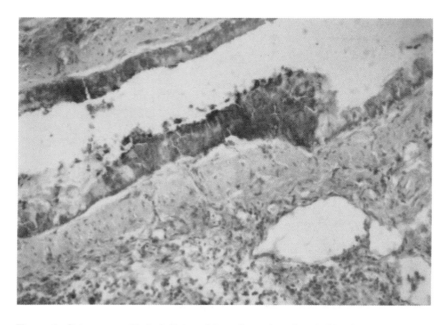

Figure 4. Columnar epithelium lining of lung from plutonium-induced dog lung tumor specifically stained for epidermal growth-factor receptor (EGFR).

Table 2. Expression of epidermal growth-factor receptor (EGFR), epidermal growth factor (EGF), transforming growth factor-α (TGF-α), and bombesin in a radon-induced squamous carcinoma of a rat lung.

Tissue Type	EGFR	EGF	TGF-α	Bombesin
Squamous carcinoma	+	+	+	+
Normal lung	-	-	-	-

DISCUSSION

We have demonstrated that EGFR binding in radiation-induced lung tumors is significantly elevated compared to that in normal lung tissue in the dog. The significant increase observed is most likely the result of increased receptor numbers rather than increased binding affinity. Immunocytochemical analysis revealed that the abnormally high expression of

EGFR, EGF, TGF-α, and bombesin was predominantly associated with squamous carcinoma of the plutonium-induced tumors in dogs and of radon-induced tumors in rats. This suggests that abnormal expression of GF/GFR is involved in radiation-induced lung tumors.

Data that describe the involvement of GF and GFR in animal lung tumors are limited; however, our findings that GF/GFR levels are abnormally high in radiation-induced lung tumors in dogs and rats agree with data on human non-small-cell carcinoma of the lung (non-SCCL). Sherwin et al. (1981) reported that EGFR binding was higher than normal in 5 of 6 non-SCCL cell lines examined. They also reported no detectable EGFR binding in 8 of 8 SCCL cell lines examined. Haeder et al. (1988) recently reported that 8 of 8 non-SCCL cell lines examined had specific EGFR binding sites and that only 5 of 11 SCCL cell lines bound EGF. The molecular weight of the EGFR protein found in the non-SCCL cell lines was similar to the weight of the protein found in SCCL cell lines. There were 3 to 10 times more receptor binding sites in the non-SCCL compared to the SCCL, and 10 to 100 times higher protein kinase activity (by *in vitro* autophosphorylation) in the non-SCCL compared to the SCCL.

Gamou et al. (1987) determined by Southern blot analysis that the EGFR gene in non-SCCL was apparently in an intact and unarranged form. Using a monoclonal antibody to EGFR, Cerny et al. (1986) reported that 80% of 48 non-SCCL tissue samples examined stained positively and that all 15 SCCL samples were negative. More specifically, abnormally high expression of EGFR has been associated more often with squamous cell carcinoma than with other types of lung tumors, and EGFR was not expressed in SCCL. Hwang et al. (1986) reported that EGFR binding and receptor autophosphorylation were elevated in primary human lung tumors.

Our observations that radiation-induced lung tumors in dogs and rats have abnormally high expression of EGF and TGF-α agree with published information concerning human lung tumors. Siegfried (1987) found EGFR binding activity proteins in the serum-free conditioned medium collected from culturing a human bronchioloalveolar carcinoma of the lung. He found these same proteins in newly cultured cells from human solid lung tumor and established human lung-tumor cell lines. These proteins suggest the presence of EGF and/or TGF-α in the conditioned medium and imply that the autocrine/paracrine functions of GF/GFR are involved in oncogenesis in human and animal lungs.

It has been generally accepted that animal lung tumors are not suitable for studying human SCCL. However, we observed abnormal expression of bombesin in both plutonium- and radon-induced dog and rat lung tumors. Previously, abnormally high expression of bombesin was found only in human SCCL cell lines. Yamaguchi et al. (1983) reported that 17 to 20 of primary human squamous cell carcinoma and adenocarcinoma specimens examined had elevated expression of gastrin-releasing peptide, a bombesin-like peptide known to be present in mammalian tissues. Data showing bombesin expression in both SCCL and non-SCCL support results of recent studies that have identified antigenic, ultrastructural, and bio-chemical similarities between SCCL and non-SCCL. Even though no morphologically distinct SCCL have been observed in most animal lung tumors, the high levels of bombesin found in our dog and rat lung tumors suggest that these tumors share similarities with biochemical mechanisms with respect to GF/GFR expression in human lung tumors. Taken to-gether, these observations suggest that animal lung tumors are suitable for studying human lung cancer. The findings also support the view that all lung tumors share a common pluripotent progenitor cell and that the different histopathological types of lung carcinoma represent a contin-uum of differentiation.

The fact that EGFR was determined in "normal" and hyperplastic bronchial epithelium in plutonium-induced dog-lung tumors suggests that EGFR expression may be a differentiating biochemical marker associated with squamous cell carcinoma. Sobol et al. (1987) reported similar findings, that a monoclonal AB against EGFR stained normal bronchial epithelium identified within the human lung-tumor sections. These data suggest that genetic and biochemical alterations may precede morphological changes during oncogenesis. There may be specific profiles of GF/GFR expression that give rise to different histopathological tumor types, or the sequence of expression may differentiate among tumor types. Alternatively, there may be unique, specific GF/GFR expression in spon-taneous, radiation-, and chemical-induced lung tumors, respectively.

In conclusion, our results demonstrate that there are abnormal expressions of GF/GFR found in radiation-induced lung tumors in dogs and rats, and that there are similarities in GF/GFR expressions between animal lung tumors and human lung tumors. Our findings also suggest that animal lung tumors are a suitable experimental model for studying human lung cancer. Further investigation will be required to elucidate the biological significance of GF/GFR expression in radiation-induced lung tumors and to determine whether abnormal GF/GFR expression is an important factor in radiation-induced lung tumors.

ACKNOWLEDGMENTS

This work was supported by the U.S. Department of Energy under Contract DE-AC06-76RLO 1830. We thank Ms. D. Felton for expert editing and Ms. M.E. Mericka and Ms. H. B. Crow for their wordprocessing assistance.

REFERENCES

Abe, K, T Kameya, K Yamaguchi, K Kikuchi, I Adachi, M Tanaka, S Kimura, T Kodama, Y Shimosato, and S Ishikawa. 1984. Hormone-producing lung cancers, pp. 549-595. In: *The Endocrine Lung in Health and Disease* , KL Becker and AF Gazdar (eds.). W. B. Saunders Co., Philadelphia, PA.

Cerny, T, DM Barnes, P Hasleton, PV Barber, K Healy, W Gullick and N Thatcher. 1986. Expression of epidermal growth factor receptors (EGF-R) in human lung tumors. Br J Cancer 54:265-269.

Di Fiore, PP, JH Pierce, TP Fleming, R Hazan, A Ullrich, CR King, J Schlessinger, and SA Aaronson. 1987. Overexpression of the human EGF receptor confers an EGF-dependent transformed phenotype to NIH 3T3 cells. Cell 51:1063-1070.

Gamou, S, J Hunts, H Harigai, S Hirohashi, Y Shimosato, I Pastan, and N Shimizu. 1987. Molecular evidence for the lack of epidermal growth factor receptor gene expression in small cell lung carcinoma cells. Cancer Res 47:2668-2673.

Haeder, M, M Rotsch, G Bepler, C Hennig, K Havemann, B Heimann, and K Moelling. 1988. Epidermal growth factor receptor expression in human lung cancer cell lines. Cancer Res 48:1132-1136.

Heldin, C-H and B Westermark. 1984. Growth factors: Mechanism of action and relation to oncogenes. Cell 37:9-20.

Hwang, DL, YC Tay, SS Lin, and A Lev-Ran. 1986. Expression of epidermal growth factor receptors in human lung tumors. Cancer 58:2260-2263.

Leung, FC. 1980. Relationship between radioreceptor assay and radioimmunoassay estimates of prolactin in rat pituitary tissue incubation medium and serum: Effects of dialysis on measurements of the hormone. Endocrinology 106:61-66.

Riedel, H, S Massoglia, J Schlessinger, and A Ullrich. 1988. Ligand activation of overexpressed epidermal growth factor receptors transforms NIH 3T3 mouse fibro-blasts. Proc Natl Acad Sci USA 85:1477-1481.

Sherwin, SA, JE Minna, AF Gazdar, and GJ Todaro. 1981. Expression of epidermal and nerve growth factor receptors and soft agar growth factor production by human lung cancer cells. Cancer Res 41:3538-3542.

Siegfried, JM. 1987. Detection of human lung epithelial cell growth factors produced by a lung carcinoma cell line: Use in culture of primary solid lung tumors. Cancer Res 47:2903-2910.

Sobol, RE, RW Astarita, C Hofeditz, H Masui, R Fairshter, I Royston, and J Mendelsohn. 1987. Epidermal growth factor receptor expression in human lung carcinomas defined by a monoclonal antibody. J Natl Cancer Inst 79:403-405.

Velu, TJ, L Beguinot, WC Vass, MC Willingham, GT Merlino, I Pastan, and DR Lowy. 1987. Epidermal growth factor-dependent transformation by a human EGF receptor proto-oncogene. Science 228:1408-1410.

Yamaguchi, K, K Abe, T Kameya, I Adachi, S Taguchi, K Otsubo, and N Yanaihara. 1983. Production and molecular size heterogeneity of immunoreactive gastrin-releasing peptide in fetal and adult lungs and primary lung tumors. Cancer Res 43:3932-3939.

IDENTIFICATION OF CHANGES INVOLVED IN PROGRESSION OF RESPIRATORY EPITHELIAL CELLS TO NEOPLASIA

D. G. Thomassen, A. F. Hubbs, and G. Kelly

Lovelace Inhalation Toxicology Research Institute, Albuquerque, NM 87185

Key words: *Neoplasia, respiratory epithelial cells, carcinogenesis*

ABSTRACT

The development of neoplasia is a multistep process. An understanding of the number and nature of the specific cellular changes involved in the progression of cells to neoplasia will aid in the identification of (1) markers that are predictive or diagnostic of this disease, and (2) factors that influence its development.

We have been investigating the progression of rat tracheal epithelial (RTE) cells to neoplasia and have identified at least four steps. A critical, early event in the progression of RTE cells to neoplasia is an alteration in cellular responsiveness to calcium-mediated (squamous) differentiation. Cells capable of continued proliferation in the presence of signals that result in differentiation of normal cells have a greater probability of accumulating additional, transformation-related changes. Preneoplastic variants of RTE cells have been isolated and shown to have reductions, compared to normal cells, in the number of growth factors required for proliferation. This reduced their responsiveness to factors normally involved in regulating cell proliferation. Two preneoplastic stages of RTE cell transformation have been identified, based on the susceptibility of cells to (transfected) v-Ha-*ras*-induced neoplastic transformation. Some variants are transformed neoplastically by a transfected v-Ha-*ras* oncogene; other variants require additional oncogenes. The acquisition of responsiveness to transfected v-Ha-*ras* correlates with additional changes in the responsiveness of the cell to growth factors, suggesting that *ras*-responsive cells are at least one step closer to neoplasia than *ras*-nonresponsive cells. Finally, neoplastic, but not normal or preneoplastic cells, are resistant to transforming growth factor beta-induced (squamous) differentiation, suggesting that this is a very late change in the development of neoplasia.

These studies are useful in identifying specific changes involved in multistep progression to neoplasia.

INTRODUCTION

Neoplastic transformation *in vivo* and *in vitro* is a multistep process. However, the nature, origin, and number of specific cellular changes required for the development of most tumors are undefined. To understand the cellular and molecular basis of carcinogenesis, specific cellular phenotypic changes essential for neoplastic transformation need to be identified and characterized. We have examined the multistep progression of rat tracheal epithelial (RTE) cells to neoplasia and have identified changes associated with at least three stages of progression to neoplasia: (1) an early, carcinogen-induced change associated with increased proliferative potential; (2) changes associated with preneoplastic stages of carcinogenesis, including reductions in growth-factor requirements and variable responsiveness to v-Ha-*ras*-induced neoplastic potential; and (3) a late change associated with the conversion of preneoplastic to neoplastic cells, characterized by an increased resistance to transforming growth-factor beta (TGF-β).

The proliferation and preneoplastic transformation of RTE cells in culture have previously been described (Pai et al., 1983; Thomassen et al., 1983, 1986). The RTE cell transformation system in our laboratory exposes cells to a carcinogen using a serum-free medium developed for normal RTE cells (Thomassen et al., 1986). After time has been allowed for expression of carcinogen-induced changes, the culture medium is replaced with a serum-containing medium permissive for proliferation of preneoplastic, but not normal, RTE cells (Thomassen et al., 1983). The first detectable stage in progression of RTE cells to neoplasia is the formation of large colonies of altered cells, termed enhanced growth variants (EGV). The cell populations that comprise these colonies exhibit an enhanced proliferative potential when compared to normal cells but do not form tumors when injected into nude mice.

The role of calcium in the proliferation and transformation of RTE cells was investigated because calcium has been shown to play a role in the regulation of epithelial cell transformation, proliferation, and differentiation in other systems (for example, see Yuspa, 1987). Cultures of RTE cells were exposed to the carcinogen N-methyl-N'-nitro-N-nitrosoguanidine (MNNG) and were selected for preneoplastic variants using serum-containing selective medium with variable concentrations of calcium. Increasing the concentration of calcium in selective medium from 0.3 mM (concentration normally used) to 1.6 mM reduced the frequency of MNNG-induced variants by a maximum of 50% (Figure 1). In contrast, increasing the calcium concentration resulted in a significantly greater reduction (75% to 90%, $p < 0.05$) in the frequency of variants in cultures not exposed to carcinogen. Furthermore, the proliferation of preneoplastic RTE cell lines in serum-containing selective medium was unaffected by the same range of calcium concentrations. This difference between treated and control cultures suggests a direct role for MNNG in the development of an altered responsiveness to calcium and also suggests that this may be one of the earliest changes involved in the preneoplastic transformation of RTE cells.

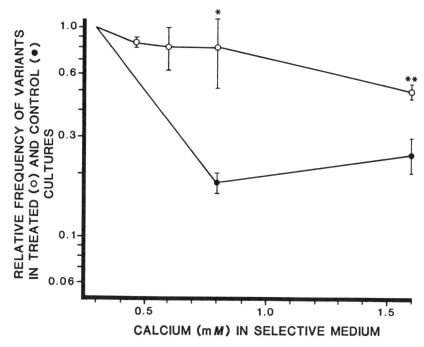

Figure 1. Relative frequency of preneoplastic variants of rat tracheal epithelial (RTE) cells in N-methyl-N′-nitro-N-nitrosoguanidine- (MNNG-) treated and untreated control cultures after selection with medium containing variable calcium. Relative frequencies of transformation in treated and control cultures were calculated based on the values obtained in cultures with medium containing 0.3 mM calcium. Levels of significance were calculated between treated and control cultures at each calcium concentration: *, $p < 0.1$; **, $p < 0.05$.

Alterations in cellular responsiveness to growth factors are common in the development of neoplasia (Goustin et al., 1986). Normal RTE cells exhibit clonal proliferation in a culture medium consisting of Ham's F12 medium supplemented with bovine serum albumin, bovine pituitary extract, cholera toxin, epidermal growth factor, hydrocortisone, and insulin. Deletion of individual factors from this medium results in 60% to >99% reduction of colony formation of normal RTE cells. Simultaneous deletion of more than one factor results in >99% reduction in colony-forming efficiency for all 57 combinations of multiple deletions. In contrast, preneoplastic variant cell lines were much less sensitive to deletion of single or multiple factors. The reduced responsiveness of preneoplastic RTE cells to some factors in serum-free medium required for proliferation of normal RTE cells suggests that an early change in the development of these variants may result in a reduced requirement for, or an independence from, certain growth factors.

To identify differences or similarities between preneoplastic RTE cell lines with respect to their ability to progress to neoplasia, variants were transfected with v-Ha-*ras* or polyoma virus DNA and injected into nude mice for a determination of their oncogene-induced tumorigenicity. Differences in responsiveness to *ras*, but not to polyoma virus, were observed among four cell lines tested. All four cell lines exhibited an increase in their tumorigenicity after transfection with polyoma DNA. In contrast, only two of four cell lines transfected with *ras* exhibited increased tumorigenic potential. These data demonstrate that epithelial cells, unlike many fibroblastic cells described in the literature, require changes in addition to immortality to be susceptible to *ras*-induced neoplastic transformation. The data also suggest that cells at different stages of preneoplastic progression can be characterized by their susceptibility to *ras*-induced progression to neoplasia.

Most neoplastic, but not normal, human bronchial epithelial cells are resistant to TGF-β-induced differentiation (Jetten et al., 1986; Masui et al., 1986). The timing of the acquisition of this resistance is not known, however, because preneoplastic human bronchial cells have not been readily available. Normal, preneoplastic, and neoplastic RTE cells were examined for their sensitivity to TGF-β inhibition of colony formation (Figure 2). Normal and preneoplastic RTE cells exhibited similar dose-response relationships for TGF-β inhibition of colony formation; neoplastic RTE cells were more resistant at all concentrations. These data suggest that acquisition of resistance to TGF-β is a late change in progression to neoplasia.

Our studies have identified several cellular changes associated with the progressive development of neoplastic respiratory epithelial cells. An early change in RTE cell carcinogenesis is an alteration of the responsiveness of cells to agents or conditions that induce a nonproliferative, terminal state in normal cells. Preneoplastic cells that develop from these carcinogen-altered cells have reduced requirements, compared to normal cells, for growth factors. Variants representing different stages of preneoplastic progression can also be characterized on the basis of their responsiveness to *ras*-induced progression to neoplasia. Finally, neoplastic transformation is associated with an increased resistance to the inhibitory effects of TGF-β. Future studies defining the biochemical and/or molecular basis of these changes will prove useful for understanding critical events in the progression of respiratory cells to neoplasia.

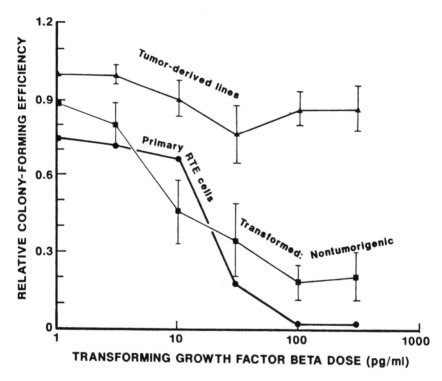

Figure 2. Relative colony-forming efficiency of normal rat tracheal epithelial (RTE) cells or of tumorigenic or nontumorigenic RTE cell lines in serum-free medium containing variable concentrations of transforming growth-factor beta (TGF-β). Relative colony-forming efficiencies were calculated based on values in cultures with no TGF-β.

ACKNOWLEDGMENT

Research was sponsored by the U.S. Department of Energy Office of Health and Environmental Research under Contract No. DE-AC04-76EV01013.

REFERENCES

Goustin, AS, EB Leof, GD Shiplely, and HL Moses. 1986. Growth factors and cancer. Cancer Res 46:1015-1029.

Jetten, AM, JE Shirley, and G Stoner. 1986. Regulation of proliferation and differentiation of respiratory tract cells by TGF-β. Exp Cell Res 167:539-549.

Masui, T, LM Wakefield, JF Lechner, MA LaVeck, MB Sporn, and CC Harris. 1986. Type β transforming growth factor is the primary differentiation-inducing serum factor for normal human bronchial epithelial cells. Proc Natl Acad Sci USA 83:2438-2442.

Pai, SB, VE Steele, and P Nettesheim. 1983. Neoplastic transformation of primary tracheal epithelial cell cultures. Carcinogenesis 4:369-374.

Thomassen, DG, ME Kaighn, and U Saffiotti. 1986. Clonal proliferation of rat tracheal epithelial cells in serum-free medium and their response to hormones, growth factors, and carcinogens. Carcinogenesis 7:2003-2039.

Thomassen, DG, TE Gray, MJ Mass, and JC Barrett. 1983. High frequency of carcinogen-induced, early preneoplastic changes in rat tracheal epithelial cells in culture. Cancer Res 43:5956-5963.

Yuspa, SH. 1987. Cellular and molecular mechanisms of carcinogenesis in lining epithelia. Symp Fundam Cancer Res 39:3-15.

QUESTIONS AND COMMENTS

Q: M. E. Frazier, PNL, Richland, WA

Your data suggest that *ras* activation is a late event in the progression to carcinogenesis, while the research of Balmain et al. in a classic skin-painting model (using TPA/DMBA) showed that *ras* activation is an early event.

Recognizing that these are indeed different model systems, could you provide any additional insights into the "apparent" conflict between your findings and those of Allen Balmain?

A: Thomassen

Although some of our preneoplastic cell lines could be converted into neoplastic lines by a transfected *ras* oncogene, we do not propose that changes in cellular *ras* are regular or essential events in rat tracheal cell carcinogenesis. However, we do propose that some change(s) induced by a transfected *ras* gene, which may also be caused by non-*ras* cellular genes, are regularly involved in progression to neoplasia.

Studies by **Schorschinsky** and Mass (Proc. Am. Assoc. Cancer Res. 29:137, **1988**) at EPA and **Walker et al.** (Proc. Natl. Acad. Sci. USA 84:1804-1808, **1987**) at NIEHS have suggested that changes in Ha-*ras* methylation or expression may be involved in the transformation of rat tracheal cells in culture. Although these results are consistent with those of Balmain, the fact remains that some preneoplastic variants of rat tracheal cells do respond to transfection with an activated *ras* oncogene. Inappropriate expression or activation of *ras* could play a role at different times during multistage carcinogenesis. In addition, different levels of *ras* expression (provided by transfected *ras* oncogenes) could also be important. For example, it could be argued that *myc* genes are critical early changes based on cell culture studies where *myc* + *ras* will transform some normal cells. However, many *in vivo* studies suggest that *myc* is important at very late stages of progression, e.g., development of metastatic potential in some lung tumors. Thus, until the actual roles of oncogenes in carcinogenesis are determined, we really have no basis for assuming a role for a given oncogene at specific stages of carcinogenesis in different tissues or cell types.

GENETIC AND CYTOGENETIC INSTABILITY: PRIMARY DRIVER OF THE NEOPLASTIC PROCESS

P. M. Kraemer

Los Alamos National Laboratory, Los Alamos, NM 87545

Key words: *Carcinogenesis, genomic instability, flow cytometry, fluctuation analysis*

ABSTRACT

Normal Chinese hamster cells sequentially acquire neoplastic changes when carried in culture. We have used this spontaneous process to determine the relationship between chromosome changes and *in vitro* transformation, immortalization, and tumorigenicity. Methods have been developed at the molecular, cellular, and *in vivo* levels for characterizing and quantifying these four categories of neoplastic change. They include: (1) DNA fingerprinting, to generically assess genomic stability and heterozygosity in cell lineages; (2) flow cytometry and flow cytogenetics, for following the emergence of specific stemlines during the neoplastic process; (3) immortalization rate assays, determined by fluctuation analysis; and (4) a retrievable sponge method for studying cell populations during tumorigenesis in nude mice.

In general, our studies show that an ongoing, generalized genetic instability underlies the entire multistep neoplastic process. Numerous phenotypic and cytogenetic variants are generated continuously, and neoplastic progression results from selections of variants with favorable changes of oncogenes and other cancer-related genes.

The multistep nature of carcinogenesis raises two categories of questions. First, what genes and cellular systems of phenotypic control are involved in each step of the process? Alternatively, does a single change serve to drive the entire process? Such a change would have to occur early, be heritable at the cellular level, and be capable of causing subsequent heritable changes in other genes dispersed throughout the genome. We have favored the latter inquiry, and for this purpose have utilized *in vitro* models of carcinogenesis. Appropriate cell culture models of carcinogenesis, in our view, include only those that (1) are initiated with normal cells directly obtained from normal mammals; (2) acquire, in stepwise fashion, various phenotypic changes associated with neoplasia; and (3) ultimately yield cell populations that are demonstrably tumorigenic in hosts such as athymic (nude) mice.

In one model that we have studied extensively (see references listed at end of article for other studies of this model), untreated Chinese hamster cells, explanted from normal adults or fetuses, routinely, inevitably, and sequentially (on serial subcultivation) became immortalized, capable of growth in medium with reduced serum growth factors, anchorage independent, and tumorigenic in nude mice. In other words, the spontaneous carcinogenesis of Chinese hamster cells constitutes an appropriate model by our criteria even though we do not know what genes or genetic alterations cause the transformed phenotypes, such as anchorage independence or immortalization. We were able to show, however, that the latter event is "mutation like" because it occurred at a rate of 2×10^{-6} per cell per generation. Immortalization is an early event in the Chinese hamster model and thus permits the early emergence of permanent sublineages within the culture that then acquire further neoplastic characters without the loss of proliferative capacity (i.e., cellular senescence) suffered by normal cells.

Ongoing cytogenetic changes were found to accompany the entire process, beginning with the earliest stages such as immortalization, and continued in cell populations that were transformed by all *in vitro* criteria and were highly tumorigenic *in vivo*. The changes, assayed by both conventional G-banding analyses and flow cytometric methods, included both numerical and structural chromosome rearrangements. Specific karyotypic changes (e.g., trisomies of chromosomes 3 and 5) were selectively favored during the evolution of numerous independently derived neoplastic cell lines. However, studies of parallel cell clones showed that numerous chromosomal abnormalities were being continuously generated, and that none of the favored changes was actually required for neoplastic progression. Thus, these studies suggested that an ongoing karyotypic instability was the underlying cause of the neoplastic process in this model (Kraemer et al., 1987a).

We have utilized "fingerprinting" probes to generically assay karyotypic instability in cell lineages undergoing neoplastic change (Kraemer et al., 1989). Such probes hybridize with minisatellite variable number tandem repeat (VNTR) DNA sequences that have a common core sequence at numerous loci throughout the genome. Ordinarily, the patterns of bands that are detected by Southern blot analysis are somatically highly stable and unique to each individual. We have found, however, that cell lineages undergoing neoplastic transformation can have extremely unstable loci that are detectable by this technique. In addition, the fingerprinting method commonly detects losses of parental alleles that accompany tetraploidization-segregation cycles of whole chromosomes. Such cycles may be important in the emergence of recessive oncogenes during neoplasia.

Chromosomal instability has also proven to be of primary importance in the transformation of human diploid fibroblasts with plasmid constructs containing the early genes of SV_{40} virus. We have achieved lineages that are transformed, immortalized, and tumorigenic in nude mice. Of particular interest has been the observation that the early transfected cells, selected with a dominant marker (neo) and shown to be T antigen positive, were not transformed by any standard criteria. Nevertheless, these cell populations showed extreme cytogenetic instability, including much cell death. Only after many passages did lineages gradually acquire, in stepwise fashion, the characteristics of neoplastic cells. By that time, the cells were blatantly aneuploid and had numerous marker chromosomes. However, the degree of chromosomal instability, although still abnormal, was reduced from that observed in the earliest phases.

Both the Chinese hamster and human fibroblast models of carcinogenesis appear to support the primary role of generalized cytogenetic instability in the neoplastic process. Heritable changes in genes that are directly related to the neoplastic phenotype (i.e., oncogenes, tumor suppressor genes, "metastasis genes," etc.) may be secondary events selected from the numerous variants produced by the cytogenetic instability. If so, an important challenge will be the identification of genes and structures that are altered when cells become cytogenetically unstable.

REFERENCES

Bartholdi, MF, FA Ray, LS Cram, and PM Kraemer. 1984. Flow karyology of serially cultured Chinese hamster cell lineages. Cytometry 5:534-538.

Bartholdi, MF, FA Ray, LS Cram, and PM Kraemer. 1987. Karyotype instability of Chinese hamster cells during in vivo progression. Somatic Cell Mol Genet 13:1-10.

Cram, LS, MF Bartholdi, FA Ray, GL Travis, and PM Kraemer. 1983. Spontaneous neoplastic evolution of Chinese hamster cells in culture: Multistep progression of karyotype. Cancer Res 43:4828-4837.

Cram, LS, MF Bartholdi, FA Ray, MS Habbersett, and PM Kraemer. Univariate flow karyotype analysis. In: Flow Cytogenetics, JW Gray (ed.). Academic Press, Orlando, FL (in press).

Goolsby, CL, JL Cooper, MF Bartholdi, LS Cram, and PM Kraemer. Early events in the SV_{40} transformation of human cells. Exp Cell Res (in press).

Kraemer, PM, GL Travis, FA Ray, and LS Cram. 1983. Spontaneous neoplastic evolution of Chinese hamster cells in culture: Multistep progression of phenotype. Cancer Res 43:4822-4827.

Kraemer, PM, FA Ray, MF Bartholdi, and LS Cram. 1987a. Spontaneous *in vitro* neoplastic evolution: Selection of specific karyotypes in Chinese hamster cells. Cancer Genet Cytogenet 27:273-287.

Kraemer, PM, EW Campbell, JL Cooper, R Stallings, and W Wharton. 1987b. Karyotypic evolution during neoplastic progression in nude mice, pp. 175-181. In: *5th International Workshop on Immune Deficient Animals*, B Rygaard, et al. (eds.). Karger, Basel, Switzerland.

Kraemer, PM, RL Ratliff, MF Bartholdi, NC Brown, and HL Longmire. 1989. Use of VNTR (minisatellite) sequences for monitoring chromosomal instability. Prog Nucleic Acid Res Mol Biol 36:187-204.

Kraemer, PM, GL Travis, GC Saunders, FA Ray, AP Stevenson, K Bame, and LS Cram. 1984. Tumorigenicity assays in nude mice: Analysis of the implanted gelatin sponge method, pp. 214-219. In: *Immune Deficient Animals in Experimental Research*, B Sordat (ed.). Karger, Basel, Switzerland.

Ray, FA, MF Bartholdi, PM Kraemer, and LS Cram. 1986. Spontaneous *in vitro* neoplastic evolution: Recurrent chromosome changes of newly immortalized Chinese hamster cells. Cancer Genet Cytogenet 21:35-51.

Schwarzacher-Robinson, T, PM Kraemer, and LS Cram. 1988. Spontaneous *in vitro* neoplastic evolution of cultured Chinese hamster cells. Nucleolus organizing region activity. Cancer Genet Cytogenet 35:119-128.

Wakshull, E, PM Kraemer, and W Wharton. 1985. Multistep change in epidermal growth factor receptors during spontaneous neoplastic progression in Chinese hamster embryo fibroblasts. Cancer Res 45:2070-2075.

Use of Multilevel Systems to Study Development

ALTERED IMPRINTING OF ACTIVATION/DETOXICATION MECHANISMS IN RATS FOLLOWING NEONATAL EXPOSURE TO DIETHYLSTILBESTROL

C. A. Lamartiniere and G. A. Pardo

Department of Environmental Health Sciences, University of Alabama at Birmingham, Birmingham, AL 35294

Key words: *Diethylstilbestrol, imprinting, enzymology*

ABSTRACT

We have previously shown, in rats, that steroid hormone and xenobiotic exposure during the perinatal period of development is capable of causing permanent, irreversible modifications on the hypothalamic-pituitary-liver axis. These modifications include alterations in endocrine secretion, morphological and sexual behavior, and hepatic metabolism. Some of these alterations can be explained on the basis of altered imprinting mechanisms. This report focuses on the effects of neonatal diethylstilbestrol (DES) exposure that result in altered hepatic activation/detoxication enzyme levels in the adult.

Neonatal exposure of male rats to DES (DES males) resulted in decreased endogenous levels of uridine diphosphate (UDP) -glucuronyltransferase, compared to those in control males. Female rats exposed neonatally to DES (DES females) had higher endogenous epoxide hydrolase and glutathione transferase activity levels than control females. Adult animals treated neonatally with DES also had altered metabolic potential following exposure to 3-methylcholanthrene and phenobarbital. The DES males treated in adulthood with 3-methylcholanthrene had higher benzo[a]pyrene (BaP) hydroxylase activities (assayed by high-pressure liquid chromatography metabolite concentrations) and lower UDP-glucuronyl transferase activity levels than control males treated in adulthood with 3-methylcholanthrene. The DES males exposed in adulthood to phenobarbital had reduced cytochrome P-450 and glutathione transferase activity levels compared with those of their respective controls. The DES females treated in adulthood with 3-methylcholanthrene had lower BaP hydroxylase and epoxide hydrolase activity levels than control females that received 3-methylcholanthrene. The DES females challenged in adulthood with phenobarbital also had decreased BaP hydroxylase, epoxide hydrolase, UDP-glucuronyltransferase, and glutathione transferase activity levels, compared with those of their respective controls.

Our results demonstrate that neonatal exposure to DES changed the endogenous levels of specific hepatic enzymes and altered the metabolic response of these animals when they were exposed, as adults, to a carcinogen or a drug, perhaps making these animals more susceptible to biochemical insult.

INTRODUCTION

Maturation or genesis of biochemical insult can be greatly influenced by genetic, physiological, and environmental factors. After conception and establishment of genotype, hormones play a pivotal role in organizational effects on the central nervous system (CNS). Organizational or imprinting effects are, in part, developmental modifications to nerve endings as a consequence of exposure to steroids during a limited critical period of fetal or early postnatal development. Biochemical imprinting effects are permanent, and the expression of this type of hormone effect does not occur until after the onset of sexual maturation, long after the effector has been metabolized and excreted.

The critical period of brain growth in human beings is primarily during the last trimester of pregnancy, but in laboratory rats the critical period is primarily during the last few days of pregnancy and the first week after birth (Dobbing and Sands, 1979). The fetus and newborn are consequently susceptible to numerous factors that can have deleterious effects on the developing organism. Work by us and others has demonstrated the role of neonatal androgen and estrogen for the determination of sex-differentiated hepatic metabolism (Gustafsson et al., 1980; Lamartiniere et al., 1979; Lamartiniere and Lucier, 1983). We have also shown that perinatal exposure to hormones and estrogenically active xenobiotics can alter the ontogeny of hepatic metabolism (Lamartiniere and Lucier, 1983; Lamartiniere et al., 1982; Lamartiniere and Pardo, 1988). This report is concerned with the potential of neonatal diethylstilbestrol (DES) exposure to alter activation/detoxication mechanisms in adult rats.

For these studies, neonatal male and female Sprague-Dawley rats (Charles River Breeding Laboratories, Raleigh, NC) were injected sc on days 2, 4, and 6 postpartum with 1.45 μmol DES or 20 μl propylene glycol (PG). At 6 months of age, these animals were treated with 0.1% phenobarbital in drinking water for 5 days or 20 mg 3-methylcholanthrene/kg ip for 3 days.

Activation/detoxication enzyme activities were measured from isolated organelles (Lamartiniere and Pardo, 1988). Aryl hydrocarbon hydroxylase, epoxide hydrolase, glutathione transferase, and UDP-glucuronyltransferase activities were determined to be higher in adult males than in adult females (Table 1). Adult male rats treated neonatally with DES (DES males) had aryl hydrocarbon hydroxylase, epoxide hydrolase, and glutathione transferase activities that were similar to those found in adult males treated neonatally with PG (PG males). However, UDP-glucuronyltransferase activities were lower in DES males as compared to PG males. Phenobarbital treatment induced all four enzyme activities in both treatment groups, but glutathione transferase was induced to a lesser extent in DES males as compared to PG males. 3-Methylcholanthrene induced all four enzymes, but aryl hydrocarbon hydroxylase activity was higher and UDP-glucuronyltransferase was lower in DES males as compared to PG males. Therefore, neonatal DES exposure resulted in lower endogenous activity levels of the conjugative enzyme, UDP-glucuronyltransferase, and altered the enzymatic response of these adult male animals to phenobarbital and 3-methylcholanthrene.

Table 1. Effects of phenobarbital and 3-methylcholanthrene on hepatic activation/detoxication enzyme activities in adult rats treated neonatally with diethylstilbestrol.

| Treatment | Activity (nmol/min/mg protein) | | | |
| | | | | |
Neonatal Adult	Aryl Hydrocarbon Hydroxylase	Epoxide Hydrolase	Glutathione Transferase (CDNB)[a]	UDP-Glucuronyl-Transferase[a]
PG males + 3-MC[a]	2.20 ± 0.22^b	7.37 ± 1.06^c	2633 ± 162^c	115.84 ± 6.14^b
PG males + PB[a]	0.93 ± 0.05^b	11.87 ± 0.52^b	4751 ± 476^b	26.23 ± 2.29^b
PG males + C.O.[a]	0.56 ± 0.04	5.55 ± 0.40	2056 ± 42	10.17 ± 0.64
DES males + C.O.[a]	0.53 ± 0.02	6.10 ± 0.28	1808 ± 123	3.19 ± 0.23^d
DES males + PB[a]	1.04 ± 0.10^e	9.80 ± 0.56^b	2711 ± 317^c	25.33 ± 3.24^b
DES males + 3-MC[a]	3.70 ± 0.26^b	8.78 ± 0.68^b	2562 ± 227^c	26.45 ± 0.50^b
PG females + 3-MC[a]	7.34 ± 0.73^b	8.18 ± 1.14^b	1950 ± 169^e	51.91 ± 4.26^b
PG females + PB[a]	1.11 ± 0.08^b	19.07 ± 3.09^b	2279 ± 120^b	17.67 ± 1.40^b
PG females + C.O.[a]	0.19 ± 0.03	2.70 ± 0.16	1383 ± 57	4.67 ± 0.51
DES females + C.O.[a]	0.19 ± 0.02	4.21 ± 0.22^d	1395 ± 114	4.04 ± 1.03
DES females + PB[a]	0.50 ± 0.07^e	8.74 ± 1.02^e	1495 ± 96	10.15 ± 0.67^b
DES females + 3-MC[a]	3.11 ± 0.28^b	5.33 ± 0.30^c	1848 ± 38^c	73.30 ± 8.30^b

[a] Abbreviations: PG, propylene glycol; DES, diethylstilbestrol; 3-MC, 3-methylcholanthrene; PB, phenobarbital; C.O., corn oil; CDNB, 1-chloro-2, 4-dinitrobenzene; UDP, uridine diphosphate.
[b] $p < 0.001$ compared to respective treatment controls.
[c] $p < 0.05$ compared to respective treatment controls.
[d] $p < 0.001$ compared to respective sex controls.
[e] $p < 0.01$ compared to respective treatment controls.

In female rats, endogenous activities of aryl hydrocarbon hydroxylase, glutathione transferase, and UDP-glucuronyltransferase were similar in DES females as compared to PG females (see Table 1). However, endogenous epoxide hydrolase activities were higher in DES females as compared to PG females. Phenobarbital treatment of PG females resulted in induction of all four enzyme systems. Diethylstilbestrol females were induced to one-half the extent of PG females for all except glutathione transferase, which was not induced at all. Exposure of adult females to 3-methylcholanthrene resulted in a lesser induction of aryl hydrocarbon hydroxylase, a greater induction of UDP-glucuronyltransferase, and similar induction of epoxide hydrolase and glutathione transferase in DES females as compared to PG males. Neonatal DES exposure therefore altered the endogenous activity of epoxide hydrolase in adult female rats. Diethylstilbestrol females also responded differently from control females exposed in adulthood to a drug and xenobiotic.

More recently, we have investigated the binding of aflatoxin B_1 (AFB_1) to liver DNA of these adult rats treated neonatally with DES. Control male rats had higher AFB_1-DNA adduct concentrations than control females. This is consistent with reports for sex-differentiated aflatoxin tumorigenesis (Newberne and Wogan, 1968; Butler and Barnes, 1968; Gurtoo and Motycka, 1976). Diethylstilbestrol males had slightly higher adduct concentrations than PG males, and DES females had significantly higher (sixfold) adduct concentrations than PG females.

In summary, adult male rats had higher activity levels of aryl hydrocarbon hydroxylase, epoxide hydrolase, UDP-glucuronyltransferase, and glutathione transferase as compared to adult females. After exposure to AFB_1 in adulthood, males had higher concentrations of AFB_1-DNA adduct than females. This may result from the balance of endogenous activation/ detoxication reactions favoring the formation of electrophiles that, in turn, bind to DNA before these electrophilic metabolites (epoxide of AFB_1) can be conjugated with glutathione. Neonatal exposure of male rats to DES resulted in lower endogenous levels of UDP-glucuronyltransferase and had no significant effect on the other enzymes measured. UDP-glucuronyltransferase does conjugate some aflatoxin metabolites (P_1, M_1, Q_1), but glutathione conjugates of AFB_1 epoxide are the primary biliary product in rat bile (Gurtoo, 1980). Hence, the reduced glucuronide conjugation would play a minor role in detoxication in DES male rats. This is reflected by only slightly higher adduct levels in DES males as compared to PG males.

Diethylstilbestrol females had higher endogenous epoxide hydrolase but similar aryl hydrocarbon hydroxylase, glutathione transferase, and UDP-glucuronyltransferase activity levels as compared to control females. The most striking effects are for higher AFB_1-DNA adduct concentrations in these DES females exposed in adulthood to AFB_1. This may be explained on the basis of induced enzyme activity levels. Exposure of adult rats to phenobarbital induced all measured enzymes except for glutathione transferase (the primary detoxication pathway) in DES females when compared to respective controls. This means, therefore, that DES females exposed to a cytochrome P-450 inducer (e. g., aflatoxin) will have less capacity for conjugating electrophiles such as AFB_1-epoxide. This may be reflected in the high AFB_1-DNA adduct levels in the DES females.

In conclusion, our results demonstrated that exposure to a hormonally active xenobiotic (DES) altered the expression of hepatic activation/deactivation enzymology in adult animals. Using measurements of carcinogen-DNA adducts as a surrogate for genotoxicity, we detected alterations after exposure to a procarcinogen (aflatoxin B_1). We suggest that these alterations occur as a consequence of altered imprinting mechanisms with DES, causing developmental modifications early in life. In adulthood, these animals are susceptible to biochemical insult long after this original effector is eliminated.

ACKNOWLEDGMENT

This research was supported by a grant from the National Institute of Environmental Health Sciences (ES 04360).

REFERENCES

Butler, WH and JM Barnes. 1968. Carcinogenic action of groundnut meal containing aflatoxin in rats. Food Cosmet Toxicol 6:135-144.

Dobbing, J and J Sands. 1979. Comparative aspects of the brain growth spurt. Early Hum Dev 13:79-83.

Gurtoo, HL. 1980. Genetic expression of aflatoxin B_1 metabolism: Effects of 3-methylcholanthrene and 2,3,7,8-tetrachlorodibenzo-p-dioxin on the metabolism of aflatoxins B_1 and B_2 by various inbred strains of mice. Mol Pharmacol 18:296-303.

Gurtoo, HL and LE Motycka. 1976. Effect of sex difference on the *in vitro* and *in vivo* metabolism of aflatoxin B_1 by the rat. Cancer Res 36:4663-4671.

Gustafsson, JA, A Mode, G Norstedt, T Hohfelt, C Sonnenscheinn, P Eneroth, and P Skett. 1980. The hypothalamo-pituitary-liver axis, a new hormonal system in control of hepatic steroid and drug metabolism, p. 47. In: *Biochemical Action of Hormones*, G Litwack (ed.). Academic Press, New York, NY.

Lamartiniere, CA and GW Lucier. 1983. Endocrine regulation of xenobiotic conjugative enzymes, pp. 295-312. In: *Organ and Species, Specificity in Chemical Carcinogenesis*, R Langeback, S Nesnow, and J Rice (eds.). Plenum Press, New York, NY.

Lamartiniere, CA and GA Pardo. 1988. Altered activation/detoxication enzymology following neonatal diethylstilbestrol treatment. J Biochem Toxicol 3:87-103.

Lamartiniere, CA, CS Dieringer, E Kita, and GW Lucier. 1979. Altered sexual differentiation of hepatic UDP-glucuronyltransferase by neonatal hormone treatment in rats. Biochem J 180:313-318.

Lamartiniere, CA, MA Luther, GW Lucier, and NP Illsley. 1982. Altered imprinting of rat liver monoamine oxidase by o,p'-DDT and methoxychlor. Biochem Pharmacol 31:647-651.

Newberne, PM and GN Wogan. 1968. Sequential morphologic changes in aflatoxin B_1 carcinogenesis in the rat. Cancer Res 28:772-781.

QUESTIONS AND COMMENTS

Q: D. L. Springer, PNL, Richland, WA

Do you think that *in vitro* assays that are closer to the whole animals (such as freshly isolated hepatocytes), as opposed to S9 preparations, will provide a more accurate measure of cytochrome P-450 imprinting?

A: Yes, assays in hepatocytes will probably yield more meaningful information than incubations with S9 fractions. Furthermore, metabolite extractions from fresh liver would probably be even better.

Q: J. Bond, Lovelace-ITRI

In terms of your DES neonatal treatment, do you expect similar changes for the other P-450 isozymes in the liver? Also, in terms of epoxide hydrolase activity, did you investigate the effects of DES neonatal treatment on cytosolic epoxide hydrolase?

A: In reference to altered imprinting effects on cytochrome P-450 isoenzymes other than aryl hydrocarbon hydroxylase, it is hard to predict. The changes we see are related to the response (induced activity) of DES males and DES females to adult exposure to 3-methylcholanthrene treatment. 3-Methylcholanthrene treatment results in higher aryl hydrocarbon hydroxylase activities in DES males and lower activity of this enzyme in DES females, compared to that of their respective controls.

There was no change in *endogenous* aryl hydrocarbon hydroxylase activities. Yet there could be changes in other specific isoenzymes that would not reflect an obvious change in total cytochrome P-450 content.

In reference to cytosolic epoxide hydrolase, no, we did not measure it. While cytosolic epoxide hydrolase may be important, the activity levels are low compared to microsomal epoxide hydrolase, and we simply do not have time to measure the cytosolic enzymes.

INFLUENCE OF IMPRINTING AGENTS ON CYTOCHROME P-450 EXPRESSION

D. L. Springer and R. C. Zangar

Biology and Chemistry Department, Pacific Northwest Laboratory, P.O. Box 999, Richland, WA 99352

Key words: *Cytochrome P-450, imprinting, gene expression, DES*

ABSTRACT

Neonatal or fetal exposure to a number of agents has been shown to alter adult enzymatic activities, including cytochrome P-450. Presumably, this is the result of permanent changes in the expression of the genes for these enzymes. Therefore, we have begun studies to better identify the molecular mechanisms involved in these effects.

Neonatal rats were treated with either diethylstilbestrol (DES), dimethylbenzanthracene, pregnenolone carbonitrile, or phenobarbital, and evaluated as adults (5-6 months of age) for changes in carcinogen binding to DNA. In addition, studies are underway to determine whether other cytochrome P-450-catalyzed activities, including those involved in steroid hormone biosynthesis and degradation, are altered.

Results indicate that male rats treated neonatally with DES and challenged with a carcinogenic dose of radiolabeled aflatoxin had smaller amounts of aflatoxin bound to DNA, relative to corresponding control animals. Neonatal exposure to the other agents did not influence aflatoxin-DNA binding levels. These results suggest that altered imprinting of cytochrome P-450 enzymes may change the susceptibility of the animals to tumor development.

INTRODUCTION

The presence of stimuli such as hormones during normal development determines the capability of mammals to express and regulate certain genes later in life. These processes, known as imprinting, occur during certain sensitive periods of development. Prenatal or neonatal contact with chemicals or radiation may cause altered imprinting, which then results in shifts in biochemical pathways. These shifts may be lethal, or in less severe cases may be manifested as physiological imbalances that may alter the animal's susceptibility to disease. For example, it is well known that some female offspring of women who were given the synthetic steroid diethylstilbestrol (DES) developed cervical adenocarcinoma. Although the mechanism for this effect has not been fully identified, data indicate that DES exposure disturbed the normal imprinting process, resulting in hormonal and other imbalances that may have contributed to tumor development.

The cytochrome P-450-catalyzed monooxygenase system appears to be involved in altered imprinting. For example, Lamartiniere and Pardo (1988) reported that neonatal subcutaneous exposure of rats to DES resulted in altered hepatic activation and detoxification enzyme activities, including those of UDP-glucuronyltransferase, epoxide hydrolase, and glutathione transferase; several other changes in cytochrome P-450-catalyzed activities were also observed when DES-treated animals were challenged as adults with phenobarbital. Bagley and Hayes (1985) reported that neonatal exposure to phenobarbital resulted in significant elevation of total cytochrome P-450, increased activities of cytochrome P-450 reductase, cytochrome c reductase, ethoxycoumarin-O-deethylase, testosterone glucuronidase, and glucuronosyl transferase; the magnitude of these increases ranged from 27% to 94%. In addition, when these animals were challenged with aflatoxin B_1, a known hepatic carcinogen, the amount of this compound that was covalently bound to hepatic DNA increased by 1.5- to 2.3 fold over that in corresponding controls. These results were consistent with those of Faris and Campbell (1983).

The foregoing observations indicate that endogenous P-450-dependent enzymes are altered by xenobiotic administration during development and that these changes may play an important role in susceptibility to cancer. Altered cytochrome P-450 levels may have other important consequences, because certain cytochrome P-450-dependent enzymes catalyze reactions in the biosynthesis and metabolism of steroids; in fact, several rate-limiting or key regulatory steps in these pathways are controlled by specific P-450 isozymes. Thus, altered imprinting could change the isozyme patterns as well as the total levels of P-450-dependent monooxygenase activities. Because these key issues have not been addressed experimentally, we studied the relationships between altered imprinting, P-450-dependent enzyme activities, and steroid biosynthesis and metabolism.

Male and female rats were injected subcutaneously with three potential imprinting agents (DES; pregnenolone-16a-carbonitrile, PCN; 7,12-dimethylbenz [a]anthracene, DMBA, dissolved in sesame seed oil) on days 1, 3, and 5 of age; control animals were given oil alone by the same route of administration. Other animals were injected with phenobarbital, another potential imprinting agent; because it is water soluble, control animals received injections of physiological saline. When the animals were approximately 23 weeks old, a number of animals from each treatment group were randomly selected and killed, and hepatic microsomes were prepared. Analyses of these microsomal preparations indicated that total cytochrome P-450 concentrations for males from all treatment groups were not significantly different from those of controls, whereas total cytochrome P-450 was increased by 21% for DES-treated females (Figure 1).

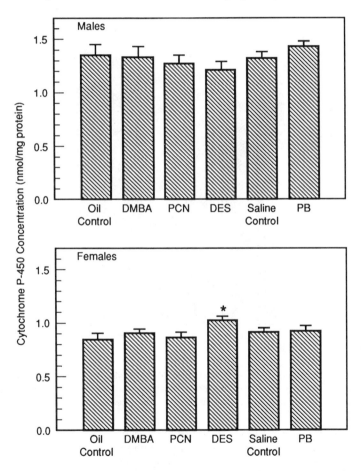

Figure 1. Concentration of protein and cytochrome P-450 from microsomes from livers of rats treated with potential imprinting agents (mean ± SEM). Top: males; bottom, females. Abbreviations: DMBA, dimethylbenz(a)anthracene; PCN, pregnenolone-16α-carbonitrile; DES, diethylstilbestrol; PB, phenobarbital; *, $p > 0.05$ (females).

Other males, randomly selected from each treatment group at 23 wk of age, were administered radiolabeled aflatoxin B_1; binding to hepatic DNA was determined after extensive DNA purification. Under these conditions, binding of aflatoxin B_1 to hepatic DNA for DES-treated males was decreased by 36% relative to binding for corresponding controls; exposure to the other test materials did not result in significant changes in aflatoxin binding (Figure 2).

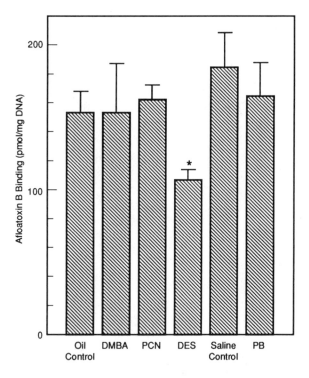

Figure 2. *In vivo* binding of aflatoxin B_1 to hepatic DNA in male rats treated with potential imprinting agents (mean ± SEM). Abbreviations: DMBA, dimethylbenz(a)anthracene; PCN, pregnenolone-16α-carbonitrile; DES, diethylstilbestrol; PB, phenobarbital; *, $p > 0.05$.

Our primary purpose is to determine the consequences of neonatal exposures on cytochrome P-450-dependent monooxygenase system at the molecular level; however, it is also important to relate changes at the molecular level to those that are manifested in the intact animal. A multilevel approach may provide molecular information to help interpret effects on intact animals. Thus, we evaluated the animals for survival and growth from the time of neonatal treatment until they were killed as adults (at approximately 23 wk of age). Few deaths occurred in the PCN-treated, phenobarbital-treated, or control groups during this time. Fifteen percent of the DMBA-treated males and approximately 12% of the females died between 20 and 23 wk of age, mainly because of tumors at the injection site or mammary tumors. Deaths also occurred in the DES treatment group, beginning around 7 wk of age. By the final sacrifice at 23 wk, 35% of the animals in this group had died; the cause of these deaths was not identified. Body weights for DES-treated females were significantly increased (15%) relative to controls; in contrast, at 12 wk of age body weights for DES-treated males were significantly decreased. These changes suggested that the growth pattern of the females had begun to resemble that of males, and vice versa; these changes were consistent with those observed by Lamartiniere and Pardo (1988).

These data suggest that neonatal exposure to DES may alter the susceptibility of animals to tumor development (and possibly other diseases), and that cytochrome P-450-dependent pathways may be involved. These changes also demonstrate the need for further evaluation, with particular emphasis on determining the cytochrome P-450 isozymes involved in aflatoxin binding for DES-treated females, because their total cytochrome P-450 concentrations were 21% higher than those of controls. Future work will focus on molecular end points, such as oligonucleotide probes for mRNA and antibodies to P-450, to identify the isozymes involved.

ACKNOWLEDGMENTS

Research was supported by the U.S. Department of Energy's Office of Health and Environmental Research under contract DE-AC06-76RLO 1830.

REFERENCES

Bagley, DM and JR Hayes. 1985. Xenobiotic imprinting of the hepatic monooxygenase system. Biochem Pharmacol 34:1007-1014.

Faris, RA and TC Campbell. 1983. Long-term effects of neonatal phenobarbital exposure on aflatoxin B_1 disposition in adult rats. Cancer Res 43:2576-2583.

Lamartiniere, CA and GA Pardo. 1988. Altered activation/detoxication enzymology following neonatal diethylstilbestrol treatment. J Biochem Toxicol 3:87-103.

QUESTIONS AND COMMENTS

Q: Gantt, NCI

What sort of mechanisms do you envision to implement the imprinting?

A: It has been postulated that imprinting of these enzymes involves gene expression and regulation and is mediated via the hypothalmic-pituitary axis.

Q: Bond, Lovelace-ITRI
DES treatment did not alter male hepatic P-450 levels, but resulted in a significant decrease in aflatoxin metabolites to hepatic DNA. How do you explain this apparent inconsistency?

A: The isozymes responsible for activation of aflatoxin may represent a small portion of the cytochrome P-450 present. Thus there could be substantial changes in the amount of aflatoxin converted to the epoxide metabolite and coresponding increases in the specific cytochrome P-450 responsible without a detectable change in total cytochrome P-450 content.

Q: Nelson, Jet Propulsion Laboratory
Is there any evidence for imprinting in this or any other system by challenge with a physical agent such as ionizing radiation, heat shock etc.?

A: Not to my knowledge.

ANALYSES OF CRITICAL TARGET CELL RESPONSES DURING PRECLINICAL PHASES OF EVOLVING CHRONIC RADIATION-INDUCED MYELOPROLIFERATIVE DISEASE: EXPLOITATION OF A UNIQUE CANINE MODEL

T. M. Seed,[1] L. V. Kaspar,[1] D. V. Tolle,[1] T. E. Fritz,[1] and M. E. Frazier[2]

[1]Biological, Environmental, and Medical Research Division, Argonne National Laboratory, Argonne IL 60439

[2]Pacific Northwest Laboratory, P.O. Box 999, Richland, WA 99352

Key words: *Chronic radiation leukemogenesis, myeloid leukemia, hematopoiesis, stem cells*

ABSTRACT

Chronic, whole-body exposure to a select range of low daily doses (1.9-12.8 cGy/day) elicits a high incidence of myeloproliferative disease (MPD), principally myeloid leukemia, in beagles. Sequential analyses of hematopoietic tissue responses during the evolution of this radiation-induced disease complex has revealed four major preclinical phase transitions: (I) suppression, (II) recovery, (III) accommodation, and (IV) preleukemic expansion. Recent work has focused on the transition between Phases I and II—a critical, early occurring event involving a broadly based hematopoietic recovery that clearly "sets the stage" for subsequent progression and expression of MPD. This critical transition of the hematopoietic system appears driven largely by acquired changes in radiosensitivity, cellular repair, and proliferative capacity of lineage-committed hematopoietic progenitors, the putative critical targets for chronic radiation-induced leukemogenesis. The magnitudes of these preclinical cellular acquisitions are proportional to the daily rate of exposure and manifest a strong "selective-pressure" effect for the outgrowth of aberrant clonal types. Although the genetic/molecular basis of these functional acquisitions by targeted stem cells remains largely unknown, site-specific chromosomal alterations and associated enhancement of DNA repair capacity have been identified in the marrow of MPD-prone dogs. The influence of selectively activated genes, in particular the N-ras and fms oncogenes, during this early transitional phase remains to be determined, although at much later stages of MPD progression (preclinical Phase IV and clinical Phase V), both appear to be activated and amplified, with high levels of expression.

Continued use of this canine model of chronic radiation leukemogenesis promises to identify not only the key cellular/molecular events within principal hematopoietic target cells but also their temporal patterns of occurrence on a realistic time scale.

INTRODUCTION

Ionizing radiation is a well-recognized and established leukemogen for both man and animals. However, the leukemogenic potency of selected types of radiation exposure regimens (e.g., low-dose/low-dose-rate or highly fractionated-type exposures) remains poorly defined. This deficit in our knowledge presents a problem in assessing health risks associated with such exposures. Further, the current process(es) of assessing risk in the low-dose/low-dose-rate region is subject to question because the radiobiological basis for leukemia induction and progression has yet to be properly defined (BEIR, 1980).

With these considerations in mind, we developed a useful canine model, along with appropriate *in vitro* target cell assays, to pursue questions involving (a) leukemic potential of chronic, low-dose/low-dose-rate exposures, and (b) the nature and mechanisms of early occurring preclinical events.

Our intent here is to briefly summarize and highlight ongoing studies on the cellular and molecular processes involved in the induction and progression of myeloid leukemia in dogs chronically exposed to low daily doses of whole-body gamma irradiation. Under such conditions, selected groups of dogs exhibited extremely high frequencies of myeloproliferative disease (MPD) (i.e., ~50%), of which myeloid leukemia was the most prominent (Seed et al., 1985).

MATERIALS AND METHODS

Beagles, ~400 days old at the start, were exposed daily to whole-body ^{60}Co gamma irradiation at dose rates from 0.3 to 26.8 cGy per 22-hr day. Nonirradiated controls were caged and handled similarly, except for being housed in a shielded anteroom. All dogs were sequentially monitored clinically and hematologically with time of exposure. Hematological tests included (1) quantitation and functional assessment of the granulocyte/monocyte- (GM-) committed progenitorial compartment of the marrow, as assayed by a modified Pike Robinson soft-agar cloning system *in vitro* (Seed et al., 1982); (2) titration of circulating plasma levels of GM-colony-stimulating activity (GM-CSA) *in vitro*, via measures of plasma-induced clonogenic response of control GM-progenitor targets (Kaspar and Seed, 1984); (3) assessment of the radiosensitivity and cellular repair capacity of GM progenitors by using either the loss or recovery, respectively, or clonogenicity, as measured end points (Seed et al., 1982, 1986a); (4) assessment of the DNA repair within GM-progenitor-enriched marrow by an akaline elution/microfluorometric technique; (5) cytogenetic analyses of both banded and nonbanded metaphase spreads in detecting numerical and structural chromosomal aberrancies; and (6) oncogene analyses by both a standard NIH 3T3 transfection assay and by Southern/Northern blot-^{32}P-probe hybridization procedures (Frazier et al., 1987).

RESULTS

Evolution of the Chronic Radiation-Induced Myeloid Leukemic Syndrome—Definition of the Preclinical Phase Sequence

Irradiated dogs in progression to overt myeloid leukemia exhibit a reproducible sequence of four preclinical hematopoietic phases: (I) radiotoxic suppression; (II) partial recovery; (III) accommodation; and (IV) preleukemic transition (Figure 1). The entire preclinical sequence requires a mean time of ~900 days at the 7.5-cGy dose rate.

Two major events have been identified within one of the key hematopoietic progenitor subpopulations (i.e., the GM-lineage-committed progenitors), which is putatively a population considered to be a principal target for the leukemogenic action of ionizing irradiation. The first event occurs early (~150-250 days) and involves the renewal of proliferative capacity in the target cell, coupled tightly with increased radioresistance. The second event occurs much later, during the preleukemic transition phase (IV), and involves the acquisition of aberrant clonal functions, including autocrine-like activities.

Circulating blood levels of GM-progenitor-specific hematopoietin (GM-CSA) are significantly elevated during the periods encompassing both the early and late target cell events. During the initial periods of exposure (preclinical phases I and II), GM-CSA levels rise and subsequently fall reciprocally with the initial decline and recovery of GM progenitors (Kaspar and Seed, 1984). In contrast, with progression into the late preleukemia transitional period, GM-CSA serum levels often rise in concert with an expanding, but aberrant, GM-progenitor population.

Hematopoietic Recovery, An Early Occurring, "Stage-Setting" Process for Leukemic Development

Hematopoietic recovery (preclinical phase II) within the leukemia-prone animal is broadly based, involving not only restoration of critically depleted circulating cell pools and marrow reserves but also recovery of vital stem cell and progenitorial marrow compartments (Seed et al., 1980, 1982). As such, the latter provides the basis for long-term hematopoietic recovery and accordingly "sets the stage" for subsequent leukemic progression. Without this recovery, there is no leukemic progression with continued exposure but only progression to aplastic anemia (Seed et al., 1985). Further, the quality of the elicited hematopoietic recovery plays a role in leukemia induction: forced hematopoietic recovery under the constant selective pressure of chronic irradiation seems to be a prerequisite for leukemia induction. Termination of irradiation before or during the recovery process disrupts pathological progression, thus lowering the leukemic frequency (Seed et al., 1985, 1986a).

Major Targeted Stem Cell Events during Progression of Chronic Radiation–Induced Myeloid Leukemia and Related Myeloproliferative Disorders in Canines

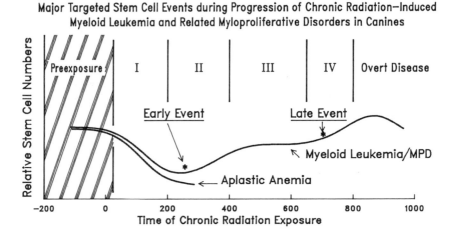

Preclinical Phases
  I. Suppressive
  II. Recovery
  III. Accommodative
  IV. Preleukemic Transition

Target Cell Events

Early – Acquired radioresistance with enhanced cell renewal
Late – Acquired autocrine functions with clonal aberrancies

Figure 1. Diagram of sequential change in key hematopoietic targets [granulocyte/ monocyte (GM) progenitors] in response to chronic, whole-body gamma irradiation (7.5 cGy/day) of beagles (~400 days old at start of exposure) and in progression to myeloid leukemia or aplastic anemia. Four preclinical phases and two major target cell events (occurring at approximate periods indicated by asterisks) served to characterize induction and progression to overt leukemia; a single phase of progressive hematopoietic decline characterizes aplasia-prone animals. "Time" on abscissa given in days. MPD, myeloproliferative disease.

Properties and Mechanisms of the "Early" Event

During the transition from the initial radiotoxic phase (I) to recovery phase (II) (150-300 days), the proliferative capacity of the targeted GM progenitors shifts from being progressively diminished to being progressively enlarged. The driving force behind this change appears to be, in part, the increased radioresistance of the target cell, a novel cellular acquisition that not only spares sterilization of vital progenitorial marrow compartments but also allows for the aberrant outgrowth and repopulation of the hypoplastic marrow with aberrant clonotypes. The radioresistance of GM progenitors nearly doubles with transition from preclinical phases I to II and remains markedly resistant with subsquent phase transitions (II/III, III/IV).

The magnitude of the radioresistance expressed by GM progenitors appears related to the daily exposure rate and, in turn, to leukemia incidence; for example, rising proportionately with rising exposure rates in the range of 0.3 to 7.5 cGy/day (Seed and Kaspar, 1988). Further, once radioresistance is acquired, it appears to be expressed in a stable manner for prolonged periods so long as daily exposure continues. There are, however, both radiological and biological factors that tend to destabilize the radioresistant state and, in turn, lower the leukemic risk; for example, by terminating chronic exposure, by reducing exposure rate, or by continuing pathological progression to an alternate, nonmalignant disease state such as aplastic anemia.

Altered Repair Function as an Underlying Basis for Acquired Radioresistance

Altered repair within targeted GM progenitors of irradiated dogs in preclinical phases II-IV appears to be, in part, a principal mediator of acquired radioresistance—the key process driving the early event. Several lines of evidence have been collected to support this contention. Evidence of modified cellular/molecular repair comes from (1) split-dose experiments, indicating markedly enhanced survival maxima (ratios) at the interfractional radiation times of 3 and 10 hr; (2) low-dose-rate experiments, indicating that the reduction of the dose rate by two orders of magnitude (i.e., from 25 to 0.25 cGy/min) markedly enhanced *in vitro* survival and radioresistance; (3) high-linear-energy-transfer (high-LET) neutron sensitivity experiments, showing that the extended sublethal damage capacity (SLD) is effectively ablated by exposure to fission neutrons (mean energy of 1 MeV); and finally (5) single-strand DNA break (SSB) repair analyses, via an alkaline elution-microfluorometric assay, demonstrating an enhancement of SSB repair capacity (Seed et al., 1986b).

Site-Specific Chromosomal Alteration Associated with Acquired Hematopoietic Repair in Preleukemic Dogs

Cytogenetic analyses of preleukemic dogs have revealed a high-frequency "lesion" within the first chromosomal pair. The lesion, defined morphologically by an elongated Q arm and hyperextended homogeneously staining distal bands, is seen consistently in all preleukemic dogs at the time of or after hematopoietic recovery. In contrast, both aplasia-prone dogs and nonirradiated controls rarely exhibit the "lesion," and then only at low frequency.

Preleukemic Transition—A Late Occurring Event

As the early event of acquired hematopoietic repair sets the stage for leukemic evolution, the second major late occurring event, namely, the elicited complex of clonal dysfunctions, provides the script for the final act—overt leukemia. Virtually all preleukemic dogs that eventually progress to overt disease express one or more types of clonal dysfunction(s) of the targeted GM-progenitor population during this late transitional period (preclinical phase IV) (Seed et al., 1981). Two of the more prominent dysfunctions are (1) high-density cluster formation (small clones with restricted growth potential *in vitro*), resulting in an overall clonal pattern termed a "lawn-type" growth pattern and accompanied commonly by a marked reduction in numbers of normal GM colonies; and (2) spontaneous colony formation in the absence of exogenous colony-stimulating factor(s) (GM-CSF). Such spontaneous cloning has been observed in about one-half of cases studied to date. Presumably, its mechanism involves acquired autocrine functions (i.e., the endogenous elaboration of GM-CSF) and, in turn, self-clonal stimulation.

Oncogenetic Alterations Associated with Leukemic Transformation

A selected number of oncogenes are activated during this "late" preleukemic transitional phase. Although clearly linked in a temporal sense to the late event, causal links remain in question and need to be elucidated. Nevertheless, results of the standard NIH 3T3 cell transfection assay consistently indicate the presence of dominant-acting transforming genes, most probably of the *ras* family (Frazier et al., 1987). Further, combined Southern and Northern hybridization analyses with a standard bank of oncogene probes (including *N-ras*, *ki-ras*, *erb-b*, *myc*, *abl*, *fms*, *sis*, *scr*, *myb*) show that *N-ras* and *fms* appear consistently activated, amplified, and overexpressed.

DISCUSSION

Chronic radiation leukemogenesis, as described in this canine model, is multistaged, with four distinct preclinical phases preceding overt leukemia. The utility of the model lies in the analyses of these early preclinical responses, especially the sequential monitoring of critical hematopoietic targets (e.g., progenitor cells, hematopoietins, and stroma) within selected "high-risk" individuals. Within the preclinical sequence, two major target cell events have been identified: (1) an early "stage-setting" event involving a coupling of acquired radioresistance and renewed proliferative capacity, and (2) a late event involving the expression of a complex of aberrant clonal patterns. The characteristics and interrelationships of the events are diagrammed in Figure 2.

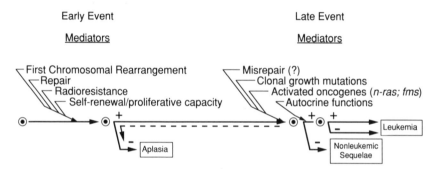

Figure 2. Schematized temporal sequence and mediators of major early and late target cell [granulocyte/monocyte (GM) progenitors in marrow] events in progression to myeloid leukemia. Effective mediator input routes symbolized by (+). Alternate pathological routes to aplastic anemia or other nonleukemic pathological sequelae are promoted by absence of appropriate mediator input symbolized by (-).

Although the temporal link between these late events is clear, the causal link is not. Several mechanisms are possible, each involving disruption of the triad of key hematopoietic elements that normally provides for functional hematopoiesis under steady-state conditions but that has gone awry under chronic irradiation.

The functional hematopoietic tissue triad consists of (1) pluripotential and lineage-committed stem cells with self-renewal capacities, (2) hematopoietins that drive progenitor populations into both proliferative and differentiative routes, and (3) the stromal network that provides the inductive ecological niche for selected hematopoietic lineages.

Myeloid leukemia may be thought of as arising from dysfunctional lineage-committed stem cells having exaggerated self-renewal capacity and, consequently, limited sensitivity to regulatory hematopoietins and thus restricted differentiative patterns. Similarly, within the preleukemic animal, the early process of acquired radioresistance (event 1) might serve to block the enhanced differentiative flow caused by daily irradiation, while simultaneously promoting the competing target cell process of self-renewal. With time, the target cell's sensitivity to external control by hematopoietin would diminish as self-renewal is enhanced, with promotion of clonal dysregulation as the consequence (event 2). In sum, the latter proposed transitional mechanism between the two target cell events is a caricature of the overt leukemic syndrome.

Because of the nature and timing of these target cell events, one might speculate that perhaps in the natural evolution of the leukemic syndrome, normal endoregulatory controls (e.g., internal regulation of self-renewal versus differentiative pathways following cell division) are first dysregulated before the advent of exoregulatory dysfunctions (e.g., gain of autocrine functions) (von Wangenheim, 1987).

It is uncertain whether oncogenes are involved in the expression of these preclinical target cell events. Clearly, during the overt leukemic phase, selected oncogenes (e.g., N-ras and fms) appear consistently rearranged [evidenced by tumor-specific restriction fragment-length polymorphisms (RFLP)], amplified, and overexpressed. However, we might speculate that selected oncogenes such as N-ras and fms with their respective gene products, GTP-binding protein and CSF surface receptor, and their well-recognized respective endo- and exoregulatory roles in cell function might well be involved in both the expression and sequence of these major preclinical target cell events (Bishop, 1987; Metcalf, 1986).

In the proposed event-linking mechanism involving disruption of endo- and exoregulatory processes, acquired radioresistance serves only to raise the radiation threshold for induced differentiative flow by targeted progenitors. We consider it likely that acquired radioresistance is involved in additional ways. For example, acquired radioresistance is mediated, in part, by altered cellular and molecular repair processes. The latter processes appear analogous to the "SOS" repair systems of prokaryotes, which serve to rescue otherwise lethally irradiated organisms but with the consequence of a greatly increased rate of mutational transformations (Witkin, 1975). Similar mammalian systems have been reported but remain poorly defined (Hart et al., 1978). In our canine model, repair processes that mediate radioresistance are esssentially constitutive in nature and clearly not error free, as indicated by the tendency of progenitors bearing such repairing systems to transform. With constant priming of the acquired repair system by continuous daily irradiation, repair-related errors in the target cell genome most likely accumulate with time, resulting in increased numbers of viable mutations, some of which probably manifest themselves in the altered clonal patterns of the transitional preleukemia phase (IV).

CONCLUSIONS

The early stage-setting event of evolving chronic radiation-induced myeloid leukemia in dogs involves a coupling of acquired radioresistance and renewed proliferative capacity by targeted GM-lineage-committed stem cells. Acquisition of modified repair functions provides, in part, the cellular basis of acquired radioresistance; the underlying genetic mechanism might involve a first chromosomal rearrangement. Such coupling of vital, endoregulatory stem cell processes and the apparently permissive but operative exoregulatory feedback controls by GM-specific hematopoietin allow for effective selection and outgrowth of aberrant clones under continuous radiation exposure.

Early occurring processes evolve, giving rise to an aberrant clonal complex—the "late event." A major component of the complex involves the loss of exoregulatory controls of clonal growth by specific hematopoietin (GM-CSA) and is temporally associated with the activation of several proto-oncogenes (e.g., *fms*, *N-ras*) with well-recognized endoregulatory cell functions, thus perhaps allowing for unrestricted clonal expansion in the absence of the normal concert of exoregulatory/endoregulatory growth controls.

Continued exploitation of this canine model of chronic radiation leukemogenesis promises to yield not only the identification of key cellular/molecular events within key hematopoietic target cells, but also their temporal patterns of occurrence on a realistic time scale.

ACKNOWLEDGMENT

This work was supported by the U.S. Department of Energy under Contract No. W-31-109-ENG-38.

REFERENCES

BEIR (National Research Council Committee on the Biological Effects of Ionizing Radiation). 1980. Leukemia, pp. 398-431. In: *The Effects on Populations of Exposure to Low Levels of Ionizing Radiation*. National Academy Press, Washington, DC.

Bishop, JM. 1987. The molecular genetics of cancer. Science 235:305-311.

Frazier, ME, TM Seed, LL Scott, and GL Stiegler. 1987. Radiation-induced carcinogenesis in dogs, pp. 488-493. In: *Radiation Research*, EM Fielden et al. (eds.). Taylor and Francis, London.

Hart, RW, KY Hall, and FB Daniel. 1978. DNA repair and mutagenesis in mammalian cells. Photochem Photobiol 28:131-155.

Kaspar, LV and TM Seed. 1984. CFU-GM colony-enhancing activity in sera of dogs under acute and chronic gamma-irradiation regimens. Acta Haematol 71:189-197.

Metcalf, D. 1986. The molecular biology and functions of the granulocyte-macrophage colony-stimulating factors. Blood 67:257-267.

Seed, TM and LV Kaspar. 1988. Acquired radioresistance of CFU-GM during chronic radiation leukemogenesis. Exp Hematol 16:523.

Seed, TM, LV Kaspar, DV Tolle, and TE Fritz. 1986a. Chronic radiation leukemogenesis: Postnatal hematopathologic effects resulting from *in utero* irradiation. Leuk Res 11:171-179.

Seed, TM, LV Kaspar, and D Grdina. 1986b. Hematopoietic repair modifications during preclinical phases of chronic radiation-induced myeloproliferative disease. Exp Hematol 14:443.

Seed, TM, LV Kaspar, TE Fritz, and DV Tolle. 1985. Cellular responses in chronic radiation leukemogenesis, pp. 363-379. In: *The Role of Chemicals and Radiation in the Etiology of Cancer*, E Huberman and SH Barr (eds.). Raven Press, New York, NY.

Seed, TM, LV Kaspar, DV Tolle, and TE Fritz. 1982. Hematologic predisposition and survival time under continuous gamma irradiation: Responses mediated by altered radiosensitivity of hemopoietic progenitors. Exp Hematol 10:232-248.

Seed, TM, SM Cullen, LV Kaspar, DV Tolle, and TE Fritz. 1980. Hemopathological consequences of protracted gamma irradiation: Alterations in granulocyte reserves and granulocyte mobilization. Blood 56:42-51.

Seed, TM, LV Kaspar, DV Tolle, CM Poole, and TE Fritz. 1981. Clonal growth patterns of granulocyte progenitors from beagle dogs with myeloid leukemia. Exp Hematol 9:68.

von Wangenheim, KH. 1987. Cell death through differentiation. Potential immortality of somatic cells: A failure in control of differentiation, pp. 130-159. In: *Perspectives on Mammalian Cell Death*, CS Potten (ed.). Oxford University Press, Oxford.

Witkin, EM. 1975. Elevated mutability of polA and uvr polA and uvr pol A derivates of *Escherichia coli* B/r at sublethal doses of ultraviolet light: Evidence for an ultraviolet error-prone repair system (SOS repair) and its anomalous expression in these strains. Genetics 79:199-213.

QUESTIONS AND COMMENTS

Q: Eastmond, Lawrence Livermore National Laboratory
What are the survival rate and the leukemia incidence rate for the dogs that develop aplastic anemia?

A: At the dose rate of 7.5 cGy/day (as used in these studies), the incidence of early deaths from aplastic anemia is ~60%, whereas the incidence of myeloid leukemia occurring in the long-surviving, leukemia-prone animals is ~20%. The remaining ~20% of the long-surviving animals die of nonleukemic pathologies.

Q: Are these myeloid leukemias acute or chronic?

A: The vast majority of these leukemias are of the acute type, with a pronounced preleukemic phase.

Q: What advantages does the dog model have over rodent models for leukemia?

A: Our canine model offers the unique and chief advantage over comparable rodent models (CBA or RF mouse models) in terms of a serial assessment of hematopoietic tissue structure and function over a given time course of exposure. The small size of the mouse precludes such serial assessments, thus necessitating serial sacrifice-type protocols that clearly present problems in sorting out critical preclinical events in individuals with differential susceptibilities to given radiation-induced hematopathologies (e.g., aplastic anemia versus myeloid leukemia).

FETAL PULMONARY DEVELOPMENT IN THE RAT: EFFECT OF CHEMICAL MIXTURES ON CELLULAR MORPHOLOGY AND GROWTH FACTORS*

T. J. Mast, R. L. Rommereim, J. R. Coleman, and F. C. Leung

Pacific Northwest Laboratory, P. O. Box 999, Richland, WA 99352

Key words: *PAH, teratogeny, pulmonary hypoplasia, EGF, TGF-α*

ABSTRACT

Complex mixtures (CM) containing polynuclear aromatic hydrocarbons (PAH) have been shown to be teratogenic in rats and mice when administered by inhalation, oral, or dermal routes. The major fetal abnormalities induced by gestational exposure to CM were pulmonary hypoplasia (the most frequent), cleft palate, edema, cutaneous syndactyly, and subcutaneous hemorrhage in the sagittal suture area. Because growth factors and their receptors are intimately involved in regulating the developmental processes, we examined the temporal sequence of the expression of several growth factors and their receptors in developing fetal lung tissue. Time-pregnant (2-hr matings) Sprague-Dawley rats were dermally exposed to CM or to a vehicle control (acetone). Groups of dams were serially sacrificed on 16-22 days of gestation (dg). Using immunocytochemical techniques, fetal lung sections were assayed for epidermal growth factor (EGF), EGF receptor (EGFR), bombesin, and transforming growth factor (TGF-α). The level of expression of EGF and TGF-α in fetal lung tissue, as well as the temporal sequence of their expression, were significantly altered by gestational exposure to CM. The early expression of both EGF and TGF-α was delayed by treatment with CM, and EGF showed a significant level of expression late in development which was not present in control fetal lungs. Thus, it appears that the fetal pulmonary hypoplasia following gestational exposure to CM either results from, or is closely correlated to, alterations in growth-factor expression.

INTRODUCTION

Coal-derived liquids (complex mixtures, CM) have been shown to be teratogenic to pregnant rats or mice when administered by either inhalation, oral, or dermal routes (Hackett et al., 1985; Hackett and Rommereim, 1986). Subsequent studies on the chemical class fractions of this mixture,

---

*This work was supported by the U.S. DOE under Contract No. DE-AC06-76RLO 1830.

obtained by liquid chromatography, showed that the teratogenic activity resided almost entirely in the polynuclear aromatic hydrocarbon fraction (Mast et al., 1987). Although a variety of major malformations resulted from exposure to these materials, the most prevalent was pulmonary hypoplasia (Figure 1). This malformation has also been reported in the offspring of rats exposed to cigarette smoke during pregnancy (Collins et al., 1985). Ultrastructural examination of the hypoplastic lungs at various times during the course of development and comparison with electron micrographs of corresponding control fetal lungs showed that gestational exposure to CM resulted in precocious differentiation and maturation of the fetal lung alveolar tissue. This early maturation occurred in the absence of adequate pulmonary growth; however, mesenchymal tissue continued to proliferate, which resulted in very thick and disorganized septal walls at the time of birth (Figure 2; Mast et al., 1988).

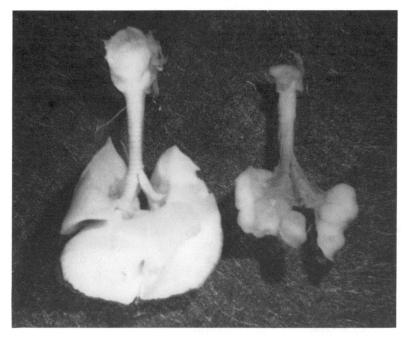

Figure 1. Fetal rat lungs at 20 days of gestation (dg). Left: fetal lung from control animal; right: hypoplastic fetal lung after *in utero* exposure to coal-derived complex mixture (CM).

The precocious differentiation of the hypoplastic lungs and the continued proliferation of the mesenchymal tissue indicated that gestational exposure to CM may have caused altered expression of the growth factors that regulate cellular differentiation and maturation. To determine if this was the case, the expression of three growth factors and one growth-factor receptor was evaluated in the lungs of rat fetuses, control and treated, during the course of development. Because the administration of triamcinolone (TAC), a synthetic glucocorticoid, during pregnancy has also been shown to cause fetal pulmonary hypoplasia (Mast et al., 1988), another group of dams was treated with this compound, and the lungs of their fetuses were evaluated for growth-factor expression.

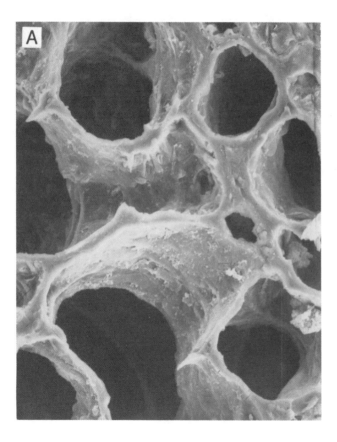

Figure 2. Scanning electron micrographs (SEM) of distal alveolar region of fetal rat lungs at 22 days of gestation (dg). A, Control. (Continued on following page.)

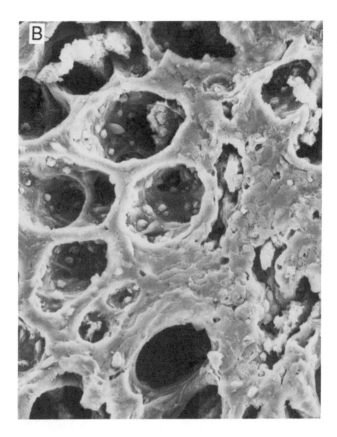

Figure 2 (continued). Scanning electron micrographs (SEM) of distal alveolar region of fetal rat lungs at 22 days of gestation (dg). B, Hypoplastic lung following *in utero* exposure to coal-derived complex mixture (CM). Note thickened septal wall and small alveoli in lung of treated fetus.

MATERIALS AND METHODS

Timed-pregnant (2-hr matings) Sprague-Dawley rats were dermally exposed to CM in acetone (500 mg/kg in a constant dosing volume of 1 ml/kg) or to a vehicle control (acetone; 1 ml/kg) on days 11 to 14 of gestation (dg). Another group of animals were injected intramuscularly with TAC (0.25 mg/kg). Groups of dams were sacrificed daily from 15 to 22 dg; the fetal lungs were perfused *in situ* with 10% neutral-buffered formalin and fixed in paraffin blocks. Paraffin sections were then evaluated for expression of EGF, EGF receptor (EGFR), bombesin, and transforming growth factor-α (TGF-α), using immunocytochemical techniques. The results are presented as the mean "stain intensity" observed for each growth factor or receptor. The intensity of the stain for each lung was graded qualitatively and assigned a number between 0 and 4. The responses were averaged for each litter, and the mean response per litter was calculated for each experimental group. The number of litters per data point, 1 to 3, was too small to permit statistical analyses.

RESULTS AND DISCUSSION

Epidermal growth-factor expression was observed in mesenchymal cells, but not in the columnar epithelial cells in both treated and control lungs (Figures 3A and 3B). The EGF expression in the mesenchyme of control fetal lungs was detected on 15 and 16 dg and at a lower level on 21 dg. Gestational exposure to either TAC or CM altered both the intensity and the temporal sequence of EGF expression in the fetal lung. Exposure to CM caused a decrease in the expression of EGF on 15 dg relative to that of the controls. However, the expression of EGF in treated lungs was nearly equivalent to that of controls on 16 dg, and exceeded that of controls by 20 dg. Beginning on 19 dg, there was a continual rise in EGF expression

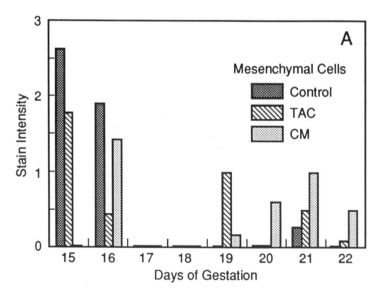

Figure 3A. Response to immunocytochemical staining for epidermal growth factor (EGF) in fetal lung mesenchymal cells, and in columnar epithelial cells. Amount of EGF present is directly proportional to stain intensity.

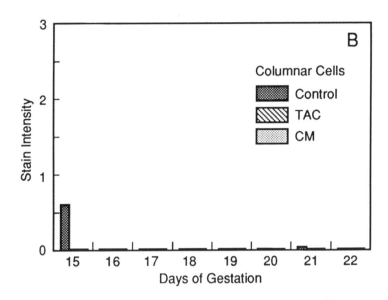

Figure 3B. Response to immunocytochemical staining for epidermal growth factor (EGF) in fetal lung mesenchymal cells, of untreated (control) fetuses and fetuses after *in utero* exposure to triamacinolone (TAC) or complex mixture (CM). Amount of EGF present is directly proportional to stain intensity.

in the treated fetuses through the end of gestation, 22 dg. In the case of TAC, the 16-dg EGF expression was depressed with respect to the control lungs; however, a significant level of expression was observed on 19 dg. The late EGF expression (21 dg) in TAC-treated lungs was similar to the EGF expression in the control lungs.

Preliminary evaluation of fetal pulmonary EGFR expression following gestational exposure to CM or TAC indicated that the level of expression of the receptor was affected less than the expression of EGF (Figure 4). Further evaluation of these slides will enable us to localize expression to either the mesenchymal or epithelial tissue. Bombesin, the nonmammalian peptide hormone homologous to gastrin-releasing peptide, was expressed in mesenchymal cells from 15 to 18 dg and in columnar cells on 15 and 16 dg (Figures 5A and 5B). Expression of this peptide in fetal lungs, although relatively intense, was variable, and definitive statements as to treatment-related effects are not possible.

Expression of the growth factor TGF-α was maximal in control fetal lungs on 15 and 16 dg and, as with EGF, was found primarily in mesenchymal tissue (Figure 6). Gestational exposure of the fetuses to either CM or TAC considerably altered both the temporal sequence and the magnitude of TGF-α expression. Gestational exposure to CM or TAC had similar effects on both EGF and TGF-α expression on 15 and 16 dg; both toxicants appeared to reduce the overall quantity of the growth factors, and CM appeared to delay the onset of expression. However, effects of the toxicants on the levels of these two growth factors late in gestation differed. There was little or no detectable TGF-α on 20 through 22 dg in the lungs of either treated or untreated fetuses; however, the late expression of EGF was substantial on 20 through 22 dg. Mesenchymal tissue in the lungs of fetuses exposed to either toxicant exhibited a distinct expression of both growth factors on 19 dg that was not present in control fetuses. Although it has been reported that EGF and TGF-α have substantial structural homology and bind to the same receptor (Nexo et al., 1980; Twardzik et al., 1982), the results from our study indicate that their expression during development differs considerably, especially late in gestation.

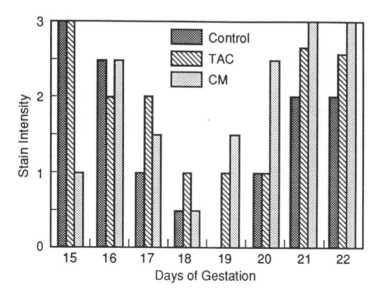

Figure 4. Response to immunocytochemical staining of fetal lungs for epidermal growth-factor receptor (EGFR) from fetuses of untreated dams (control), and following *in utero* exposure to triamacinolone (TAC) or complex mixture (CM). Amount of EGFR present is directly proportional to stain intensity.

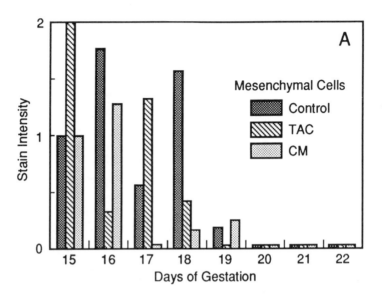

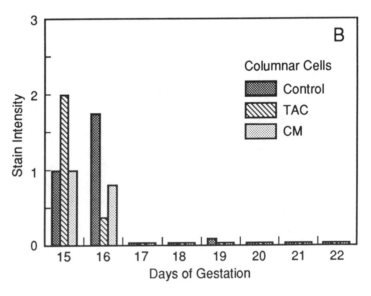

Figure 5. Response to immunocytochemical staining for bombesin in fetal lung mesenchymal cells (A), and in columnar epithelial cells (B), of untreated (control) fetuses, and fetuses after *in utero* exposure to triamacinolone (TAC) or complex mixture (CM). Amount of bombesin present is directly proportional to stain intensity.

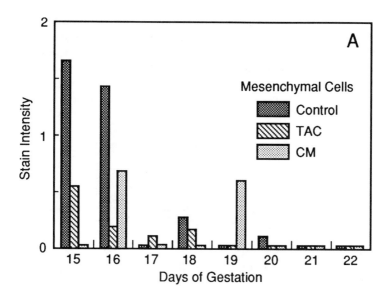

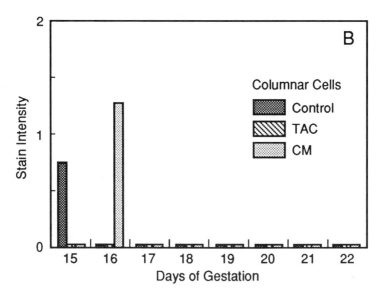

Figure 6. Response to immunocytochemical staining for transforming growth factor-α (TGF-α) in fetal lung mesenchymal cells (A), and in columnar epithelial cells (B), of untreated (control) fetuses, and fetuses after *in utero* exposure to triamacinolone (TAC) or complex mixture (CM). Amount of TGF-α present is directly proportional to stain intensity.

In summary, it appears that the fetal pulmonary hypoplasia following gestational exposure to either CM or TAC results from, or may be closely correlated to, alterations in growth-factor expression. Furthermore, because the altered growth-factor expression that followed exposure to CM differed from the alterations in expression following gestational exposure to TAC, it may be conjectured that the mechanisms of action of these two toxicants are dissimilar. The results of this study will be used as the basis for further inquiry into the molecular mechanisms regulating fetal pulmonary development during normal and abnormal development.

REFERENCES

Collins, MH, AC Moessinger, J Kleinerman, J Bassi, P Rosso, AM Collins, LS James, and WA Blanc. 1985. Fetal lung hypoplasia associated with maternal smoking: A morphometric analysis. Pediatr Res 19:408-412.

Hackett, PL and RL Rommereim. 1986. Teratology of complex mixtures, pp. 61-62. In: *Pacific Northwest Laboratory Annual Report for 1985 to the Department of Energy Office of Energy Research, Pt. 1, Biomedical Sciences*, PNL-5750. NTIS, Springfield, VA.

Hackett, PL, DD Mahlum, and RL Rommereim. 1985. Teratology of complex mixtures, pp. 59-63. In: *Pacific Northwest Laboratory Annual Report for 1985 to the Department of Energy Office of Energy Research, Pt. 1, Biomedical Sciences*, PNL-5500. NTIS, Springfield, VA.

Mast, TJ, RL Rommereim, and JS Young. 1988. Molecular control of lung development, pp. 67-70. In: *Pacific Northwest Laboratory Annual Report for 1985 to the Department of Energy Office of Energy Research, Pt. 1, Biomedical Sciences*, PNL-6500. NTIS, Springfield, VA.

Mast, TJ, PL Hackett, RL Rommereim, and DL Springer. 1987. Teratology of complex mixtures, pp. 65-69. In: *Pacific Northwest Laboratory Annual Report for 1985 to the Department of Energy Office of Energy Research, Pt. 1, Biomedical Sciences*, PNL-6100. NTIS, Springfield, VA.

Nexo, E, MD Hollenberg, A Figuero, and RM Pratt. 1980. Detection of EGF-urogastrone and its receptor during fetal mouse development. Proc Natl Acad Sci USA 77:2782-2785.

Twardzik, DR, JE Ranchalis, and GJ Todaro. 1982. Mouse embryonic transforming growth factors related to those isolated from tumor cells. Cancer Res 42:590-593.

QUESTIONS AND COMMENTS

Q: Gantt, NCI

    Do the late stages of treated lungs resemble in any way aged lung tissue?

A: I don't know.

ETHYLNITROSOUREA-INDUCED GROWTH INHIBITION AND CELL CYCLE PERTURBATIONS IN MICROMASS CULTURES OF RAT EMBRYONIC MIDBRAIN CELLS

P.L. Ribeiro[1] and E.M. Faustman[2]

[1]Departments of Environmental Health and Pathology, University of Washington, Seattle, WA 98195

[2]Department of Environmental Health, and Child Development and Mental Retardation Center, University of Washington, Seattle, WA 98195

Key words: *Embryonic, cell cycle, teratogen, ethylnitrosourea*

ABSTRACT

Ethylnitrosourea (ENU) is a proven animal teratogen, but the mechanism of its toxicity is unknown. The micromass rat embryo midbrain (CNS) culture system was applied in an effort to determine the mechanism by which ENU exerts its teratogenic effect. When cultivated at high cell densities, rat CNS cells undergo several rounds of replication while organizing and differentiating into discrete foci containing neuronal cells. Neuronal differentiation was monitored after 5 days in culture by staining the differentiated foci with hematoxylin. The objectives of this study were to: (1) define the population kinetics of the micromass culture system (cellular proliferation, cell cycle compartmentation, and differentiation); and (2) determine how ENU disrupts the normal growth and differentiation of these cultures. Studies with this culture system have demonstrated concentration-dependent decreases in cell attachment and viability within the first 24 hr after the addition of ENU to the medium. Exposed cultures have also exhibited significant growth inhibition as determined by cell counts. Cell cycle analysis of these affected cultures has revealed an accumulation of cells in late G_1/early S phase. Our examination of the cultures suggests that the ultimate effects of ENU on neuronal differentiation are related to both its early effects on cell attachment and its effects on proliferation.

INTRODUCTION

During the past two decades, numerous culture techniques have been developed and applied to the study of normal developmental biology as well as to developmental toxicity (Neubert, 1982; Kochhar, 1975, 1982; Shepard et al., 1983; Faustman, 1988). As Neubert (1982) stated, if a test system is to be applicable to the study of developmental toxicity it must be able to mimic certain processes that occur during embryonic/fetal development. Even though no *in vitro* system to date has been able to mimic the entire developmental process, a given culture system can nevertheless serve as a useful model for certain aspects of prenatal development. In particular, cultures derived from embryonic tissues have yielded considerable information when applied to the definition of basic mechanisms of normal development and developmentally toxic action.

The micromass cell culture method for rat embryonic neural cells (CNS) developed by Flint (1983), an adaptation of the culture method presented by Umansky (1966) and Ahrens et al. (1977), has received much attention in recent years. When cultured for 5 days under conditions of high cell density, embryonic CNS cells organize into discrete cell masses, proliferate, and ultimately differentiate into foci of neuronal cells that stain differentially with hematoxylin. Neuronal differentiation has been confirmed using a variety of histological (silver staining, neuronal cell morphology) and biochemical (^{3}H-γ-aminobutyric acid uptake, expression of neuronal ganglioside) end points (Flint, 1983, 1986; Flint et al., 1984).

In previous validation studies using both known teratogens and nonteratogens, Flint and his coworkers combined the CNS micromass cell culture with a similar culture for limb bud cells (LB) into a test system with a high success rate in predicting teratogenic potential (Flint and Orton, 1984; Flint et al., 1984). In one study in which the cultures were derived from embryos exposed transplacentally to 18 known teratogens, 17 compounds caused inhibition of *in vitro* differentiation (Flint et al., 1984). When both culture systems were used in a wholly *in vitro* application (the agent was added directly to the culture medium), 85% and 90% of the known teratogens inhibited differentiation in the CNS and LB cultures, respectively (Flint and Orton, 1984). When results from both systems were considered, 25 of the 27 teratogens and only 2 of the 19 known nonteratogens inhibited differentiation in either system. For the study of agents that require metabolic activation, Brown et al. (1986) demonstrated that the embryonic cell cultures have the potential to metabolize xenobiotics as indicated by the presence of cytochromes P-450. Studies by Faustman and Flint (1988) used this culture system to examine the role of glutathione modulation in the developmental toxicity of chlorambucil and niridazole.

Ethylnitrosourea (ENU) is a proven animal carcinogen and teratogen. Depending on the developmental stage at which it is administered transplacentally (Druckery, 1973), this chemical is capable of producing CNS tumors or a number of teratogenic effects that include the CNS system

(Diwan, 1974; Alexandrov and Napalkov, 1976; Ivankovic and Druckery, 1968). Much effort has been devoted to studying the mechanism of carcinogenicity of this and related compounds (Goth and Rajewsky, 1974; Veleminsky et al., 1970; Loveless, 1969), but much less attention has been directed to the actual mechanism(s) of its developmental toxicity. In our study, the micromass rat embryonic midbrain culture system was used to understand further the effects of ENU on susceptible embryonic cell populations. The objectives of our study were to: (1) define the population kinetics of the micromass culture system (cellular proliferation, cell cycle dynamics and differentiation); and (2) determine how ENU disrupts these processes.

MATERIALS AND METHODS

Pregnant (12.5-day post-coitum) Sprague-Dawley albino rats (Tyler Laboratories, Bellevue, WA) were used as the source of embryos for these experiments. All tissue culture reagents [Earle's balanced salt solution (EBSS), heat-inactivated horse serum, fetal bovine serum, Ham's F-12, calcium- and magnesium-free EBSS (CMF-EBSS), Dulbecco's phosphate buffered saline (DPBS), streptomycin, penicillin, and L-glutamine] were obtained from Life Technologies, Staten Island, NY (Gibco). Trypsin (1:250) was obtained from DIFCO Labs, Detroit, MI.

Cell Isolation and Culture Conditions

The rats were killed and the gravid uteri obtained aseptically. Cell cultures were prepared according to Flint (1983). Briefly, the embryos were removed in 50% solution (v/v) of EBSS/horse serum and the midbrains collected. After several washes in CMF-EBSS, the tissues were incubated in a fresh volume of the same solution at 37°C for 20 min. After this incubation, the CMF-EBSS was removed and replaced with 1% trypsin (w/v) in CMF-EBSS. After another 20-min incubation at 37°C, the trypsin was removed and the tissues washed with complete culture medium [CM; F-12 Ham's supplemented with 10% fetal bovine serum, penicillin (50 IU/ml), streptomycin (5 μg/ml), and L-glutamine (5.8 mg/ml)]. A fresh volume of CM was added to the tissues, which were dissociated by gentle trituration through a 0.7-mm-bore (i.d.) Pasteur pipet. The resultant cell suspension was then passed through a 10-μm nylon mesh to remove cell clumps. The cell density of the single-cell suspension was determined with a hemacytometer and adjusted to a final cell density of 5×10^6 cells/ml. The cells were plated as five 10-μl aliquots per 35-mm-diameter plastic culture dish

(Primaria, Falcon, Becton Dickinson Labware, Lincoln Park, NJ). The cultures were incubated at 37°C in a 5% CO_2/95% air atmosphere with 100% relative humidity for 2 hr to allow for cell attachment. After this attachment period, CM (with or without test compound) was added to a final volume of 2 ml. Cultures were maintained until analysis in this medium, according to the conditions previously described.

Exposure Conditions

A working stock solution of ENU (20 mg/ml) was prepared in 0.1 M sodium acetate buffer, pH 6.5, immediately before use. Dilutions were made from this working stock in the same buffer, with the final dilution occurring in the prewarmed and CO_2-equilibrated culture medium. Appropriate vehicle controls were included, and all cultures received the same concentration of vehicle (0.5 mM sodium acetate). Because ENU is labile at physiological pH, the final dilution into culture medium was followed immediately by addition of the solution to culture dishes. Each dilution into culture medium was added to dishes before the next stock was added to culture medium. Exposure occurred after the 2-hr attachment period, and cells were cultured until analysis. Because it is hazardous, ENU was weighed in a glove box, and all dilutions were made in closed containers in a safety hood. All containers, pipets, and stock solutions were inactivated with saturated sodium hydroxide and neutralized before disposal or washing.

Cell Counts/Growth Studies

On days 1, 2, and 5, the cultures were harvested using a dilute trypsin/EDTA solution (0.05%/0.02%, respectively, in calcium-/magnesium-free PBS). As the cultures matured over the course of the 5 days, the time in this solution had to be increased slightly. This treatment produced a uniform, single-cell suspension that was then counted using a hemacytometer. An aliquot of cells was diluted 1:1 with an isotonic 0.4% trypan blue stain (Sigma Chemical Co., St. Louis, MO), and the percentage of viable cells was determined by dye exclusion using a light microscope.

Cell Cycle Analysis

At days 1, 2, and 5, cultures were harvested as described and the cells collected by centrifugation. The cell pellets were washed with 0.5 ml of DPBS and resuspended in 0.2 ml of DPBS containing 1% dimethyl sulfoxide. Cells were frozen at -70°C until all samples of an experiment were accumulated. Immediately before analysis, the cells were quickly thawed in a 37°C waterbath, 0.4 ml of 4,6-diamidino-2-phenyl indole (DAPI) (Accurate Chem. Co., Westbury, NY), 10 μg/ml in Tris saline, pH 7.4, containing 0.1% NP-40 (Sigma Chemical Co., St. Louis, MO) was added, and a nuclear suspension was prepared by passing the mixture through a 25-gauge needle five times. Cell cycle analysis was performed using a Phywe ICP-22 flow cytometer (Ortho Diagnostic Systems, Westwood, MA) coupled with a Digital DEC PDP 11/23 Computer (Digital Equipment Co., Maynard, MA), according to the method of Koch et al. (1984). The DAPI fluorescence emission (λ_{em}:400-600 nm) was monitored using a long band-pass filter after illumination at λ_{ex} 365 nm. The data were fitted to the Multicycle program (written by Dr. Peter S. Rabinovitch, Phoenix Flow Systems, San Diego, CA).

Staining/Differentiation

At selected times, cultures were fixed and stained according to the method described by Flint (1983). Briefly, after aspiration of the medium, the cultures were fixed in 10% formaldehyde for 20 min at room temperature. The fixative was removed, and the cells were rinsed with tap water. Cells were stained for 1 min with Delafield's hematoxylin (Carolina Biological Supply, Burlington, NC), washed with tap water, and air-dried.

Statistical Analysis

The cell count data (Figures 1 and 3) were subjected to a one-way ANOVA (Duncan's test for significance) (Number Cruncher Statistical System, Version 2.1, Dr. Jerry L. Hintze, Kaysville, UT). Ordered χ^2 analysis was performed on the trypan blue viability data (Figure 2) and the cell cycle data (Figure 4) (Everitt, 1977). The level of significance used for all these evaluations was $p \leq 0.05$.

RESULTS

Figure 1 shows the plating efficiency for the CNS cultures. Cells of the control cultures exhibited an attachment efficiency of 43% (± 12.3%) (mean ± 1 SD) at 24 hr after plating. Figure 1 also shows that ENU treatment produced a concentration-dependent reduction in attachment efficiency in which the value for the highest concentration used was 40% of that for the untreated control cultures.

Figure 2 shows total cell viability (attached and detached cells) as determined by trypan blue exclusion at 24 hr after exposure. Cell viability decreased in a concentration-dependent manner ($p < 0.05$, χ^2 test), primarily because of the large number of detached cells. Viability of detached cells ranged from 70% for untreated cultures to 40% for cells in the highest treatment group (854 μM) (data not shown).

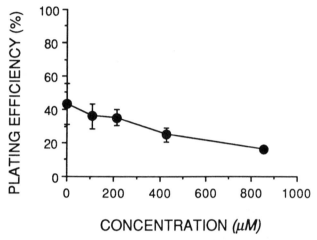

Figure 1. Effect of ethylnitrosourea (ENU) on plating efficiency of CNS cells. At 24 hr after exposure, cultures were washed and attached cells were dissociated with trypsin/EDTA, harvested, and counted. Plating efficiency was determined as a percentage of the total number of cells plated at day 0. Each point represents average of three experiments.

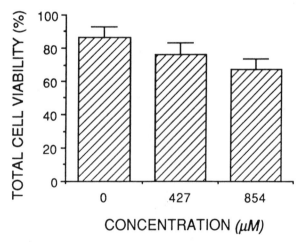

Figure 2. Effect of ethylnitrosourea (ENU) on total cell viability at 24 hr after exposure. Both floating and attached cells were harvested; viability was determined by trypan blue exclusion.

During days 2 to 5, the untreated cells underwent two to three cell dou-blings (Figure 3). A significant concentration-dependent decrease in cell number at all days after exposure was seen for ENU-treated cells at the two highest treatment groups (427 and 854 μM) ($p \leq 0.01$, Duncan's test). At 427 μM, a sharp initial reduction in cell number was evident with no further increases in cell number during culture. At the highest dose (854 μM), overt cell death was indicated by a steady decrease in cell number during the 5-day culture period.

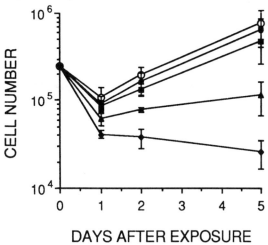

Figure 3. Effect of ethylnitrosourea (ENU) on the growth of CNS micromass cultures. During the 5-day culture period, cultures were dissociated with trypsin/EDTA and cells harvested and counted. Symbols: 0 μM, $\bigcirc$; 107 μM, $\bullet$; 213 μM, $\blacksquare$; 427 μM, $\blacktriangle$; 854 μM, $\blacklozenge$.

Cell cycle analysis was performed with DAPI-stained DNA in a nuclear suspension. The fluorescence of the DAPI/DNA complex is directly propor-tional to the amount of DNA present in the nucleus, thereby enabling one to determine the location in the cell cycle for each cell (cells in G_2 and M phases have as much as twice the amount of DNA as cells in G_0/G_1). Figure 4 shows the percentage of total cells in each cell cycle stage during 5 days of culture. A gradual accumulation of cells in the G_0/G_1 compartment (54% ± 10%, day 1; 78% ± 1.6%, day 5) ($p < 0.05$, χ^2 test) appeared to occur at the expense of the S and G_2 + M compartments, because both decreased during this time.

When the cells from the two most severely affected cultures, 427 and 854 μM, were submitted for cell cycle analysis, an extra peak that was evident at 2 days after exposure suggested a cell cycle block in late G_1/early

S phases. Figure 5 shows a representative series of cell cycle profiles illustrating the concentration-dependent nature of this extra peak ($p < 0.05$). The appearance of these peaks corresponded with the onset of cellular proliferation in the cultures (see Figure 3) and with parallel decreases in the S-phase compartments. The percentage of total cells arrested at the G_1/S border is shown for each treatment. The appearance of these arrested cells was transitory: they were not usually present at day 5 if they were evident at day 2.

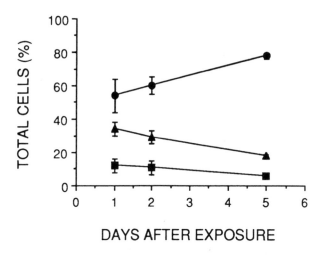

DAYS AFTER EXPOSURE

Figure 4. Cell cycle kinetics of untreated cultures during 5-day culture period. At times shown, cells were harvested for flow cytometric cell cycle analysis after staining nuclei with 4,6-diamidino-2-phenyl indole (DAPI). Changes that occur in each cell cycle compartment during 5-day culture period are seen. Each point represents the average of six separate experiments. Symbols: G_1, ●; S, ▲; G_2 + M, ■.

As shown in Figure 6, the cells in the unexposed cultures initially aggregated into discrete cell bundles or pre-foci (day 1), which then proliferated (days 2 to 5) and eventually differentiated into foci of neuronal cells that stain preferentially with hematoxylin. Figure 7 shows a comparison of the fixed and stained cultures of ENU-exposed cells and visually demonstrates ENU-induced inhibition of both cell growth and differentiation. The effects of ENU on neuronal cell differentiation, as monitored by the presence of stained foci, parallel the results of the cell count data.

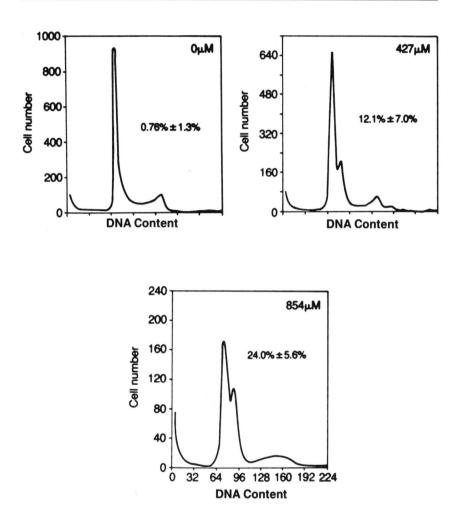

Figure 5. Cell cycle kinetics of ethylnitrosourea- (ENU-) exposed cultures analyzed by 4,6-diamidino-2-phenyl indole (DAPI) flow cytometry. Values given for each treatment concentration represent percentage of total number of cells arrested at the G_1/S border in each culture ($\bar{x} \pm$ SD) and are averages of at least four experiments. Representative cell cycle profiles are shown for control, and for 427 μM and 854 μM ENU-exposed cell cultures.

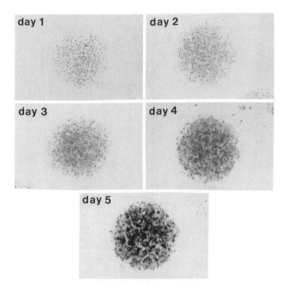

Figure 6. Staining pattern in fixed and hematoxylin-stained control cultures from each of 5 days in culture reveals progressive changes that resulted from cellular proliferation and neuronal differentiation. Note appearance of densely stained neuronal foci at days 4 and 5.

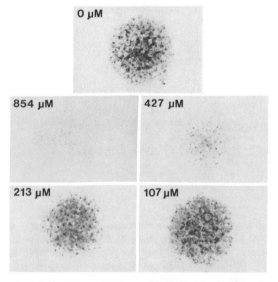

Figure 7. Effect of ethylnitrosourea (ENU) on differentiation of CNS micromass cultures. Both untreated and treated cultures were maintained for 5 days, then washed, fixed, and stained. Photograph demonstrates strong concentration-dependent reduction in number of differentiated foci as well as total cell number present in cultures at day 5.

DISCUSSION

One aim of this project was to characterize the CNS micromass culture in terms of cell growth, cell cycle kinetics, and differentiation during a 5-day culture period. Within the first 24 hr after plating, untreated CNS cells exhibited an average plating efficiency (percentage cell attachment per total cells plated) of 43% ± 12.3%, similar to the 30% reported by Flint (1983). In contrast to Flint's methods, we used a dilute solution of trypsin/EDTA to dissociate the cultures into a single-cell suspension that facilitated cell counting and our analysis by flow cytometry. During the 5-day culture period, the cells underwent two to three cell population doublings, increasing in cell number from 1.09×10^5 cells/dish (day 1) to 7.72×10^5 cells/dish (day 5).

The flow cytometric method of Koch et al. (1984) was employed to study the cell cycle kinetics of these cultures. In this method, the DNA dye DAPI (which specifically binds to the adenine-thymine-rich regions) was used to determine the cell cycle profile during the 5-day culture period. The cell cycle analysis demonstrated a gradual enrichment of the G_1/G_0 compartment, which increased during the culture period at the expense of the S and $G_2 + M$ compartments. We believe that this enrichment is the result of the gradual withdrawal of the CNS cells from the cell cycle as they commit to neuronal differentiation, and will try to confirm this idea with the bromodeoxyuridine/Hoechst staining method of Latt et al. (1977), which allows for a more comprehensive study of cell cycle withdrawal in cultured cells. Giaretti et al. (1988) used a similar approach to examine the cell cycle in differentiating chondrocytes.

Analysis of fixed and stained cultures during the 5-day culture period demonstrated a sequence of events that is in agreement with the observations of Flint (1983). After cell attachment, the cells organized into discrete colonies within each cell island, followed by several rounds of replication as evidenced by the expansion of the colonies. This observation concurs with the gradual increase in cell numbers from days 1 to 5. During the culture period, the cells within each colony differentiated into neurons producing discrete foci that stained intensely with hematoxylin. The appearance of the differentiated foci was consistent with the enrichment of the G_1/G_0 compartment over the same time period. Terminal differentiation of various stem cell types (epithelial, hematopoietic, muscle, and neural) is associated with the irreversible withdrawal from the cell cycle (loss of proliferative capacity) (Wier and Scott, 1986). Currently available evidence suggests that the expression of the terminally differentiated phenotypes is preceded by the growth arrest in the G_1 phase of the cell cycle (Scott et al., 1982).

The second aim of our project was to study how the cellular processes, as defined here, were affected by a known chemical teratogen, ENU. In exposed cultures, an effect was seen as early as 24 hr after exposure as a concentration-dependent decrease in plating efficiency (43%-16.4%) over the concentration range studied (0-854 μM). This decreased plating efficiency, which was especially evident at the two highest treatment groups (427 and 854 μM), was followed by a strong concentration-dependent decrease in the normal pattern of increase in cell number. At the highest dose (854 μM), overt cytotoxicity was observed.

The cell cycle analysis of the ENU-exposed cultures produced interesting findings. The cultures of the two highest treatment groups (427 and 854 μM) demonstrated a concentration-dependent arrest in the early S phase in the form of a well-defined peak appearing first at day 2. This aberrant peak appeared at the expense of the S-phase compartment, which prematurely decreased (day 2) to the levels that the control cells attained at the end of the culture period (day 5). The temporary nature of this peak is consistent with findings in the literature (Tobey et al., 1979) in that other alkylating agents, like ENU, can produce a transitory block in the S phase of the cell cycle that results from a prolongation of the DNA synthetic phase.

Examination of the fixed and hematoxylin-stained cultures (day 5) demonstrated a strong concentration-dependent inhibition of differentiation. The stained cultures also paralleled the ENU-induced inhibition on cell growth demonstrated by the cell count data. The effects of ENU exposure on these cultures can be summarized as follows: (1) during the early period of culture, ENU cytotoxicity was quite evident in the form of a concentration-dependent cellular detachment; (2) in the two highest treatment groups, the cells that remained attached showed no increase in cell number and appeared to be replicatively inactive, an observation supported by our flow cytometric studies; and (3) these findings, in conjunction with an assessment of the fixed and stained cultures, suggest that cell proliferation and differentiation in these cultures are closely associated during the developmental/differentiating process.

We believe that the micromass culture system is ideally suited for the study of the molecular and cellular processes in normal development. In the course of this project, flow cytometry has proven to be a very useful tool, increasing our understanding of ENU-induced CNS developmental toxicity. In our continuing studies, we will, first, use flow cytometry to study the relationship between cell cycle traverse, cell cycle withdrawal, and neuronal differentiation, and the possible effects of ENU on these processes. Second, we will characterize the effects of other structurally related N-nitroso compounds in this culture system.

ACKNOWLEDGMENTS

The authors express sincere appreciation to Azure Morgan Skye, who prepared this typed document, and to Zamyat Kirby, whose critical review of this manuscript was invaluable. We thank NIEHS (ES-03157 and ES-07032) and the University of Washington, Department of Environmental Health, Industrial Hygiene Research Fund for their support. We also thank Mike Shen and Dr. Ann Adams, of the University of Washington Department of Pathology, for advice and assistance with the flow cytometric determinations.

REFERENCES

Ahrens, PB, M Solursh, and RS Reiter. 1977. Stage-related capacity for limb chondrogenesis in cell culture. Dev Biol 60:69-82.

Alexandrov, VA and NP Napalkov. 1976. Experimental study of relationship between teratogenesis and carcinogenesis in the brain of the rat. Cancer Lett 1:345-350.

Brown, LP, OP Flint, TC Orton, and GG Gibson. 1986. *In vitro* metabolism of teratogens by differentiating rat embryo cells. Food Chem Toxicol 24:737-742.

Diwan, BA. 1974. Strain-dependent teratogenic effects of 1-ethyl-1-nitrosourea in inbred strains of mice. Cancer Res 34:151-157.

Druckery, H. 1973. Specific carcinogenic and teratogenic effects of 'indirect' alkylating methyl and ethyl compounds, and their dependency on stages of teratogenic development. Xenobiotics 3:271-303.

Everitt, BS. 1977. *The Analysis of Contingency Tables.* Chapman and Hall, London.

Faustman, E.M. 1988. Short-term tests for teratogens. Mutat Res 205:355-384.

Faustman, EM and OP Flint. 1988. Developmental toxicity of niridazole and chlorambucil on limb and midbrain cells *in vitro:* Influence of glutathione modulation. Teratology 37:455.

Flint, OP. 1983. A micromass culture method for rat embryonic neural cells. J Cell Sci 61:247-262.

Flint, OP. 1986. An *in vitro* test for teratogens: Its practical application. Food Chem Toxicol 24:627-631.

Flint, OP and TC Orton. 1984. An *in vitro* assay for teratogens with cultures of rat embryo midbrain and limb bud cells. Toxicol Appl Pharmacol 76:383-395.

Flint, OP, TC Orton, and RA Ferguson. 1984. Differentiation of rat embryo cells in culture: Response following acute maternal exposure to teratogens and non-teratogens. J Appl Toxicol 4:109-116.

Giaretti, W, G Moro, R Quarto, S Bruno, A Di Vinci, E Geido, and R Cancedda. 1988. Flow cytometric evaluation of cell cycle characteristics during *in vitro* differentiation of chick embryo chondrocytes. Cytometry 9:281-290.

Goth, R and MF Rajewsky. 1974. Molecular and cellular mechanisms associated with pulse-carcinogenesis in the rat nervous system by ethylnitrosourea: Ethylation of nucleic acids and elimination rates of ethylated bases from the DNA of different tissues. Z Krebsforsch 82:37-64.

Ivankovic, S and H Druckery. 1968. Transplacental induction of malignant tumors of the nervous system. Z Krebsforsch 71:320-360.

Koch, H, T Bettecken, M Kubbies, D Salk, JW Smith, and PS Rabinovitch. 1984. Flow cytometric analysis of small DNA content differences in heterogeneous cell populations: Human amniotic fluid cells. Cytometry 5:118-123.

Kochhar, DM. 1975. The use of *in vitro* procedures in teratology. Teratology 11:273-288.

Kochhar, DM. 1982. Embryonic limb bud organ culture in assessment of teratogenicity of environmental agents. Teratog Carcinog Mutagen 2:303-313.

Latt, SA, YS George, and JW Gray. 1977. Flow cytometric analyses of bromodeoxyuridine-substituted cells stained with 33258 Hoechst. J Histochem Cytochem 25:927-934.

Loveless, A. 1969. Possible relevance of O^6 alkylation of deoxyguanosine to the mutagenicity and carcinogenicity of nitrosamines and nitrosamides. Nature 223:206-207.

Neubert, D. 1982. The use of culture techniques in studies of prenatal toxicity. Pharmacol Ther 18:397-434.

Scott, RE, DL Florine, JJ Wille, and K Yun. 1982. Coupling of growth arrest and differentiation at a distinct state in the G_1 phase of the cell cycle: G_0. Proc Natl Acad Sci USA 79:845-849.

Shepard, TH, AG Fantel, PE Mirkes, JC Greenaway, E Faustman-Watts, M Campbell, and MR Juchau. 1983. Teratology testing. Prog Clin Biol Med 135:147-164.

Tobey, RA, MS Oka, and HA Crissman. 1979. *Analysis of Effects of Chemotherapeutic Agents on Cell-Growth Kinetics in Cultured Cells.* Wiley, New York.

Neubert, D. 1982. The use of culture techniques in studies of prenatal toxicity. Pharmacol Ther 18:397-434.

Scott, RE, DL Florine, JJ Wille, and K Yun. 1982. Coupling of growth arrest and differentiation at a distinct state in the G_1 phase of the cell cycle: G_0. Proc Natl Acad Sci USA 79:845-849.

Shepard, TH, AG Fantel, PE Mirkes, JC Greenaway, E Faustman-Watts, M Campbell, and MR Juchau. 1983. Teratology testing. Prog Clin Biol Med 135:147-164.

Tobey, RA, MS Oka, and HA Crissman. 1979. *Analysis of Effects of Chemotherapeutic Agents on Cell-Growth Kinetics in Cultured Cells.* Wiley, New York.

Umansky, R. 1966. The effect of cell population density on the developmental fate of reaggregating mouse limb bud mesenchyme. Dev Biol 13:31-56.

Veleminsky, J, S Osterman-Golkar, and L Ehrenberg. 1970. Reaction rates and biological action of N-methyl- and N-ethyl-N-nitrosourea. Mutat Res 10:169-174.

Wier, ML and RE Scott. 1986. Regulation of the terminal event in cellular differentiation: Biological mechanisms of the loss of proliferative potential. J Cell Biol 102:1955-1964.

QUESTIONS AND COMMENTS

Q: Wilson, Monsanto Co.
It is well known that mutagens like ethyl nitrosourea frequently induce mutations affecting expression of *ras* and related oncogenes. A consequence of increased expression of these oncogenes is inhibition of differentiation. Have you considered looking for oncogene activation, with an eye toward relating this to the retarded differentiation seen?

A: Dr. Wilson, that's a very interesting point to bring up. As you have suggested, oncogene activation is a proven characteristic of N-nitroso compounds as well as alkylating agents in general. The idea that you propose would be quite interesting to pursue since several proto-oncogenes have demonstrated expression during different times of development in intact rat embryos. Some of these proto-oncogenes have been positively associated with cellular differentiation as well. Our new NIEHS grant is directed toward this aim.

MECHANISTIC EXPLANATIONS FOR THE ELEVATED SUSCEPTIBILITY OF THE PERINATAL THYROID GLAND TO RADIOGENIC CANCER

M. R. Sikov, D. D. Mahlum, G. E. Dagle, J. L. Daniel, and M. Goldman

Biology and Chemistry Department, Pacific Northwest Laboratory, P.O. Box 999, Richland, WA 99352

Key words: *Carcinogenesis, thyroid, perinatal irradiation, radioiodine, rats*

ABSTRACT

Results from laboratory experiments and epidemiological studies suggest that the thyroid gland is more susceptible to radiogenic cancer during the late prenatal or early postnatal periods than in adulthood. We have evaluated several end points in experiments in which rats were exposed to graded doses of ^{131}I at ages ranging from late gestation to adulthood. Morphological responses at sequential times after exposure were evaluated in one series of experiments. Cell death, degeneration, and fibrosis of the gland were the predominant findings after exposure of weanlings or adults, but inhibition of thyroid growth and differentiation was the characteristic change after perinatal exposure. Degree of maturation as well as dosimetric factors are involved in this differential morphological response, which also results in age-dependent physiological differences in the postexposure period.

It appears that these differences also play roles in the observed patterns of tumor incidence, as observed in our studies of thyroid carcinogenesis. The predominant neoplasm in control rats was the C-cell tumor; its incidence was unaffected at lower doses but decreased at higher doses in all age groups. The incidence of follicular tumors, the primary histological type in exposed animals, increased after administration of lower doses to rats of all age groups. Incidence continued to increase progressively with dose in groups exposed in the prenatal or neonatal period but decreased at higher doses in older animals.

Thyroid cell proliferation was studied more recently to examine possible amplification phenomena because other workers suggested that higher proliferation rates in the prenatal mouse thyroid gland lead to shorter tumor latency. We found that the peak of follicular cell proliferation occurred during the second week of postnatal life, although there was a proliferating population of interfollicular cells that subsequently appeared to give rise to more follicles. Combinations of age-related differences in radiogenic thyroid injury, delayed effects, and reparative processes, and their early and prolonged interactions with the thyroid-pituitary feedback processes seemed to be involved in the elevated perinatal sensitivity to thyroid tumorigenesis by radiation.

INTRODUCTION

Several early studies found that irradiation of the thyroid gland during the perinatal period could lead to increased incidences of tumors, but the sensitivity of this process relative to that in the adult was not quantified. Our subsequent studies provided data that demonstrated that the thyroid of the rat is more susceptible to the induction of cancer by exposure to ^{131}I in the late prenatal or early postnatal periods than in weanlings or during adulthood, and later provided some details of the response (Sikov et al., 1973, 1984; Sikov, 1989). In these experiments, groups of weanling and adult rats, pregnant rats at 17 days of gestation (dg), and others that were nursing newborn litters were gavaged with carrier-free ^{131}I on 5 successive days. Each age group received vehicle solution or adjusted activity ranges of three dosage levels that would produce similar spectra of subacute effects in the adult and weanling rats and in offspring. Some animals of each group were killed sequentially to measure tissue concentrations and establish dosimetry, but most were kept until spontaneous death or 30 months of age. At necropsy, the thyroid and pituitary glands were removed, and skip-serial histological sections were prepared and examined. The groups exposed at weaning or as adults showed an initial increase in overall thyroid tumor incidence in the 5- to 8-Gy dose range, but incidence decreased at higher doses as the result of marked parenchymal cell destruction. The prenatal group showed a progressive increase in incidence at all radiation doses (0.4, 4.25, and 34 Gy); the neonatal groups had an intermediate pattern. Postnatal exposure increased mammary tumor incidence, but incidence was not affected by prenatal exposure.

In contemporaneous experiments, other workers have observed comparable differences after irradiation of prenatal and adult mice with x rays, exposure to ^{131}I , or combinations of the two modalities. Walinder and Sjöden (1972) compared the carcinogenic effects of combined prenatal irradiations with radioiodine β particles and maternal x-ray exposure of CBA mice at 18 dg with those produced in noncontemporaneous experiments using adults. They found thyroid tumors produced by both types of radiation at both ages of exposure and a sharp inflection in the dose-response curves at an intermediate dose, after which the slope was markedly greater. Dose at inflection, lifetime thyroid tumor incidences at each dose level, and minimum doses for detectable incidences of thyroid tumors were lower for prenatal than adult exposures. Walinder and Sjöden (1973) subsequently used a similar design for contemporaneous exposures of fetuses and adults, but the mice were necropsied at 1 year of age to avoid losses through spontaneous deaths. No thyroid tumors were found among any group of mice exposed as adults after this relatively short interval. In contrast, tumors were detected in offspring from dams that had received the highest ^{131}I level, which resulted in a 78-Gy β dose to the perinatal thyroid, or 1.8 Gy of maternal x-irradiation plus 47 Gy of β-irradiation.

It appears that similar age-related differences in thyroid sensitivity may also pertain after clinical procedures or accidents that result in irradiation of the immature human thyroid gland with x rays or radioiodine, although the quantitative relationships are less clear. No systematic examinations of the various explanations have been offered for these age-dependent differences in the oncogenic susceptibility of the thyroid gland. This gap in our understanding led us to perform the evaluations presented here.

Dosimetric Considerations

The importance of stage of gestation on the potential for tissue localization and the resulting radiation dose has been recognized ever since Speert et al. (1951) demonstrated that ^{131}I did not concentrate in the fetal mouse thyroid gland until follicles were observable. Subsequently, investigators found a similar physiological dependence during development of the human thyroid, as well as quantitative changes during the prenatal and postnatal development of several animal species.

Many details concerning the age-dependent uptake, retention, and dosimetry of the several radioiodine isotopes have been compiled by Book (1978). It is clearly necessary to consider administered dosage, concentrations in the thyroid gland, and radiation doses as a function of time after administration when interpreting data from studies of age-dependent effects of radioiodines. As might be expected, the quantitative relationships among these factors differ with age, and tissue dose may be further affected by radiation-induced changes in the gland. We have found that rapid radionecrosis after larger ^{131}I dosages to mature rats shortened the biological half-life of ^{131}I in the thyroid so that it delivered a lower time-integrated radiation dose than did the next lower dosages administered (Sikov, 1969).

These analyses illustrate the possibility of reaching quantitatively erroneous conclusions regarding dose-response relationships unless all factors are considered. The concentrations of ^{131}I in the thyroid gland were measured at sequential times after administration in our studies on the radiation response of the thyroid relative to the prenatal or postnatal age of the rat (to be discussed). The effects were analyzed relative to the resulting radiation doses, which were calculated for each individual group in these studies. Similar dosimetric determinations were performed as part of the comparisons of carcinogenesis by prenatal and adult exposures of mice to x rays and/or [131]I. Accordingly, major errors in the expressions of average radiation doses to the thyroid do not appear to be an important consideration in the observed age-related differences in the organ's oncogenic susceptibility.

A potentially important caveat remains, however, in that average radiation doses were used in these calculations although the pattern of microscopic distribution of radiation doses from radioiodines is known to vary with age. This phenomenon has been evaluated primarily in terms of the age-dependent size distribution of the thyroid follicles, the path length of the β particles, and the associated doses to the cells on the periphery of the follicles. This problem assumes greater significance when considered relative to the developmental pattern in the perinatal thyroid. A significant but progressively decreasing fraction of the cell population (including stem cells) that eventually will organize to constitute follicles is located in the areas between follicles during the initial phases of development of the gland. These are generically designated "interfollicular cells" to provide a semantic basis for distinguishing them from the specific perifollicular or C cells, which are located in the same areas. On the basis of current concepts of developmental physiology, these undifferentiated cells have progressively increasing capacities for incorporating iodine and producing organic iodides. The greatest fraction of the radiation dose is thought to derive from iodides contained in the colloid, however, so that these interfollicular cells of the perinatal thyroid may receive proportionately lower radiation doses than those of the functional follicle.

Comparative dose-response data are not available for the most prominent instances of oncogenesis by perinatal irradiation of the human thyroid gland. The two situations best documented—clinical x-irradiations of the thymus and accidental radioiodine exposures of young children—both led to increased incidences of thyroid tumors and apparently involved dosimetric factors, although the details remain obscure. There are reasonable estimates of thyroid dose for the thymic irradiation cases, but there is no similarly exposed adult population for comparison. The behavior patterns that are characteristic of childhood apparently meant that the children who were exposed to fallout in the Marshall Islands received both internal and external exposures greater than the doses to adults. Tumor incidence has been greater among those exposed as children, but accurate dose-response comparisons have not been possible, precluding unqualified statements about greater sensitivities.

Initial Responses

In the previously cited experiment, Speert et al. (1951) observed that injection of pregnant mice at stages subsequent to onset of fetal thyroid function resulted in fibrosis, compensatory hyperplasia, and adenomatous change of the offspring's thyroid glands, a pattern that has been corroborated by others. In later studies to compare several measures of age-related sensitivities in rats, we found that there were major differences in the early responses of thyroid cells, as well as parallel changes in other end points (Sikov, 1969; Sikov et al., 1972). In these experiments, rats were intraperitoneally injected with graded doses of [131]I (as much as 111 kBq/g) as young adults, weanlings, or newborns, or were exposed as fetuses by injection of their dams. Thyroid radiosensitivity, which was quantified in terms of the thyroid radiation dose required to produce a 50% reduction in iodine-trapping capacity at 4 months after exposure, progressively decreased with age at exposure (Sikov, 1969). Histopathological evaluations showed that cell death was the initial morphological response in the weanlings and adults and was followed by degeneration and fibrosis of the gland. In the two groups exposed in the perinatal period, however, growth of the thyroid gland was inhibited in a dose-related manner, and complete differentiation into definitive follicles failed to occur even by 4 months of age (Sikov et al., 1972). Walinder and Sjöden (1973) and Walinder and Rönnbäck (1984) likewise found that, at equal doses, cell killing was a more predominant feature of irradiation of the mouse thyroid during adulthood than prenatally.

Specific Cell Populations and Differential Proliferation

It has been speculated that an increased mitotic rate in the perinatal period might amplify radiogenic changes and thus be involved in the elevated susceptibility to neoplasia. The determinations previously indicated by Walinder and Sjöden (1973) and Walinder and Rönnbäck (1984) extended their reports on the greater thyroid tumor frequency and shorter latent period in mice that had been irradiated *in utero* relative to those irradiated as adults. These studies also compared the effects of prenatal and adult irradiation on thyroid cell cycle, kinetics, and regeneration. They found that there were higher proliferation rates in the prenatal mouse thyroid gland than in adult mice, in which epithelial cells are long lived, which they interpreted as suggesting that the primary carcinogenic event was independent of age. The apparently increased sensitivity of the prenatal thyroid might therefore result from an accelerated rate of tumor development associated with age-related differences in proliferation rates, and the ultimate incidences might be independent of age at exposure. Moreover, the results of these experiments indicated that prenatal irradiation also decreased latency to development of lung tumors but did not increase its overall incidence. Despite the similarity of patterns, it is not clear whether this observation has relevance to the thyroid question.

The foregoing considerations led us to examine cell proliferation and kinetics as part of a study of thyroid development. Rats of graded ages between birth and weaning were injected with pulses or with repeated doses of tritiated thymidine. They were killed at sequential times thereafter; their tracheas, with thyroid glands attached, were removed, and autoradiographs were prepared and evaluated. An important finding relative to the relationships between age and cell proliferation parameters was that the period of greatest proliferation of follicular cells, indicated by percent of labeled cells, occurred during the middle of the second postnatal week (Figure 1). This was primarily related to a concomitant increase in the number of follicles containing proliferating cells (Figure 1), whereas the percent of labeled cells in labeled follicles was largely unchanged. Until near the time of weaning, an even greater fraction of cells in the areas between the follicles were labeled than in the follicles themselves (Figure 2). The specific identity of the cells incorporating thymidine could not be established, but several lines of evidence indicated that these interfollicular cells were not perifollicular or C cells. The overall size of this population relative to the number of cells constituting follicles, and the fraction of these cells that were labeled, also declined toward the time of weaning.

Histological evidence from these studies and reports in the literature strongly suggest that these cells progressively become organized into definitive follicles, most likely through secretion of hormone into a central volume that becomes the lumen as it fills with colloid. Thus, these results failed to demonstrate differences in cell kinetics that explain the age-related differences in sensitivity to radiogenic thyroid tumors. As is considered next, however, these morphological and physiological relationships and the subsequent progression of events offer alternative explanations related to physiological interactions.

Histopathological Tumor Types and Response Curve Shape

We previously reported that the weight of the thyroid gland was less among the surviving ^{131}I-exposed rats of the carcinogenesis study than in the controls when they were terminally evaluated at 30 months of age. A tracer dose of ^{125}I was administered 24 hr before sacrifice of these animals; thyroid uptake decreased with increasing radiation dose in animals of all age groups. This is in agreement with our results, in which a similar spectrum of morphological and physiological deficits were found at 4 months after similar exposures and were preceded by a comparable series of pathogenic events.

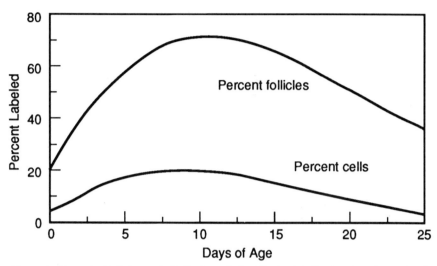

Figure 1. Percent of follicles and of follicular cells that display labeling in autoradiographs of thyroid glands after tritiated thymidine injection in rats during suckling period.

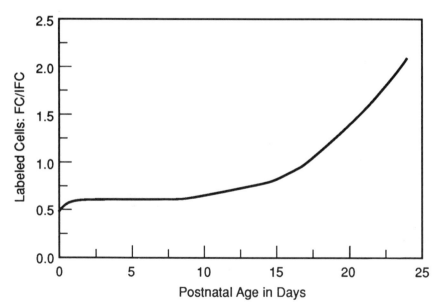

Figure 2. Age dependence of ratio of numbers of labeled follicular (FC) to intrafollicular (IFC) cells in autoradiographs of thyroid glands after tritiated thymidine injection in rats during suckling period.

As just discussed, the response curves for overall incidence of thyroid tumors in our carcinogenesis studies were complex. Because many aspects of the patterns of tumor types associated with the overall elevation in tumor incidence could evolve from differences in initial responses and their sequelae, these phenomena warrant consideration. When the age-related responses were examined relative to histological type of tumor, the picture that emerged was clearer and mechanistically more informative. In this study, the predominant thyroid neoplasm in control animals of all age groups was the C-cell tumor, which is consistent with the pattern reported by others. As indicated, however, the incidence of C-cell tumors was unaffected in groups exposed to lower doses of ^{131}I but was decreased by exposure to higher radiation doses in all age groups. These findings are consistent with the observation of Feinstein et al. (1986) that ^{131}I leads to marked destruction of C cells, with no histological indications of recovery during the 40-day period after exposure.

Few follicular tumors were detected among control animals but were the primary histological type in exposed animals. Consistent with results reported from other studies of adult rats exposed to ^{131}I , we found that their incidence increased at lower doses, irrespective of age at administration. Incidence continued to increase progressively with dose in groups exposed in the prenatal or neonatal period but decreased at higher doses in the older animals.

Secondary Interactions

It is necessary to consider another related possibility before integrating this evidence into a tentative picture. As an example, strontium was found to deposit in the sella turcica and selectively irradiate the developing pituitary, leading to pituitary tumors during later life (Schmahl and Kollmer, 1981). Because of the close proximity of the fetal thyroid and pituitary, the radiation dose that the latter would receive from ^{131}I in the former must be considered. Calculations show that β particles do not reach the pituitary and that the gamma dose is negligible, so that thyroidal changes mediated through direct radiation effects on pituitary development would not seem to play a role. Beyond direct radiation-induced effects, however, it is more likely that the differences are involved with age-dependent relationships between morphological alterations and their physiological interactions.

Our understanding of the thyroid-pituitary axis suggests that we must consider its potential contribution to the overall phenomenon, especially in the sense of the hormonal feedback mechanisms involved in pituitary interactions with the developing and mature thyroid gland. The close relationships between the thyroid and pituitary glands are compatible with the several patterns observed throughout our experiments and those of others. The C cells, which are not involved in the production of thyroid hormone, are independent of thyroid-stimulating hormone (TSH) from the pituitary. As was indicated, the incidence of tumors of these cells was unaffected at lower radiation doses, but their incidence was decreased by exposure to higher radiation doses in all age groups.

There are specific feedback relationships between levels of thyroid hormone and TSH secretion, and the several elements of evidence presented here are in good agreement with the age-related differences in morphology. Such potential interactions were also suggested by Walinder (1973); Konermann (1987) demonstrated reduced follicular colloid densities and serum thryoid hormone levels as a result of prenatal radioiodine exposures. We would expect that a reduction of functional thyroid tissue at lower doses would lead to reduced thyroid hormone levels, then to increased TSH. This, in turn, would overstimulate the remaining thyroid glandular tissue and lead to increased tumor incidence. When the gland becomes essentially fibrotic through exposure to higher doses, however, few functional cells remain to respond to the stimulation.

Because of their responses and the resulting design factors, the perinatal animals actually received a lower range of radiation doses. However, these doses seemed to be sufficient to causes a dose-dependent interference with the differentiation of the interfollicular cells into definitive follicles. Presumably, this also reduced thyroid hormone production, or at least the amount secreted into the circulation, and so also increased TSH secretion. Although this is speculative, it seems quite possible that continued TSH stimulation of the viable but incompletely differentiated interfollicular cells leads to their involvement in the progressive increase in follicular tumor incidence with dose.

CONCLUSIONS

Other factors, including the possibility of damage at the molecular level and the influence that repair and restoration might have on them, remain possibilities for speculation and investigation. If the various suppositions or suggestions are correct, however, there would be no need to invoke any inherently greater or special sensitivities *per se*; furthermore, there is a difference in the subsequent fate and role of the various populations of cells at various ages. It thus tentatively appears that much of the elevated responsiveness of the perinatal thyroid gland to oncogenesis by ^{131}I irradiation is related to the presence of incompletely differentiated interfollicular cells and the resulting microscopic distribution of radiation dose. In turn, these factors affect the patterns of cell killing and regeneration capacity and lead to differential reactions of the thyroid-pituitary axis.

ACKNOWLEDGMENTS

These studies were performed under U.S. Department of Energy Contract No. DE-AC06-76RLO 1830. We gratefully acknowledge fellowships from NORCUS, which provided the support for participation by J. L. Daniel and M. Goldman in these research activities. We also express our appreciation to W. J. Clarke for performing the initial histopathological evaluations of thyroid tumors, to R. L. Buschbom for statistical analyses, to R. J. Traub for calculating radiation doses to the pituitary gland, and to several members of the PNL technical staff who participated in the various phases of these studies.

REFERENCES

Book, SA. 1978. Age-related variation in thyroidal exposures from fission-produced radioiodines, pp. 330-343. In: *Developmental Toxicology of Energy-Related Pollutants*, DD Mahlum, MR Sikov, PL Hackett, and FD Andrew (eds.). Proceedings of the 17th Hanford Life Sciences Symposium, October 17-19, 1977, Richland, WA. CONF-771017, NTIS, Springfield, VA.

Feinstein, RE, EJ Gimeno, M El-Salhy, E Wilander and G Walinder. 1986. Evidence of C-cell destruction in the thyroid gland of mice exposed to high ^{131}I doses. Acta Radiol Oncol 25:199-202.

Konermann, G. 1987. Differences between the effectiveness of [131]J and [125]J in producing developmental effects in mice, pp. 355-362. In: *Age-Related Factors in Radionuclide Metabolism and Dosimetry, Proceedings of Workshop by the Commission of the European Communities*, GB Gerber, H Metivier, and H Smith (eds.). Martinus Nijhoff, The Netherlands.

Schmahl, W and WE Kollmer. 1981. Radiation-induced meningeal and pituitary tumors in the rate after prenatal application of strontium-90. J Cancer Res Clin Oncol 100:13-18.

Sikov, MR. 1969. Effect of age on the iodine-131 metabolism and the radiation sensitivity of the rat thyroid. Radiat Res 38:449-459.

Sikov, MR. 1989. Tumorigenesis following perinatal radionuclide exposure, pp. 403-419. In: *Perinatal and Multigenerational Carcinogenesis*, NP Napalkov, JM Rice, L Tomatis, et al. (eds.). IARC, Lyon.

Sikov, MR, DD Mahlum, and WJ Clarke. 1973. Effect of age on the carcinogenicity of ^{131}I in the rat—Interim report, pp. 25-32. In: *Radionuclide Carcinogenesis*,

CL Sanders, RH Busch, JE Ballou, and DD Mahlum (eds.). Proceedings of the 12th Hanford Biology Symposium, May 10-12, 1972, Richland, WA. CONF-72050, NTIS, Springfield, VA.

Sikov, MR, DD Mahlum, and GE Dagle. 1984. Relationships between age at exposure to iodine-131 and thyroid tumor incidence in rats, p. 79. In: *Abstracts of Papers for the 32nd Annual Meeting of the Radiation Research Society*, Orlando, Florida.

Sikov, MR, DD Mahlum, and EB Howard. 1972. Effect of age on the morphologic response of the rat thyroid to irradiation by iodine-131. Radiat Res 49:233-244.

Speert, H, EH Quimby, and SC Werner. 1951. Radioiodine uptake by the fetal mouse thyroid and resultant effects in later life. Surg Gynecol Obstet 93:230-242.

Walinder, G. 1973. Radiation-induced neoplasia and impairment of epithelial regeneration, two antagonistic effects, p. 33. In: *Radionuclide Carcinogenesis*, CL Sanders, RH Busch, JE Ballou, and DD Mahlum (eds.). CONF-720505, NTIS, Springfield, VA.

Walinder, G and C Rönnbäck. 1984. Neoplastic effects after prenatal irradiation, pp. 101-115. In: *Effects of Prenatal Irradiation with Special Emphasis on Late Effects* (EUR-8067). Commission of the European Communities, Luxembourg.

Walinder, G and AM Sjöden. 1972. Late effects of irradiation on the thyroid gland in mice. II. Irradiation of mouse foetuses. Acta Radiol Ther Phys Biol 11:577-589.

Walinder, G and AM Sjöden. 1973. Late effects of irradiation on the thyroid gland in mice. III. Comparison between irradiation of foetuses and adults. Acta Radiol Ther Phys Biol 12:201-208.

TRANSGENIC MICE AS MODELS IN WHICH TO STUDY TUMORIGENESIS ASSOCIATED WITH SV-40 T-ANTIGEN, *ras,* AND/OR *myc* EXPRESSION

C. Quaife,[1] E. Sangren,[2] R. Brinster,[2] and R. Palmiter[1]

[1]Howard Hughes Medical Institute, Department of Biochemistry, University of Washington, Seattle, WA

[2]School of Veterinary Medicine, University of Pennsylvania, Philadelphia, PA

Key words: *Oncogenes, SV-40, ras, myc, transgenic mice*

ABSTRACT ONLY

Integration of foreign DNA into the genome of mice, followed by its eventual tissue-specific expression, provides models in which to study the effects of onco-genes, both *in vivo* and in a wide variety of cell types. We have used sequences derived from the rat elastase-1 or the mouse albumin gene to direct expression of an SV-40 T-antigen (T-ag), and a mutated *ras* or *myc* gene to the liver parenchyma or pancreatic acinar cells. The expression of T-ag in the liver or pancreas resulted in neoplastic transformation of both organs.

Tumor progression has been examined in different lines of mice, and the results support a multistep pathogenesis. In contrast to T-ag, directing expression of a mutated *ras* gene to the pancreas or liver resulted in abnormalities that were apparent during early development. These organs became extremely hyperplas-tic, and death occurred in the perinatal period. However, although mechanisms that regulate proliferation and differentiation were perturbed, there was no evi-dence for aneuploidy or metastasis. Expression of a transgenic *myc* gene in the pancreas or liver produced only mild changes and did not result in neoplasia.

These models are useful for identifying processes involved in tumorigenesis.

HORMONAL REGULATION OF GROWTH AND DIFFERENTIATION IN AN *IN VITRO* MODEL SYSTEM

W. Wharton

Los Alamos National Laboratory, Los Alamos, NM 87545

Key words: *BALB/c-3T3 cells, PDGF, EGF, IGF-I, primary response genes*

ABSTRACT ONLY

The growth and differentiation of mesenchymal cells are regulated by multiple hormone-like factors that act in a parallel and sequential manner. In density-arrested BALB/c-3T3 cells, the initial events in G_0/G_1 are regulated by platelet-derived growth factor (PDGF). Subsequently, epidermal growth factor (EGF) and insulin-like growth factor (IGF-I) regulate traverse of the cells into S-phase. The phorbol ester myristate acetate can replace the combination of PDGF and EGF and, together with IGF-I, stimulate 3T3 cells to divide. The second-messenger systems that mediate the action of specific growth factors, which are beginning to be understood, clearly are both complex factors and interactive.

We have evidence that the initial events in G_0/G_1 are regulated by a combination of tyrosine kinases and calcium-mediated events, some of which are independent of calmodulin. In addition, we are isolating primary response genes that are either hormonally regulated or are cell cycle dependent. The mechanistic relationships between specific second messengers and families of genes that potentially share common promoter regions are being investigated using a combination of mitogenically variant cell lines and standard cloning techniques.

We present a model of sequential expression of clusters of genes that regulate cell cycle traverse. The model allows predictions concerning the type of processes that lead either to higher stages of differentiation or to neoplastic transformation.

Molecular Markers for Cell Damage

TWO-DIMENSIONAL GEL ELECTROPHORESIS OF CYTOPLASMIC PROTEINS IN CONTROL AND TRANSFORMED 10T$\frac{1}{2}$ AND CVP CELLS AFTER BENZO[a]PYRENE TREATMENT

J. K. Selkirk,[1] B. K. Mansfield,[1] D. J. Riese,[2] A. Nikbakht,[2] and R. C. Mann[3]

[1]Division of Toxicology Research and Testing, Carcinogenesis and Toxicology Evaluation Branch
National Institute of Environmental Health Sciences, Research Triangle Park, NC 27709

[2]Biology Division, Oak Ridge National Laboratory, Oak Ridge, TN 37831

[3]Engineering Physics and Mathematics Division, Oak Ridge National Laboratory, Oak Ridge, TN 37831

Key words: *Two-dimensional gel electrophoresis (2-DGE), benzo[a]pyrene (BaP), 10T$\frac{1}{2}$ cells, protein modulation*

ABSTRACT

It is generally accepted that environmental chemical carcinogens require metabolic activation to reactive intermediates to express their carcinogenic effect. In recent years, the metabolism of different chemical carcinogens has been carefully characterized with the result that the metabolite profile is essentially identical in all species and cells for a given carcinogen. These metabolite profiles are independent of the relative susceptibility to malignant transformation. To understand the relative transformation potential, it is necessary to develop new strategies to comprehend the critical biochemical differences that determine carcinogen susceptibility between cell types and in humans and experimental animals.

We have used two-dimensional gel electrophoresis to characterize gene products in various cell types, including those undergoing differentiation and in transformable cells treated with benzo[a]pyrene (BaP). Utilizing Friend erythroleukemia cells undergoing differentiation, we have observed a number of induced and repressed gene products with image analysis methodology on digitized fluorographs of two-dimensional electrophoresis gels of cytoplasmic proteins.

We have begun a series of experiments to study the metabolic differences among the transformable C3H 10T$\frac{1}{2}$ mouse fibroblast line, a transformed clone (C1), and a C3H fibroblast line (CVP) derived from adult mouse prostate that is highly resistant to malignant transformation. Cell cultures were treated with BaP for

24 hr, while the proteins were radiolabeled with ^{14}C amino acids. Fluorographic exposures were made to monitor those polypeptides, which rapidly accumulated the amino acids. Master composite images were constructed by means of image analysis algorithms for each cell type, so that polypeptides unique to the control cells (repressed by treatment) and those unique to the BaP-treated cells (induced by treatment) could be viewed together spatially.

Eventually, the polypeptide data base will be large enough so that it can be probed for possible elucidation of the cascade of subtle biochemical events that result in cellular commitment to malignancy following exposure to chemical carcinogens.

INTRODUCTION

It is generally accepted that environmental chemical carcinogens require metabolic activation to reactive intermediates to express their carcinogenic effect. In recent years, the metabolism of different chemical carcinogens has been carefully characterized with the result that the metabolite profile is essentially identical in all species and cells for a given carcinogen. These metabolite profiles are independent of the relative susceptibility to malignant transformation. To understand the relative transformation potential, it is necessary to develop new strategies to comprehend the critical biochemical differences that determine carcinogen susceptibility among cell types and in man and experimental animals.

We have utilized three fibroblast cell lines derived from the C3H mouse in this experiment. The polycyclic aromatic hydrocarbon- (PAH-) transformable embryonic fibroblast $10T\frac{1}{2}$ line (clone 8) was developed and kindly supplied to us by Reznikoff et al. (1973). The 3-methylcholanthrene $10T\frac{1}{2}$ transformed clone C1 was developed in our laboratory and exhibits heavy staining because of piling up of cells and positive growth in soft agar. The malignant transformation-resistant CVP line was derived from C3H mouse ventral prostate by Gehly and Heidelberger (1982).

Each of the three cell lines was seeded at 50,000 cells per 60-mm tissue culture dish in Dulbecco's modified Eagle's medium containing 10% heat-inactivated fetal calf serum supplemented with glutamine and gentamycin. After 6 days of growth, 2 μmol benzo[a]pyrene (BaP) in dimethyl sulfoxide (DMSO) was added for a 6-hr incubation. The medium was removed and replaced with fresh medium containing 7.25 μCi/ml of ^{14}C-labeled amino acids plus 2 μmol BaP. Control dishes received DMSO- and ^{14}C-labeled amino acids. After a 30-hr labeling period, the cells were harvested, lysed by homogenization, and the nuclei removed by centrifugation. The cytoplasmic fraction was dialyzed against water to remove unincorporated amino acids.

Total protein was determined by the fluorescamine assay (Weigele et al., 1972), and aliquots were taken for radioactivity measurement to ascertain the level of amino acid incorporation into proteins. The samples were lyophilized, suspended in urea-NP40 lysis buffer, and separated by two-dimensional polyacrylamide gel electrophoresis (2D-PAGE) (O'Farrell, 1975) using a 10% to 20% linear polyacrylamide gradient. Five replicate gels were prepared for each sample and infused with the fluorographic enhancer Amplify (Amersham, Arlington Heights, IL), and dried; fluorographs were prepared using Kodak type SB x-ray film at -80°C during a 4-day exposure. The x-ray films were digitized on an Optronics P-1000 scanner (Optronics International, Chelmsford, MA) and analyzed according to the method of Mann et al. (1986). Master images or "fingerprint" polypeptide patterns were created by merging the qualitative data from the replicate gel fluorographs for each of the cell types under each of the BaP treatment and control conditions. For each of the six master images created in this experiment, the polypeptide profile was composed of the most rapidly accumulating polypeptides under each of the specific experimental conditions. The control and BaP master images were merged for each of the three cell lines into three separate master composite images, resulting in the depiction of qualitative expression of treatment and control polypeptides relative to each other in the same display for a given cell line. Polypeptides present in both, and/or unique to each, of the two master images (treatment or control conditions) became readily evident (see Table 1).

Table 1. Master composite summary of benzo[a]pyrene effects in C3H cell lines.

	C1	$10T_2^{\frac{1}{2}}$	CVP
Present	273	173	260
Repressed	22	11	60
Induced	32	37	18
Modulated proteins	54	48	78

The number of proteins detected in this experiment does not represent the absolute total of cytoplasmic proteins in the cell, but it does indicate those proteins most actively incorporating labeled amino acids under the conditions of this experiment. It is clear that there are marked differences both in the total number and identities of proteins observed among the three cell lines and in the number and identities of repressed and induced proteins after treatment with BaP. Although the ratio of induced to repressed polypeptides is similar for the C1 line, the ratio of induced versus repressed in the $10T_2^1$ is approximately 3:1. In contrast, the CVP line shows the reverse ratio (3:1) for repressed versus induced polypeptides in response to BaP treatment.

Against a background of 124 polypeptides found to be common to all three cell lines, only 5 polypeptides induced in both the $10T_2^1$ and C1 lines were identical. There were 2 commonly induced polypeptides between the $10T_2^1$ and CVP lines; however, no polypeptides were commonly induced by BaP in all three cell lines. Only one spot was commonly repressed by the $10T_2^1$ and the CVP cells, and no spots were commonly repressed between either the $10T_2^1$ and C1 or CVP and C1 cells. Interestingly, a large number of spots that were present under both BaP treatment and control conditions in the C1 cells were repressed by BaP in the CVP cells.

Although it might be assumed that three cell lines derived from the same genetic background would respond to enzyme induction by the same chemical in a similar fashion, these results clearly suggest that, on the basis of subtle genotypic differences between the cell lines, distinct differences in the metabolic response to a chemical carcinogen may influence the mode of activation and detoxification of the chemical. It may be speculated, since all eukaryotes metabolize carcinogenic chemicals to the same family of derivatives, that variable responses such as these play a role in the relative resistance or susceptibility to malignant transformation. Subtle differences in the induction of detoxifying systems may play an important role in directing an activated carcinogen toward or away from critical target sites for malignant transformation within the cell.

REFERENCES

Gehly, EB and C Heidelberger. 1982. Metabolic activation of benzo(a)pyrene by transformable and nontransformable C3H mouse fibroblasts in culture. Cancer Res 42:2697-2704.

Mann, RC, BK Mansfield, and JK Selkirk. 1986. Automated analysis of digital images generated by two-dimensional electrophoresis gels, pp. 301-312. In: *Pattern Recognition in Practice II*, ES Gelsema and LN Kanal (eds.). Elsevier North-Holland, Amsterdam.

O'Farrell, PH. 1975. High resolution two-dimensional electrophoresis of proteins. J Biol Chem 250:4007-4021.

Reznikoff, CA, JS Bertram, DW Brankow, and C Heidelberger. 1973. Quantitative and qualitative studies of chemical transformation of cloned C3H mouse embryo cells sensitive to post-confluence inhibition of cell division. Cancer Res 33:3239-3249.

Weigele, M, S DeBernardo, J Tengi, and WA Leimgruber. 1972. A novel reagent for the fluorometric assay of primary amines. J Am Chem Soc 94:5927-5930.

QUESTIONS AND COMMENTS

Q: Tenforde, PNL

How sensitive are the differences in proteins observed for normal versus transformed cells to their growth phase? In other words, do the proteins change significantly when cells are in an early exponential growth phase as compared to cells from cultures appproaching confluence?

A: Selkirk

We haven't resolved this question yet because our experiments to date have dealt with single time points even though the cells are in exponential growth. Time-course experiments such as you suggest need to be done to approach an answer to qualitative and quantitative protein changes during the various growth stages. We have planned these experiments.

Q: Tenforde

A second question is whether you have examined the proteins from revertant cell lines that have phenotypically normal growth properties?

A: Selkirk

We have not yet had the opportunity to research revertant cell lines. It is a very interesting question, and I would be anxious to collaborate with anyone in the audience who may have cell variants of this type.

Q: Gantt, NCI

This was an impressive report. It looked as though you detect protein to be either present or absent. For the future you might consider trying to record rough concentration differences, which may reflect gene dosage (0, 0.5, 1 relative values). This may prove important for homozygous functional, heterozygous, and homozygous defective changes that appear to be important in the mechanism of transformation.

A: Selkirk

We hope to obtain stocks of cells that are genetically characterized so that we can begin to approach this problem. We have developed internal gel calibration standards that contain known amounts of radioactivity and can be used to convert gray values on the x-ray film to disintegrations

per minute (dpm) present in a given spot on the plate. We have succeeded in measuring hemoglobin formation in Friend erythroleukemia
cells (**Mansfield** et al., Cancer Res. 48:1110-1118, **1988**) after onset of
differentiation, but have not yet attempted to correlate gene dosage to
relative amounts of protein formed. At present, there are also practical
obstacles to accurately measuring the amount of protein in a single spot
on the gel.

USE OF MAMMALIAN CELLS TO INVESTIGATE THE GENETIC CONSEQUENCES OF DNA DAMAGE INDUCED BY IONIZING RADIATION*

T. L. Morgan,[1] E. W. Fleck,[1] B. J. F. Rossiter,[2] and J. H. Miller[1]

[1]Pacific Northwest Laboratory, Richland, WA 99352

[2]Institute for Molecular Genetics, Baylor College of Medicine, Houston, TX 76703

Key words: *Ionizing radiation, DNA damage, HGPRT locus, deletion breakpoints*

ABSTRACT ONLY

Induction of cancer is the most important health risk associated with exposure of human populations to low doses of ionizing radiation. A great deal is known about the cytotoxic and carcinogenic properties of radiation insult from cellular and whole-animal studies, but our understanding of the subcellular effects of the damage is much more limited. To connect the physical and chemical properties of radiation damage with the observed biological response, it is important to investigate the molecular nature of the damage produced in the cell's genetic material.

We have studied the effect of dose, dose fractionation, and DNA repair on the spectrum of mutations induced at the HGPRT locus in Chinese hamster ovary cells irradiated in plateau phase. The cells were either subcultured immediately or held in a nonproliferative state for 24 hr before replating. Using a hamster HGPRT cDNA probe, the molecular structure of the HGPRT gene in 89 thioguanine-resistant clones was analyzed by Southern blot analysis.

Although about 90% (79/89) of the observed mutations were caused by a detectable loss or alteration of genomic sequences binding to this probe, the specific proportion of deletions encompassing the entire gene (full deletions) depended on how the radiation dose was administered. For cells irradiated by 4 Gy and replated immediately, 69% (20/29) showed a complete deletion of the HGPRT gene; 24% (7/29) were determined to have altered banding patterns, indicating the presence

---

*Work supported by the U.S. DOE Office of Health and Environmental Research under Contract DE-AC06-76RLO 1830 and the Northwest College and University Association for Science (University of Washington) under Contract DE-AM06-76-RLO2225.

of partial deletions or rearrangements. For a dose of 2 Gy, only 43% (9/21) showed full deletions while the proportion of mutants having altered banding patterns rose to 38% (8/21). Cell populations irradiated with a split dose of 4 Gy (2 Gy + 24 hr + 2 Gy) or held in plateau phase for 24 hr following a dose of 4 Gy showed no significant difference in the mutation spectrum compared to that observed for the cells treated with 4 Gy and replated immediately. The difference between the fraction of mutant cell lines showing full deletions when irradiated by 2 Gy (9/21) as compared with the same fraction in all other treatment groups (45/68) was statistically significant at the $p = 0.056$ level. Thus the dose-effect trend appears to be toward more large-scale events at higher doses and indicates that exposure level can affect the mutation spectrum. Because the cells used in this study exhibited a low background mutation frequency ($5/10^6$ viable cells), we believe that it is unlikely that this dose effect results from contamination by mutants arising spontaneously in the population of cells irradiated with 2 Gy.

These results demonstrate that deletions are the most common lesion induced by ionizing radiation. These data also suggest that enzymatic processes associated with the repair of sublethal and potentially lethal damage acted uniformly across all types of premutational lesions.

Using a restriction-site map of the hamster HGPRT locus, we have determined the location of deletion breakpoints in 14 mutants that showed partial deletions. In 12 of these cell lines, one or both of the breakpoints was found to be located near the center of the gene, suggesting that this region of the HGPRT gene is abnormally sensitive to radiation damage, or that repair systems have more difficulty in recognizing or repairing damage in this region.

CHROMOSOMAL BINDING AND CLEARANCE OF BENZO[a]PYRENE-DIOL-EPOXIDE

A. L. Brooks and W. C. Griffith

Lovelace Inhalation Toxicology Research Institute, P.O. Box 5890, Albuquerque, NM 87185

Key words: *Benzo[a]pyrene, carcinogen distributions, chromosomes*

ABSTRACT

We have conducted research to help define, in molecular terms, the "genetic dose" after exposure to chemical carcinogens. To do this, the amount of carcinogen binding to the chromosomes was used as an index of dose, and the rate of loss of carcinogen was used as an index of repair. Chinese hamster ovary cells were exposed for 3 hr to ^{3}H-labeled ± *anti*-benzo[a]pyrene-7,8-diol-9,10-epoxide (^{3}H-BPDE), or ^{3}H-thymidine, and serially harvested. Autoradiographs were prepared, and the frequency of silver grains over metaphase chromosomes was counted as a measure of binding and removal of the carcinogen from the cells. The silver grains were randomly distributed down the length of the chromosomes, with no apparent "hot spots" at any harvest time. The ^{3}H-BPDE was lost from the chromosomes, as a linear function of time, for the first 9 hr; only 60% of the original label remained associated with the chromosomes by that time. An apparent nonrandom distribution of silver grains was observed between chromatids. This was quantitated by derivation of a distribution index, which determined whether the probability that the next silver grain was on the same chromatid was equal to the probability that the next grain was on the sister chromatid. If the grains were randomly distributed, the distribution index would be 0.5.

The incorporation of ^{3}H-thymidine was used as a positive control. Cells exposed to ^{3}H-thymidine that had undergone a single S phase of the cell cycle before metaphase had a distribution index of 0.48 ± 0.02, which was not different from random incorporation; cells that had undergone two rounds of DNA replication had an index of 0.84 ± 0.04. This demonstrated that, in control cells, one chromatid had excess label relative to that of its sister. The distribution indices for cells exposed to ^{3}H-BPDE were 0.52 ± 0.03, 0.59 ± 0.04, and 0.60 ± 0.04, respectively, at 0, 3, and 6 hr after the end of exposure. The values observed at 3 and 6 hr after exposure were significantly different ($p < 0.05$) from an expected random distribution.

These data suggest that, at early times after carcinogen exposure, there is differential loss or removal of the carcinogen from one chromatid relative to that of its sister. Additional studies to help understand the mechanisms involved in this preferential repair are discussed.

Extensive research has been conducted to determine the relationships between DNA adducts and their biological effects (Yang et al., 1982). The concept of "chemical dose" (Wogan and Gorelick, 1985) has been evaluated by determining the number of DNA adducts formed, the chemical nature of the adducts, and the repair or removal of the adducts from DNA. Evidence has accumulated that chemical dose is not uniform in DNA. It has been determined that there is a nonrandom binding of ± *anti*-benzo[a]pyrene (BaP)-7,8-diol-9,10 epoxide (BPDE) in the nuclei of epithelial cells (Poirier et al., 1982) as well as in linker DNA regions (Jack and Brookes, 1982). Nonuniform distribution of chemical dose can also be produced by DNA repair. Preferential repair occurs in regions of the DNA that are transcriptionally active (Mellon et al., 1986; Hanawalt, 1987).

Our research was carried out to determine if nonuniform distribution and repair of BPDE adducts could be detected at the chromosome level. Two different batches of the radiolabeled carcinogen, (±)r-7,T-8-dihydroxy-T-9,10-epoxy-7,8,9,10-tetrahydro-[1,3-^{3}H] BaP (*anti*-BPDE), were used in this study. The batches were from Amersham Corp., Arlington Heights, IL (batch number analysis H/7268) and Chemsyn Science Laboratories, Lenexa, KA (lot CSL-88-55-48T). The first batch was used for our initial studies on distribution and clearance of BPDE and the second for studies on distribution of BPDE between chromatids. ^{3}H-thymidine was obtained from New England Nuclear Corp. (Boston, MA).

We conducted studies to measure the binding and removal of BPDE from chromosomes of Chinese hamster ovary (CHO) cells. First, cell cycle kinetics were determined using ^{3}H-thymidine. Second, the distribution and clearance of ^{3}H-BPDE were measured as a function of chromosome location. Finally, the distribution of silver grains from ^{3}H-BPDE or ^{3}H-thymidine between the sister chromatids was scored as an index of difference in repair rates. Differential repair was measured with and without adding 5-bromodeoxyuridine (BrdU) to label the chromatid containing the newly synthesized DNA.

For studies of cell kinetics and distribution and retention of BPDE, cells were exposed to ^{3}H-thymidine and ^{3}H-BPDE for 3 hr and harvested at 0, 3, 6, 9, and 21 hr after exposure. To study BPDE distribution between chromatids, the cells were labeled with BrdU (10 μM final concentration) 24 hr before harvest and exposed to ^{3}H-BPDE (1.25 μCi/ml) for 0.5 hr at 3, 6, 9, 12, and 24 hr before harvest. Cytogenetic preparations were made using standard techniques. Slides were then coated with Ilford-L4 autoradiographic emulsion and exposed for 15-30 days to expose the film and accumulate silver grains. Differential staining of chromatids used the methods of Minkler et al.

(1978). Photographs were taken before and after differential staining to ensure that the staining procedure did not alter the distribution of silver grains.

To determine the uniformity of carcinogen distribution, four marker chromosomes were divided into segments of approximately equal lengths and the frequency of silver grains recorded in each segment. No significant "hot spots" or areas with high chemical doses were observed along the chromosomes at any harvest time (data not shown). However, the sensitivity of the method used to detect nonuniform distribution of label was limited because of the rather large areas of chromosome being evaluated and the difficulty in defining the exact size and location of the silver grains in each area.

To define cell cycle kinetics, we determined the frequency of metaphase cells with label in zero, one, or two chromatids as a function of time after ^{3}H-thymidine labeling. This study made it possible to determine the stage of cell cycle at which repair or loss of the BPDE occurred. By 9 hr after labeling, all cells had incorporated ^{3}H-thymidine into both chromatids; by 24 hr, 80% of the cells had label in a single chromatid, suggesting that the cells had gone through a single S phase by 9 hr and two S-phase periods by 24 hr. Nine and 24 hr were then used to determine the distribution of silver grains between the two different chromatids. The ^{3}H-thymidine thus served as positive and negative controls for studying the random distribution of BPDE label. For cells harvested at 9 hr after ^{3}H-thymidine labeling, each chromatid should be equally labeled; in cells harvested at 24 hr, all the label should be on the light-staining chromatid.

Clearance of label from the interphase nuclei was rapid during the first 9 hr, with only 60% of the label retained. The labeling over the interphase nucleus was constant between 9 and 24 hr after exposure, similar to the results reported by Eastman et al. (1981), in which 50% of bound BaP was still associated with DNA after 48 hr.

The distribution of label beween chromatids after exposure to BPDE appeared to be nonrandom, with some areas of label on one chromatid and little label observed on the sister chromatid. In Figure 1, the distribution index (DI) is plotted as a function of treatment and harvest time. The DI of 0.5 indicates that the silver grains are randomly distributed between the two chromatids, and numbers larger than 0.5 indicate that one chromatid has more label than the other. The DI and the standard error for the null hypothesis of DI = 0.5 is DI = $N(d)/[N(d) + N(a)] \pm \sqrt{1/4[N(d) + N(a)]}$, where $N(d)$ is the number of silver grains which have their nearest neighbor located on the same chromatid and $N(a)$ is the number of silver grains that have their nearest neighbor on the opposite sister chromatid. In ^{3}H-thymidine-labeled cells harvested at 9 hr, the label was randomly distributed (DI = 0.48 ± 0.03); cells harvested at 24 hr after ^{3}H-thymidine had a DI of 0.80 ± 0.04. ^{3}H-BPDE treatment DI values were 0.52 ± 0.03, 0.59 ± 0.03, and 0.60 ± 0.04 for cells harvested at 0, 3, and 6 hr, respectively, after the end of a 3-hr exposure. These data demonstrated, at a 95% level of confidence, that silver grains associated with BPDE were not randomly distributed between the chromatids 3 and 6 hr after exposure.

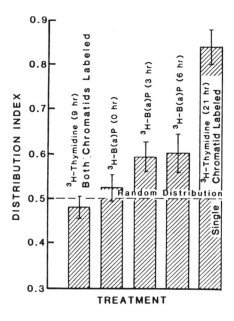

Figure 1. Distribution index (DI) for silver grains on the chromatids of cells exposed to either ^{3}H-thymidine or ^{3}H-benzo[a]pyrene-diol-epoxide. Random distribution is represented by DI = 0.5; presence of all grains on a single chromatid is shown by DI = 1.0. Bars represent 95% confidence interval for null hypothesis of DI = 0.5.

Cells were labeled with BrdU before treatment with BPDE. Double labeling made it possible to determine the potential magnitude of the error associated with scoring silver grains on chromatids, and also to determine if nonrandom distribution of silver grains between the chromatids is associated with unifilarly and bifilarly substituted DNA. The frequency of silver grains over the chromatid with unifilarly and bifilarly substituted DNA (light- and dark-staining chromatid) was measured at 5.5 hr after the end of a 0.5-hr exposure to BPDE. Figure 2 shows that cells exposed to ^{3}H-thymidine and harvested at 9 hr have a uniform distribution of silver grains between chromatids; at 24 hr, 72% of the grains are on the light-staining chromatid. Because the predicted distribution of grains would be 100% on the light-staining chromatid at 24 hr, the observed value provides an estimate of the degree of error associated with assigning silver grains to a given chromatid. For cells exposed to BPDE, 52% of the label was classified as being over the light chromatid; only 37% of the grains were scored over the dark chromatid.

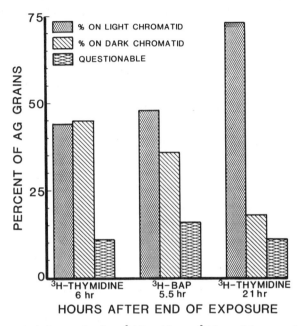

Figure 2. Percent of silver grains from ^{3}H-thymidine or ^{3}H-benzo[a]pyrene-diol-epoxide on the unifilarly and bifilarly substituted chromatids.

Cell cycle data reported here suggest that differential repair between the two chromatids is possible at the time when cells are in G_2 and S stages of the cell cycle. Our data also indicate that during repair, when BPDE adducts were removed from a chromatid, the probability that repair would occur on the same chromatid was higher than that for an adduct being lost from the opposite chromatid. We have additional data that suggest the DNA rate of repair may be higher in unifilarly substituted chromatids than in the bifilarly substituted chromatids. This difference in repair rate may account for the difference in the distribution index for chromatids exposed to BPDE.

Additional studies on the time course of BPDE removal from chromatids are necessary to understand these observations. It will be important to determine if the observed nonrandom repair process is related to the carcinogen studied and to the loss of adduct from linker DNA. Finally, it is important to evaluate whether the nonrandom repair process is related to the observed nonrandom distribution of genetic damage.

ACKNOWLEDGMENTS

The authors acknowledge the expert technical assistance of Ms. Mary Jo Waltman and Ms. Kathy McLeod. We also thank the ITRI staff and Dr. T. Coons for technical review of this manuscript. Research was conducted under U.S. Department of Energy/OHER Contract No. DE-AC04-76EV01013.

REFERENCES

Eastman, A, BT Mossman, and E Bresnick. 1981. Formation and removal of benzo-(a)pyrene adducts of DNA in hamster tracheal epithelial cells. Cancer Res 41:2605-2610.

Hanawalt, PC. 1987. Preferential DNA repair in expressed genes. Environ Health Perspect 76:9-14.

Jack, PL and P Brookes. 1982. Mechanism for the loss of preferential benzo(a)pyrene binding to the linker DNA of chromatin. Carcinogenesis 3:341-344.

Mellon, I, VA Bohr, CA Smith, and PC Hanawalt. 1986. Preferential DNA repair of an active gene in human cells. Proc Natl Acad Sci USA 83:8878-8882.

Minkler, J, D Stetka, and AV Carrano. 1978. An ultraviolet light source for consistent differential staining of sister chromatids. Stain Technol 53:359-360.

Poirier, MC, JR Stanley, JB Beckwith, IB Weinstein, and SH Yuspa. 1982. Indirect immunofluorescent localization of benzo(a)pyrene adducted to nucleic acids in cultured mouse keratinocyte nuclei. Carcinogenesis 3:345-348.

Wogan, GN and NJ Gorelick. 1985. Chemical and biochemical dosimetry of exposure to genotoxic chemicals. Environ Health Perspect 62:5-18.

Yang, LL, VM Maher, and JJ McCormick. 1982. Relationship between excision repair and the cytotoxic and mutagenic effect of the "anti" 7,8-diol-9, 10-epoxide of benzo(a)pyrene in human cells. Mutat Res 94:435-447.

QUESTIONS AND COMMENTS

Q: Morgan, PNL, Richland, WA
Dr. Hanawalt's work demonstrated a difference between genes being actively transcribed versus those which are not transcribed. Do you have any evidence that one chromatid is more active than the other?

A: Brooks
We have no evidence for differential activity of the genes between chromatids.

Q: Gantt, NCI
Might the preferential strand repair reported by Hanawalt be related to your preferential chromatid repair?

A: Brooks
It is interesting to make such a speculation. At the present time we have no evidence that our observation is related to that made by Hanawalt.

ANALYSIS OF COOKED-FOOD MUTAGENS BY HPLC/IMMUNOASSAY

B. E. Watkins, M. Vanderlaan, and J. S. Felton

Biomedical Sciences Division, University of California, Lawrence
Livermore National Laboratory, P.O. Box 5507, Livermore, CA 94550

Key words: *Immunoassay, analysis, PhIP, cooked-food mutagens*

ABSTRACT

Cooking meat at the temperatures usually used in domestic cooking produces a family of 2-amino-3-methylimadazoazaarene (AIA) mutagens. These mutagens have been implicated as a major contributor to dietary-induced cancers in humans.

To separate and quantify each of the six AIA known to be present in a cooked meat sample requires an elaborate scheme involving many high-pressure liquid chromatography (HPLC) columns, and there are many AIA-like compounds. In our studies, 15 monoclonal antibodies have been isolated which bind, to varying extents, with each of the AIA. Some are compound-specific and bind only one of the closely related AIA. Others are class-specific and bind, for example, to the quinoline-like AIA rather than to the quinoxaline-like AIA. These antibodies have been incorporated in an HPLC immunoassay that operates as a compound-specific detector after chromatographic separation. The resulting data are referred to as immunograms.

We are validating this technique for the analysis of AIA in cooked meat and in the urine of people who have eaten it. The detection limit, which is dependent on the specific AIA being detected and the antibody used, varies between 0.1 and 10 ng.

INTRODUCTION

When meat is cooked at normal household temperatures, mutagenic compounds are produced (Bjeldanes et al., 1982a,b); five of these compounds have been shown to be highly mutagenic 2-amino-3-methylimidazoazaarenes (AIA) (Felton et al., 1984). These mutagens have been implicated as a major contributor to dietarily induced cancers in humans (Sugimura et al., 1981). To determine the relative importance of these chemicals in the human diet, accurate quantitation of exposure must be correlated with epidemiological data. Many high-pressure liquid chromatography (HPLC) columns are required to separate and quantify each of the five AIA known to occur in a cooked-meat sample. Quantitation of these mutagens is difficult because other heterocyclic compounds that may or may not be mutagenic, particularly other AIA-like compounds, are present. Thus, this HPLC/mass spectrometry (HPLC/MS) analysis requires about 1 man-month of effort per sample (Felton et al., 1984).

In search of methods for analyzing these AIA that have a higher throughput and are less costly, we have developed a set of monoclonal antibodies that selectively bind to each AIA (Vanderlaan et al., 1988). 6-Phenyl-2-amino-1-methylimidazo[4,5-b]pyridine (PhIP) (Felton et al., 1986) was selected for the initial assay development because it is the most mass-abundant AIA present in cooked meat and the most genotoxic AIA in mammalian-cell short-term bioassays. It is, however, the least active AIA in the Ames *Salmonella* mutagenesis assay (Thompson et al., 1987). We recently developed a set of four monoclonals that bind to PhIP; they were produced by standard methods (Vanderlaan et al., 1988) and were derived from the immunogen described previously (Watkins et al., 1987). Each antibody has been well characterized as to its binding specificity (Vanderlaan et al., in press). The most specific antibody, PhIP-1, binds to PhIP itself with a 50% inhibition point (I_{50}) of 30 ng, but does not bind to any other AIA mutagen or to any synthetically produced derivative of PhIP, such as iso-PhIP [3-methyl-2-amino-6-phenylimidazo(4,5-b)pyridine]. However, PhIP-1 does bind with 2-deamino-PhIP and 2-deamino-2-nitro-PhIP with I_{50} of 13 and 16 ng, respectively.

Although PhIP-1 is extremely specific for PhIP as compared with other AIA mutagens and other synthetic PhIP analogs, PhIP-1 does bind with other compounds present in cooked beef. Because of the cross-reactivity, the immunoassay cannot be used to quantitate PhIP directly in crude-beef extract. However, the immunoassay can be used as a PhIP-selective detector for the HPLC, an assay format that uses the additional separation afforded by the HPLC. We refer to the data resulting from an HPLC/immunoassay as an "immunogram."

Figure 1 shows a typical immunogram of well-done beef using the PhIP-1 antibody. Fried, ground beef was extracted with $0.01M$ HCl; the extract was passed over an XAD-2 Amberlite column (Rohm and Haas), and the column eluted with acetone. The acetone was evaporated and the residue further separated by reverse-phase HPLC, as described by Felton et al. (1984); fractions were collected and subjected to enzyme-linked immunosorbent assay (ELISA) analysis (Vanderlaan et al., 1988). The immunogram shows the presence of PhIP, which is known to elute in fractions 48-51, as well as at least six other "PhIP-like" compounds. The structures of these compounds, which are yet to be determined, are assumed to be quite similar to PhIP because they bind to the antibody; they either have a much higher affinity for PhIP-1 than PhIP or are present in much higher amounts than PhIP. Work is in progress to identify these compounds and to determine their mutagenicity.

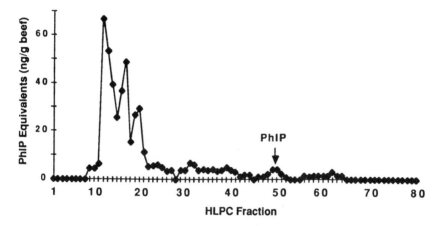

Figure 1. Immunogram of well-done cooked beef monitored using 6-phenyl-2-amino-1-methylimidazo[4,5-b]pyridine (PhIP-1). Each data point (♦) is number of PhIP g/equivalents, as determined by immunoassay, in each 1-min fraction.

To validate this assay for the quantitation of PhIP, the XAD extract was spiked with 20 and 80 ng PhIP/g of beef, compared with the 15 ng/g expected in fried beef (Felton et al., 1986). Figure 2 shows an expanded region of three immunograms in the window in which PhIP elutes. The area under the the peaks is in good agreement with the added spike.

Figure 3 shows the correlation between immunoassay data obtained using two PhIP-specific antibodies (PhIP-1 and PHIP-4) and the Ames/*Salmonella* assay. All these measurements are in good agreement with the added spike, and the measured PhIP concentration in the fried beef (12 ng/g) is in good agreement with the value previously determined by HPLC alone (Felton et al., 1986). We are currently validating this immunoassay for PhIP and the other four known AIA.

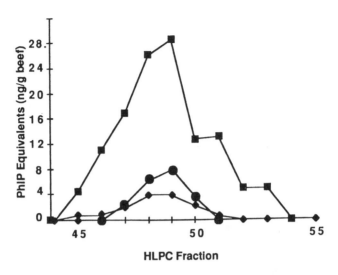

Figure 2. Immunograms of well-done cooked beef monitored using 6-phenyl-2-amino-1-methylimidazo[4,5-b]pyridine (PhIP-1). Scale is expanded to show region where PhIP elutes. Extracts were spiked with 0 (◆), 20 (●), and 80 (■) ng of PhIP/g of beef. HPLC, high-performance liquid chromatography.

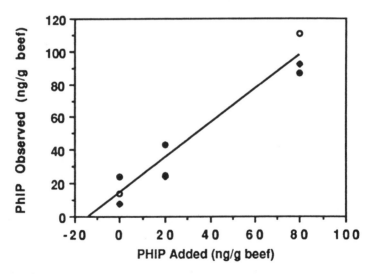

Figure 3. Correlation between amount of 6-phenyl-2-amino-1-methylimidazo[4,5-b]pyridine (PhIP-1 and PhIP-4) added to beef extract and amount determined by immunoassay. Symbols: O, PhIP-1; ◆, PhIP-4; ●, Ames/ *Salmonella* mutagenesis assay (ng/g).

ACKNOWLEDGMENTS

We thank Mona Hwang and Nancy Shen for assistance with immunoassays and *Salmonella* assays, and Mark G. Knize and Anna Marie Adams for assistance with the HPLC separations. Funding was provided by the National Cancer Institute (CA48446-01) and the U.S. Department of Energy; the work was performed at the Lawrence Livermore National Laboratory under the auspices of the U.S. Department of Energy contract W-7405-ENG-48.

REFERENCES

Bjeldanes, F, MM Morris, JS Felton, S Healy, D Stuermer, P Berry, H Timourian, and FT Hatch. 1982a. Mutagens from the cooking of food. II. Survey by Ames/ *Salmonella* test of mutagen formation in the major protein-rich foods in the American diet. Food Chem Toxicol 20:357-363.

Bjeldanes, LF, MM Morris, JS Felton, S Healy, D Stuermer, P Berry, H Timourian, and FT Hatch. 1982b. Mutagens from the cooking of food. III. Secondary sources of cooked dietary protein. Food Chem Toxicol 20:365-369.

Felton, JS, MG Knize, NH Shen, PR Lewis, BD Andresen, J Happe, and FT Hatch. 1986. The isolation and identification of a new mutagen from fried beef: 2-amino-1-methyl-6-phenylimidazo[4,5-b]pyridine (PhIP). Carcinogenesis 7:1081-1086.

Felton, JS, M Knize, C Wood, B Wuebbles, SK Healy, DH Stuermer, LF Bjeldanes, BJ Kimble, and FT Hatch. 1984. Isolation and characterization of new mutagens from fried ground beef. Carcinogenesis 5:95-102.

Sugimura, T, T Kawachi, M Nagao, and T Yahagu T. 1981. Mutagens in food as causes of cancer. Prog Cancer Res Ther 17:59-57.

Thompson, LH, SA Stewart, JD Tucker, EP Salizar, JL Minkler, AV Carrano, and JS Felton. 1987. Evaluating compounds from cooked beef for genotoxicity in repair-deficient CHO cells. Environ Mutagen 9 (Suppl 8):108.

Vanderlaan, M, BE Watkins, M Hwang, MG Knize, and JS Felton. 1988. Monoclonal antibodies for the immunoassay of mutagenic compounds produced by cooking beef. Carcinogenesis 9:53-160.

Vanderlaan, M, BE Watkins, M Hwang, MG Knize, and JS Felton. Monoclonal antibodies to 6-phenyl-2-amino-1-methylimidazo [4, 5-b] pyridine (PhIP) and their use in the analysis of well-done fried beef. Carcinogenesis (in press).

Watkins, BE, MG Knize, CJ Morris, BD Andresen, J Happe, M Vanderlaan, and JS Felton. 1987. The synthesis of haptenic derivatives of the aminoimidazoazaarene cooked-food mutagens. Heterocycles 26:2069-2072.

A RECOMBINANT DNA METHOD FOR UNDERSTANDING THE MECHANISM OF *Salmonella* REVERSE MUTATIONS: ROLE OF REPAIR

J. S. Felton,[1] R. Wu,[1] N. H. Shen,[1] S. K. Healy,[1] and J. C. Fuscoe[2]

[1]Biomedical Sciences Division, Lawrence Livermore National Laboratory, Livermore, CA 94550

[2]Center for Environmental Health, University of Connecticut, Storrs, CT 06268

Key words: *Frame-shift mutation, Ames/Salmonella, DNA sequence analysis, environmental, mutagens, food mutagens*

ABSTRACT

We have investigated the specific sequence changes in the DNA of *Salmonella* *hisD3052* revertants induced by a set of frameshift-specific mutagens. They include benzo[a]pyrene (BaP), aflatoxin B_1, and the cooked-food mutagens, IQ, MeIQ, and PhIP. Sequencing was accomplished by cleaving the *Salmonella* DNA with restriction enzymes *Sau*3A, *Eco*RI, *and Alu*I to give a 650-bp fragment. After the fragments were size fractionated, they were ligated to the bacteriophage vector *M13mp8*. After transformation into *Escherichia coli*, the recombinants were screened with a nick-translated *hisD* gene probe, and the isolated single-stranded DNA sequenced, using the Sanger/dideoxynucleotide chain termination method. In the strain TA1538, all IQ (13), MeIQ (3), PhIP (5), and aflatoxin B_1 (3) -induced revertants isolated had a 2-base (CG dinucleotide) deletion situated 10 bases upstream from the original *hisD3052* C deletion. In contrast, 9 of 24 revertants induced by BaP had extensive deletions, varying from 8 to 26 nucleotides in length and located at various sites along a 45-base sequence, beginning at nucleotide 2085 of the *his* operon. The other 15 revertants had a CG deletion at the same location as the other mutagens.

To understand which of the many mutagenic metabolites might be responsible for the large deletions, we analyzed the metabolites of BaP. This showed clearly that the "anti" 7,8-diol-9,10-epoxide was a major inducer of large lesions. (More than 50% of those induced were large deletions, compared to 38% for those induced by BaP alone.) The 4,5-epoxide showed no large deletions, only CG dinucleotide deletions in the hot spot. This effect with the diol-epoxide is in marked contrast to that for the aromatic amines from cooked food, where only the single type of lesion (dinucleotide) was seen in more than 20 revertant colonies.

The effect of intact *uvrB* repair was examined with both BaP and IQ in *Salmonella* strain TA1978. The BaP showed no CG deletions, compared to 63% with the *uvrB*-inactivated strain TA1538. Even more remarkable was the IQ response: 42% large deletions and insertions in TA1978, compared to none in TA1538. The effect of error-prone repair (pKM101 plasmid) on BaP-induced mutations was similar to *uvrB* inactivation, with the exception of two unique lesions, each with a deletion and insertion at the same mutation site.

Understanding the types of DNA base changes induced by both a mutagen and its metabolites can elucidate not only the mutational process and repair mechanisms but also the potency and mode of action of specific metabolites and their corresponding DNA adduct(s). This type of study is the beginning of a mechanistic approach to understanding chemically mediated frameshift mutations.

INTRODUCTION

The specific sequence changes in the DNA of *Salmonella* revertants that are induced by environmental mutagens and their metabolites were investigated. The compounds tested were chosen because they specifically induce frameshift lesions in strains TA1538 and TA98 (Ames et al., 1973; Felton et al., 1986). DNA lesions in these strains, analyzed in the *hisD* gene, can lead to reversion of histidine dependence by either deletions, insertions, or suppressor mutations. The understanding of the types of DNA-base changes induced by both a mutagen and its metabolites can elucidate not only the mutational process and repair mechanisms but also the potency and mode of action of specific metabolites and their corresponding DNA adduct(s). The detailed development of the methods used for this research and the original findings with benzo[a]pyrene (BaP) were recently published (Fuscoe et al., 1988).

METHODS

The compounds used in our study were BaP, BaP diol-epoxide, BaP 4,5-epoxide, aflatoxin B_1, and the food mutagens, 2-amino-3-methylimidazo[4,5-f]quinoline (IQ), 2-amino-3,4-dimethylimidazo[4,5-f]-quinoline (MeIQ), and 2-amino-1-methyl-6-phenylimidazo[4,5-b]-pyridine (PhIP). The DNA of the *Salmonella* revertants induced by these compounds was extracted and cleaved with restriction enzymes (*Sau*3A and *Eco*RI) so that the portion of the *hisD* gene of interest was incorporated in a 650-bp fragment (Figure 1). The 600- to 700-bp fragments produced after enzyme cleavage were purified from the smaller and larger fragments by agarose gel electrophoresis. These size-fractionated fragments were ligated to the bacteriophage vector *M13mp8*, and this mixture was used to transform *Escherichia coli*. The recombinants were screened with a nick-translated *hisD* gene probe to identify the revertant gene sequence. Single-stranded DNA from the recombinants was sequenced using the Sanger/dideoxy-nucleotide chain termination method (Sanger et al., 1977).

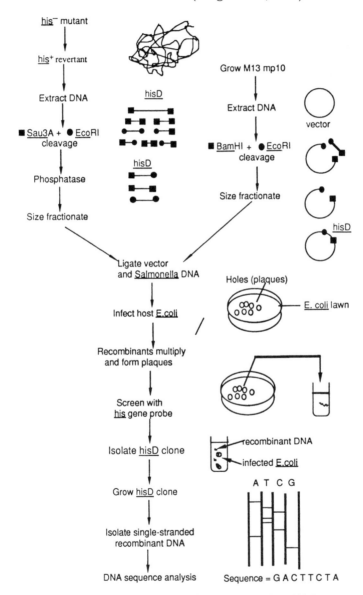

Figure 1. Flow diagram showing steps in cloning and sequencing of *hisD* revertant alleles.

RESULTS AND DISCUSSION

uvrB Excision Repair-Deficient Strains

All revertants induced by IQ (13), MeIQ (3), PhIP (5), and aflatoxin B_1 (3) that were isolated had a 2-base (-CG- dinucleotide) deletion. This deletion is situated in a run of 4-CG- dinucleotide pairs (a hot spot) ending 10 bases upstream from the original mutation in strain TA1538 (Figure 2). It is a single-C deletion designated hisD3052 that confirms the auxotrophic behavior of these strains.

```
HisD3052   GluLeuPro ArgAlaAspT hrAla GlyA rgProEND
           GAACTGCCG CGCGCGGACA CCGCC_GGCA GGCCCTGAGC GCCAGT


TA1538     GluLeuP    roArgGlyHi sArgA rgGl nAlaLeuSer AlaSer
BP-1       GAACTGC__  CGCGCGGACA CCGCC_GGCA GGCCCTGAGC GCCAGT
IQ-1


TA98       GluLeuPro ArgAlaAspT hrAla GlyA rgProLeuSer AlaSer
BP-11      GAACTGCCG CGCGCGGACA CCGCC_GGCA GGCCCT_AGC GCCAGT
                                                   ^
                                                   CT


TA98       GluLeuPro Hi   sGlyHi sArgA rgGl nAlaLeuSer AlaSer
BP-13      GAACTGCCG C___CGGACA CCGCC_GGCA GGCCCTGAGC GCCAGT
                      ^
                      A
```

Figure 2. Description of the base changes in TA1538 and TA98. Both nucleotide sequence and predicted amino acid sequence are given. Bars indicate extent of deletion.

In contrast, 9 of 24 revertants induced by BaP had extensive deletions varying from 8 to 26 nucleotides in length and located at various sites along a 45-base sequence beginning at nucleotide 2085 of the histidine operon. No pattern could be determined for either the 3' or 5' deletion sites associated with the deletions. The other 15 BaP-induced mutations had a -CG- deletion at the same location (-CG- 4-base run) as the other mutagens. In the case of one large deletion of 14 bases, 5 amino acids are not translated because of the deletion, and 8 more are mistranslated because of the change in reading frame that occurs up to the correction at the hisD3052 single-base deletion. The ability of the enzyme histidinol dehydrogenase (the product of the *hisD* gene) to continue to function with 13 amino acids either deleted or miscoded suggests two possibilities: either the enzymatic active site is quite distant or independent from this region or domain of the protein, or possibly the deletion and subsequent miscoding occur in a looped-out region of the peptide.

The amino acid sequence of this portion of the peptide suggests that the secondary structure is primarily alpha helical. Measurement of the histidinol dehyrogenase activity of individual revertants was not clearly related to the size or the location of the deletion. All revertants had decreased activity from the wild type, and varied from 11% to 89% of control. As might be expected, smaller colonies tended to have a higher percentage of large deletions, suggesting that the synthesis of histidine may have been slightly more impaired in the revertants with large deletions. These smaller colonies remained small when subcloned, thus supporting the conclusion that a genetic event is responsible for the slow growth. It is interesting that all revertants sequenced in strain TA1538 are deletions. One might expect a certain number of 2-base insertions to appear, because they could correct the reading frame just as easily as the 1-base deletions.

Repair-Competent Strain TA1978

The effect of a functional *urvB* repair gene was examined with both BaP and IQ in strain TA1978. Interestingly, BaP showed no 2-base -CG- deletions compared to 63% in the *uvrB*-inactivated TA1538. Even more remarkable was the IQ response, which showed 42% large deletions and insertions (1- and 4-base) in TA1978 compared to 0% of these types of mutations in TA1538. The mutation frequency is approximately 100-fold lower in this strain with these compounds, suggesting that the intact repair system must be selectively removing the DNA lesions responsible for the -CG- deletions. It is possible that the deletions and insertions seen in TA1978 are present in TA1538 but are masked by the 100-fold-higher mutation frequency that resulted from failure to remove the lesions causing the high frequency of -CG- deletions.

Error-Prone Repair

The effect of error-prone repair (plasmid pKM101) was examined in strain TA98. This strain has deficient *uvrB* repair activity, as does TA1538, and thus should show a similar spectrum of lesions except for the contribution from the error-prone repair system. In two BaP revertants, very unusual lesions were found; the remainder were as expected for a deficient *uvrB* system with some large deletions and 70% deletions of -CG-. The unique lesions showed a deletion and insertion at the same mutational site, and both resulted in a corrected reading frame downstream at the *hisD3052* -C- deletion (see Figure 2). In one case, an -A- was inserted adjacent to a -GCG- deletion for a net 2-base deletion. In the other, -CT- was inserted adjacent to a -G- deletion, resulting in a net 1-base addition. The intriguing mechanism by which the error-prone system leads to these unique lesions is under further study.

BaP Metabolites

Analyzing BaP metabolites to determine which of many mutagenic metabolites may be responsible for the large deletions clearly showed that the "anti" 7,8-diol-9,10-epoxide was an inducer of large lesions; more than 50% were large deletions compared to 38% for BaP alone. The 4,5-epoxide showed no large deletions, but CG dinucleotide deletions occurred in the hot spot. This effect with the diol-epoxide is in marked contrast to that for the aromatic amines from cooked food, in which case only the single-type (dinucleotide) lesion was seen in more than 20 revertant colonies analyzed. Interestingly, the BaP diol-epoxide-induced revertants in TA98 showed two additional unique revertants. In both cases, an -A- insertion occurs adjacent to a 3-base deletion.

The mechanisms for induction of the dinucleotide deletion, the larger deletions, the insertions, and the unique double insertion/deletions are not clear. However, the aromatic amines and the BaP have been shown to form C-8 adducts, which could lead to a -CG- deletion. Studies are in progress to determine further the role of repair in the types of lesions induced by PAH, aromatic amines, and other environmental chemicals.

ACKNOWLEDGMENTS

The authors thank Dr. Wayne Barnes for suppling the histidine operon DNA sequence and Professor Bruce Ames for suppling the *Salmonella* strains. The work was performed under auspices of the U.S. Department of Energy (DOE) by the Lawrence Livermore National Laboratory under contract No. W-74050ENG-48 and supported by IAG No. 222-01-ES-10063 between NIEHS and U.S. DOE.

REFERENCES

Ames, BN, WE Durston, E Yamasaki, and FD Lee. 1973. Carcinogens are mutagens: A simple test system combining liver homogenates for activation and bacteria for detection. Proc Natl Acad Sci USA 70:2281-2285.

Felton, JS, MG Knize, NH Shen, BD Andresen, LF Bjeldanes, and FT Hatch. 1986. Identification of the mutagens in cooked beef. Environ Health Perspect 67:17-24.

Fuscoe, JC, R Wu, NH Shen, SK Healy, and JS Felton. 1988. Base-change analysis of revertants of the *hisD3052* allele in *Salmonella typhimurium*. Mutat Res 201:241-251.

Sanger, F, S Nicklin, and AR Coulson. 1977. DNA sequencing with chain-terminating inhibitors. Proc Natl Acad Sci USA 74:5463-5467.

IMPROVED METHODOLOGY FOR DNA FILTER ELUTION TECHNIQUES

E. R. Blazek, J. G. Peak, and M. J. Peak

Biological, Environmental, and Medical Research Division, Argonne National Laboratory, 9700 S. Cass Ave, Argonne, IL 60439-4833

Key words: *Alkaline elution, nondenaturing (neutral) elution, DNA strand breaks, DNA-protein covalent cross-links, assay calibration*

ABSTRACT

We describe improvements in filter elution methods for quantitation of both DNA-protein covalent cross-links in the presence of strand breaks and of DNA double-strand breaks. The dose-response relationship for induction of double-strand breaks by gamma radiation, as determined by the latter method, is discussed. Finally, we report an observation that is important to the correct use of elution assays and explore its implications for the physical mechanisms underlying the elution phenomenon.

The filter elution techniques introduced by Kohn and colleagues (Kohn and Grimek-Ewig, 1973) are now the most frequently used of the ultrasensitive hydrodynamic assays of DNA damage (more than 115 publications since 1986), in part because of their versatility. Elution can be performed so as to detect total strand (usually called single-strand) breaks (SSB; Kohn et al., 1976), double-strand breaks (DSB; Bradley and Kohn, 1979), protein-associated breaks resulting from topoisomerase activity (Ross et al., 1979), DNA-protein covalent cross-links (DPC; Kohn and Ewig, 1979), total DNA cross-links including interstrand cross-links (Ewig and Kohn, 1978), and enzyme-sensitive (Fornace, 1982) or alkali-labile sites (ALS; Ewig and Kohn, 1977). Any ALS that are converted to SSB during the collection of the first elution fraction, which we term rapidly developing alkali-labile sites (RALS), cannot be distinguished from frank SSB (FSSB). Thus total or "single-" strand breaks are quantitated as:

$$SSB = FSSB + 2(DSB) + RALS \qquad [1]$$

Because no exact theory for the elution mechanism exists, the analysis of elution data has developed empirically. We describe here our improvements in the analysis of data from two types of elution assay, as well as an observation that is important in elution methodology. This observation may illuminate the physical principles underlying the elution process.

IMPROVED QUANTITATION OF DPC IN THE PRESENCE OF STRAND BREAKS

The preferred elution method for the quantitation of DPC has been method F of Kohn et al. (1981), in which a high dose of x rays is used to separate cross-linked from free DNA fragments. In this method, DPC frequencies are calculated from a formula derived on the assumption that breakage caused by the cross-linking agent under study is negligible compared to that induced by the x-ray dose. Because this assumption is not valid for the high fluences of near-ultraviolet (UV) radiation we were studying, we removed the assumption to obtain the following equation (Peak et al., 1987):

$$P_{cd} = P_{br}[(1-p)^{\frac{1}{2}} - (1-p_0)^{\frac{1}{2}}] + P_{bd}[(1-p)^{\frac{1}{2}} - 1]] \qquad [2]$$

where p_0 (x-ray dose only) and p (x rays plus cross-linking agent) are the extrapolations to zero elution time of the slowly eluting portion of the elution profile, P_{br} is the frequency of radiation-induced breaks, and P_{bd} is the frequency of breaks caused by the cross-linking agent under study. The first term of equation (2) is identical to that in the equation used for the established method F. The second term is a correction term that is proportional to the number of strand breaks induced by the cross-linking agent.

Our generalization of the DPC analysis has an interesting consequence. The action spectrum for DPC formation in human P3 cells (Peak et al., 1985) has a minor peak at 405 nm, which led us to postulate the existence of an endogenous photosensitizer active at 405 nm but not at 365 nm. Reanalysis of our data using equation (2) (Peak et al., submitted to Radiation Research) removes this artifactual feature from the action spectrum.

IMPROVED QUANTITATION OF DSB BY NONDENATURING ELUTION

In nondenaturing ("neutral") elution experiments, semilogarithmic plots of the uneluted fraction of DNA versus elution time are generally upturning, in contrast to the straight profiles obtained from alkaline elution. Therefore, the elution time (fraction number) at which profiles are compared is important. Further, the form of the assay response function has been chosen either arbitrarily or using the questionable assumption that DSB frequency is proportional to x-ray dose. Radford and Hodgson (1985) first addressed these problems. Using the fact that ^{125}I-iododeoxyuridine incorporated in the DNA of frozen cells yields almost exactly one DSB per decay, they verified the adequacy of a linear response function and a particular evaluation time for a range of 100-2000 decays per cell, and thereby calibrated the nondenaturing elution assay. We (Peak et al., 1988) extended this work by empirically selecting both the response function and the evaluation time that yielded the strongest correlation between assay response and the number of ^{125}I decays over a broader range (200-10,000 decays per cell) at two pH values. Our calibration yields:

$$\text{for pH 7.2: } DSB/10^{10} \text{ daltons } = 94.3 \text{ (4.4) } L_9 \qquad [3a]$$
$$\text{for pH 9.6: } DSB/10^{10} \text{ daltons } = 70.7 \text{ (3.0) } L_9 \qquad [3b]$$

where $L_9 = \log_{10}[R_9(^{14}C\text{-labeled control cells})/R_9(^{125}I\text{-labeled test cells})]$, and where R_9 represents uneluted radioactivity at the ninth elution fraction (13.5 hr of elution time). One form of the response function and one evaluation time proved optimal for both nondenaturing pH values.

Conflicting results have been reported on the form of the dose-response relationship for induction of DSB in cells by external gamma radiation (reviewed by Radford, 1988). We used our calibration to study this question further in (asynchronous) Chinese hamster V79 cells (Blazek et al., 1989). When elution is performed at pH 7.2, induced DSB frequency is proportional to the square of the dose with no significant linear dependence on dose. This finding suggests that two independent absorption events are needed for one DSB, although we show that these events cannot be randomly distributed, opposed SSB. Elution at pH 9.6 resulted in a DSB yield slightly greater than that measured at pH 7.2. This excess DSB yield measured at pH 9.6 may be linearly proportional to dose, suggesting that sites labile to the more alkaline pH are induced near opposed SSB or ALS by a single absorption event. In contrast, the neutral sucrose gradient sedimentations of Bloecher (1982) indicate that the entire DSB induction is linearly proportional to dose. Further work is needed to reconcile the results of elution and sedimentation assays, thereby placing quantitation of DSB frequency on a firm foundation.

IMPORTANCE OF THE ALKALINE WASH OF THE FILTER SUPPORT

A standard procedure of elution assays is to wash the filter support with 0.4 N NaOH after removal of the filter. The amount of DNA (measured as radioactivity or fluorescence) recovered by these washes is added to that associated with the filter, and this sum is analyzed as uneluted DNA (Kohn et al., 1981). The rationale for treating the washes as if they contain uneluted DNA has not, to our knowledge, been discussed in the literature. To this end we first review proposed mechanisms underlying the elution phenomenon.

Kohn et al. (1976) suggested that each DNA strand enters many filter pores, forming an equilibrium system of loops that are elongated by the flow of elution solution (Figure 1). Escape of a strand from the filter requires a fluctuation large enough that one loop predominates over and retracts all the others. This process will require longer times for strands generating more loops, that is, for strands of greater molecular weight.

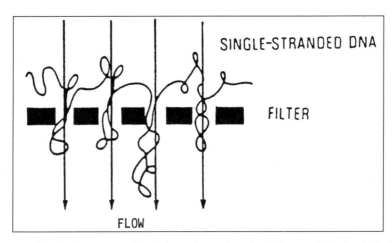

Figure 1. Mechanism proposed by Kohn and coworkers for DNA strand size discrimination by alkaline elution. The dominant (largest) loop must retract all others before the DNA strand can escape from the filter.

Models based on an entirely different concept were proposed by Nicolini et al. (1983) and Balbi et al. (1986). They envisioned the DNA strand as a random coil with a mean square end-to-end distance R that is a calculable function of molecular weight. Nicolini et al. (1983) used a simple geometric criterion for strand entry into a pore of radius r in an idealized two-dimensional membrane (Figure 2), whereas Balbi et al. (1986) used a more sophisticated thermodynamic criterion for strand entry into a three-dimensional ("thick") membrane. In both models, the ratio (R/r) determines elution behavior. Because this ratio is, in general, less than unity, once any portion of the strand exits the pore, there is no mechanism to retain the remainder of the strand.

We have performed both alkaline and nondenaturing elution, each at two pH values. Table 1 shows that the amount of uneluted DNA, defined as the sum of DNA measured on the filter and recovered in the alkaline wash of the filter support after removal of the filter, decreases only modestly when either assay is performed at the higher of its two pH values. Thus the quantity of uneluted DNA is approximately conserved despite changes in assay pH. However, the fraction of the uneluted DNA recovered on the filter itself (the filter sector) is dramatically reduced at the higher pH employed in the alkaline assay. In the nondenaturing assay, by contrast, the partitioning of the uneluted DNA is not pH dependent; instead, the filter sectors at both pH values are nearly identical for a given type and extent of DNA damage. The pH-dependent partitioning observed for alkaline elution is consistent with the looped-strand concept (Kohn et al., 1976) of the elution mechanism, provided that single-stranded DNA hanging in loops beneath the filter is more easily broken (by filter removal) at pH 12.6 than at pH 12.1. Independent measurements of the pH dependence of DNA shear degradation (Adam and Zimm, 1977) indicate that the fragility of DNA is indeed increased by elevation of pH over at least the range of pH 7 to pH 11.5 (higher pH values were not tested). However, the pH independence of partitioning for nondenaturing elution, despite apparently greater DNA fragility at pH 9.6 than at pH 7.2, suggests that substantially different physical mechanisms may govern the passage of single- and double-stranded DNA molecules through micropore filters.

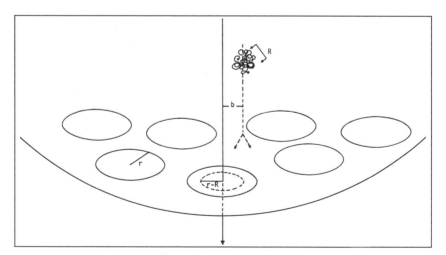

Figure 2. Mechanism proposed by Nicolini and coworkers for DNA strand size discrimination by alkaline elution. The DNA strand is idealized as a freely jointed polymer without excluded volume, of root mean square end-to-end distance R (in Å) = $3.4\,nM^{\frac{1}{2}}$, where n is the number of nucleotides in the strand and M is the number of nucleotides in a statistical segment (believed to be ≤ 100). It will traverse the filter if the impact parameter b (distance from center of strand mass to center of pore) is $< (r - R)$. Therefore, the probability of strand elution is proportional to $(r - R)^2$.

Table 1. Uneluted fractions [(F + W)/T] and filter sectors [F/(F + W)] of DNA radioactivity.[a]

| Alkaline Elution | Uneluted Fraction | | Filter Sector | |
Cell Treatment	pH 12.1	pH 12.6	pH 12.1	pH 12.6
None (control)	0.89 ± 0.02^b	0.75 ± 0.03	0.84 ± 0.04	0.49 ± 0.06
X-rays (3 Gy)	0.14 ± 0.03	0.10 ± 0.03	0.29 ± 0.05	0.07 ± 0.02
HPD (5 Gapc)^c	0.25 ± 0.05	0.14 ± 0.03	0.27 ± 0.02	0.12 ± 0.002
405 nm (2 MJm^{-2})	0.41 ± 0.08	0.21 ± 0.06	0.57 ± 0.12	0.10 ± 0.03
(4 MJm^{-2})	0.20 ± 0.07	0.09 ± 0.03	0.39 ± 0.12	0.14 ± 0.05
Nondenaturing Elution	Uneluted Fraction		Filter Sector	
Cell Treatment	pH 7.2	pH 9.6	pH 7.2	pH 9.6
None (control)	0.92 ± 0.02	0.96 ± 0.01	0.88 ± 0.02	0.90 ± 0.03
^{60}Co γ-rays (45 Gy)	0.68 ± 0.04	0.51 ± 0.03	0.62 ± 0.04	0.62 ± 0.03
^{125}I (0-2000 dpc)^d	0.75 ± 0.03	0.78 ± 0.02	0.81 ± 0.02	0.83 ± 0.02
(4000-6000 dpc)	0.66 ± 0.03	0.56 ± 0.03	0.60 ± 0.09	0.67 ± 0.04
(8000-10000 dpc)	0.51 ± 0.02	0.41 ± 0.02	0.55 ± 0.01	0.54 ± 0.08

[a] F, radioactivity recovered on filter alone; W, radioactivity recovered in filter support washes; T, total radioactivity loaded on filter.
[b] Mean $\pm$ SEM (n = 4 to 25).
[c] Hematoporphyrin derivative photosensitization (5 × 10^9 photons absorbed by intracellular hematoporphyrin derivative per cell).
[d] Disintegrations per cell of ^{125}I-iododeoxyuridine incorporated into the DNA.

Whatever physical mechanisms govern the elution process, the approximate conservation of the sum of the DNA associated with the filter and that recovered in washes of the filter support despite changes in the assay pH is compelling evidence that it is correct to regard this sum as uneluted DNA. Therefore the complete recovery (by two or more alkaline washes) of the DNA left on the filter support after removal of the filter is essential to the correct analysis of filter elution data.

ACKNOWLEDGMENTS

This work was supported by grants RO1 CA34492 and RO1 CA37848 awarded by the National Cancer Institute, U.S. Department of Health and Human Services, and by the U.S. Department of Energy Office of Health and Environmental Research, under Contract No. W-31-109-ENG-38.

REFERENCES

Adam, RE and BH Zimm. 1977. Shear degradation of DNA. Nucleic Acids Res 4:1513-1537.

Balbi, C, M Pala, S Parodi, G Figari, B Cavazza, V Trefiletti, and E Patrone. 1986. A simple model for DNA elution from filters. J Theor Biol 118:183-198.

Blazek, ER, JG Peak, and MJ Peak. 1989. Evidence from nondenaturing filter elution that induction of double-strand breaks in the DNA of Chinese hamster V79 cells by γ radiation is proportional to the square of dose. Radiat Res 119:466-477.

Bloecher, D. 1982. DNA double strand breaks in Ehrlich ascites tumour cells at low doses of x-rays. I. Determination of induced breaks by centrifugation at reduced speed. Int J Radiat Biol 42:317-328.

Bradley, MO and KW Kohn. 1979. X-ray induced DNA double-strand break production and repair in mammalian cells as measured by neutral filter elution. Nucleic Acids Res 7:793-804.

Ewig, RAG and KW Kohn. 1977. DNA damage and repair in mouse leukemia L1210 cells treated with nitrogen mustard, 1,3-bis(2-chloroethyl)-1-nitrosourea, and other nitrosoureas. Cancer Res 37:2114-2122.

Ewig, RAG and KW Kohn. 1978. DNA-protein cross-linking and DNA interstrand cross-linking by haloethylnitrosoureas in L1210 cells. Cancer Res 38:3197-3203.

Fornace, AJ. 1982. Measurement of M. luteus endonuclease-sensitive lesions by alkaline elution. Mutat Res 94:263-276.

Kohn, KW and RAG Ewig. 1979. DNA-protein crosslinking by trans-platinum(II) diamminedichloride in mammalian cells, a new method of analysis. Biochim Biophys Acta 562:32-40.

Kohn, KW and RA Grimek-Ewig. 1973. Alkaline elution analysis, a new approach to the study of DNA single-strand interruptions in cells. Cancer Res 33:1849-1853.

Kohn, KW, LC Erickson, RAG Ewig, and CA Friedman. 1976. Fractionation of DNA from mammalian cells by alkaline elution. Biochemistry 15:4629-4637.

Kohn, KW, RAG Ewig, LC Erickson, and LA Zwelling. 1981. Measurement of strand breaks and cross-links by alkaline elution, pp. 379-401. In: DNA Repair: A Laboratory Manual of Research Procedures, Vol. I, Part B, EC Friedberg and PC Hanawalt (eds.). Marcel Dekker, New York.

Nicolini, C, A Belmont, S Zietz, A Maura, A Pino, L Robbiano, and G Brambilla. 1983. Physico-chemical model for DNA alkaline elution: New experimental evidence and differential role of DNA length, chain flexibility and superpacking. J Theor Biol 100:341-357.

Peak, JG, MJ Peak, and ER Blazek. 1987. Improved quantitation of DNA-protein crosslinking caused by 405-nm monochromatic near-UV radiation in human cells. Photochem Photobiol 46:319-321.

Peak, JG, ER Blazek, CK Hill, and MJ Peak. 1988. Measurement of double strand breaks in Chinese hamster cell DNA by neutral filter elution: Calibration by ^{125}I decay. Radiat Res 115:624-629.

Peak, JG, MJ Peak, RS Sikorski, and CA Jones. 1985. Induction of DNA-protein crosslinks in human cells by ultraviolet and visible radiations: Action spectrum. Photochem Photobiol 41:295-302.

Radford, IR. 1988. The dose-response for low-LET radiation-induced DNA double-strand breakage: Methods of measurement and implications for radiation action models. Int J Radiat Biol 54:1-11.

Radford, IR and GS Hodgson. 1985. ^{125}I-induced DNA double strand breaks: Use in calibration of the neutral filter elution technique and comparison with X-ray induced breaks. Int J Radiat Biol 48:555-566.

Ross, WE, D Glaubiger, and KW Kohn. 1979. Qualitative and quantitative aspects of intercalator-induced DNA strand breaks. Biochim Biophys Acta 562:41-50.

GENETIC AND MOLECULAR ANALYSIS OF CYTOCHROME P-450IA1 INDUCTION IN A MOUSE HEPATOMA CELL LINE

O. Hankinson,[1] R. M. Bannister,[2] N. Carramanzana,[2] F.-F. Chu,[1] E. C. Hoffman,[1] H. Reyes,[1] F. Sander,[2] and A. J. Watson[3]

[1]Department of Pathology and Laboratory of Biomedical and Environmental Sciences, University of California, Los Angeles, CA

[2]Laboratory of Biomedical and Environmental Sciences, University of California, Los Angeles, CA

[3]School of Public Health and Laboratory of Biomedical and Environmental Sciences, University of California, Los Angeles, CA

Key words: *Cytochrome P-450IA1, Ah receptor, mutants, cloning*

ABSTRACT

The mouse hepatoma cell line Hepa-1 is highly inducible for cytochrome P-450IA1 (cytochrome P_1-450) by polycyclic and halogenated aromatic hydrocarbons. Hepa-1 is also sensitive to benzo[a]pyrene (BaP) toxicity. We isolated BaP-resistant mutants of the line and showed that they are defective in P-450IA1 induction; a few of the mutants are dominant; the majority are recessive. The latter were assigned to four complementation groups (i.e., genes). The A gene is the P-450IA1 structural gene. Mutations in the B, C, and D genes affect functioning of the *Ah* receptor, which is required for induction of P-450IA1.

We designed a "reverse selection" procedure for selecting P-450IA1-inducible cells from among noninducible cells. Representative recessive mutants were treated with human DNA, and transfectants in which P-450IA1 inducibility was restored were isolated using reverse selection. From a secondary transfectant of C mutant, we cloned human DNA fragments corresponding to the human C gene. The dominant mutants synthesized a transacting repressor of P-450IA1 transcription. We treated wild-type Hepa-1 cells with DNA from a dominant mutant and, by means of BaP selection, isolated transfectants defective in P-450IA1 induction. The noninducibility phenotype of these transfectants was shown to be dominant in somatic cell hybrids with the wild-type cells. We are attempting to clone the dominant gene, utilizing a strategy based on transfection of the gene.

INTRODUCTION

Certain polycyclic aromatic hydrocarbons (PAH), such as benzo[a]pyrene (BaP), and certain halogenated aromatic hydrocarbons (HAH), such as

2,3,7,8-tetrachlorodibenzo-p-dioxin (TCDD), are important environmental pollutants. Many of these compounds are extremely toxic and carcinogenic. These same compounds also bind the soluble Ah receptor and are thereby capable of inducing cytochrome P-450IA1. Cytochrome P-450IA1-dependent aryl hydrocarbon hydroxylase (AHH) activity, in turn, plays a central role in metabolism of PAH to their ultimate carcinogenic derivatives. Pathogenesis by HAH also depends on action of the Ah receptor. In the case of these compounds, however, the HAH themselves, rather than metabolites, are the pathogenic agents, and P-450IA1 activity is not involved.

The 300-kdalton mouse Ah receptor appears to dissociate, on treatment with high salt, to a 100-kdalton ligand-binding polypeptide (Denison et al., 1986a) that is the same size as the receptor detected under denaturing conditions (Poland and Glover, 1987). This suggests that the receptor is polymeric but does not shed light on whether it contains one or more than one type of subunit.

In addition to their intimate involvement in chemical carcinogenesis, cytochrome P-450IA1 and the Ah receptor are very interesting for at least two other reasons: (1) They provide a good model for studying gene regulation in mammalian cells, because P-450IA1 is highly inducible and is expressed to widely different degrees in different tissues and at different times in development; and (2) the Ah receptor appears to be involved in the regulation of cell division and cell differentiation in certain tissues (reviewed by Poland, 1984; Nebert and Gonzalez, 1987). We summarize here our studies on this system.

ISOLATION OF MUTANTS DEFICIENT IN INDUCTION OF CYTOCHROME P-450IA1

Most of our research has utilized the cultured mouse hepatoma line, Hepa-1, which is highly inducible for AHH activity by PAH and HAH. [Mutations in the cytochrome P-450IA1 structural gene abolish AHH activity in Hepa-1 cells, and therefore all AHH activity in the line can be ascribed to this form of cytochrome P-450 (Hankinson et al., 1985).] Moreover, inducible AHH activity remained stable in Hepa-1 cells during many months in culture, and there was no detectable heterogeneity in inducible AHH activity among subclones of the line (Hankinson, 1979, 1981). This stability of AHH activity augured well for a genetic analysis of P-450IA1 induction in the line.

The Hepa-1 line was found to be very sensitive to BaP toxicity, and a single-step selection procedure for isolating BaP-resistant (BaP^r) clones was designed (Hankinson, 1979). We subsequently isolated more than 100 such clones, and all have proven to be noninducible for AHH activity. We investigated whether the BaP^r clones originate by a mutational process (i.e., by a change in DNA sequence), because, along with others, we have obtained convincing evidence that loss in AHH activity can arise in some hepatoma cell lines by an epigenetic process(es) (Whitlock et al., 1976; Gudas and Hankinson, 1987). If a mutational event is responsible for loss of AHH activity, one can conclude that all the changes in phenotype probably result from a change in a single gene. Table 1 summarizes evidence we have obtained that our BaP^r clones are bona fide mutants.

Table 1. Evidence that the BaP^r, AHH-deficient clones of Hepa-1 are mutational in origin.

1. Arise at the low spontaneous frequency of 2×10^{-7} events/cell generation (Hankinson, 1979).

2. Phenotypes are stable (Hankinson, 1979, 1981).

3. Frequency is increased by the application of known mutagens (Hankinson, 1981).

4. Spontaneous reversion frequencies are low and increased by mutagens (not demonstrated for the D$^-$ mutant) (Van Gurp and Hankinson, 1984).

5. Not reverted by 5-azacytidine, which leads to demethylation of cytidine residues in DNA (not demonstrated for the D$^-$ mutant) (Van Gurp and Hankinson, 1984).

6. Defects are complemented by purified DNA.

7. In the case of two A$^-$ mutants, nucleotide substitution mutations in the P-450IA1 cDNA have been shown to be responsible for loss of AHH activity (Kimura et al., 1987).

To determine whether AHH-deficiency was dominant or recessive, somatic cell hybrids were constructed between individual BaP^r mutants and wild-type Hepa-1 cells. Five of the BaP^r mutants proved to be dominant, and 65 were recessive. Hybridizations performed between the recessive mutants demonstrated that they belonged to four complementation groups, named A to D (Hankinson, 1983; Karenlampi et al., 1988). Whitlock and coworkers used our BaP selection procedure to isolate two complementation groups of AHH-deficient variants of Hepa-1 that resemble our B$^-$ and C$^-$ mutants (Miller et al., 1983).

Biochemical Characterization of the Mutants

The results obtained with representative mutants are summarized in Table 2 (Legraverend et al., 1982; Hankinson et al., 1985; Karenlampi et al., 1988). The AHH activities correlated with the levels of P_1-450 mRNA in all mutants except some of the A^- class. The A^- mutants are heterogeneous: A^- subgroup II mutants lack P-450IA1 mRNA; subgroup IV mutants possess high levels of P-450IA1 mRNA, although they totally lack inducible AHH activity. These observations provided the initial evidence that gene A is the P-450IA1 structural gene. We also found that hybrids formed between individual dominant mutants and that the wild type lacked inducible P-450IA1 mRNA as well as AHH activity (Hankinson et al., 1985), which indicates that the dominant mutants synthesize a repressor of P-450IA1 transcription. In fact, we have shown that at least one site of repressor action lies within 1186 bp upstream of the cap site of the rat P-450IA1 gene (Chu et al., unpublished data). One possibility is that the dominant mutants arose by the activation of a gene that normally regulates tissue and/or developmental expression of P-450IA1.

Table 2. Properties of the mutants.[a]

Type of Strain	AHH-Specific Activity in TCDD-Induced Cells[b]	P-4510IA1 mRNA Levels in TCDD-Induced Cells	Ah Receptor Levels After In Vivo Treatment with [³H] TCDD		Basis
			Cytosol	Nucleus	
Hepa-1	100	100	100	100	
A⁻ subgroup II	0	0	100	100	P-450IA1 structural gene
A⁻, subgroup IV	0	100	100	100	
B⁻	2	2	2	2	Ah receptor gene?
C⁻	0	0	120	0	Ah receptor gene?
D⁻	3	3	20	3	Ah receptor gene?
Dominant	1	1	100	100	Repressor

[a]Each parameter is presented as a percentage of the same parameter in Hepa-1.
[b]TCCD, 2,3,7,8-tetra chlorodibenzo-p-dioxin.

There is some controversy as to whether the unoccupied Ah receptor, when not bound to ligand, is cytosolic or nuclear in location (Whitlock and

Galeazzi, 1984; Denison et al., 1986b). We enucleated uninduced Hepa-1 cells with cytochalasin B; with this procedure, nuclear proteins apparently do not leak into the cytosol. We found *Ah* receptor in the cytosolic fraction but not in the nuclei (Gudas et al., 1986; Gudas and Hankinson, 1986). We therefore believe that the unoccupied *Ah* receptor is cytoplasmic, and we have interpreted our *Ah* receptor assays on the mutants accordingly. The *A⁻* and dominant mutants have normal levels and functionality of the *Ah* receptor. The *B⁻* mutants have much reduced levels of the *Ah* receptor, which is nevertheless able to translocate to the nucleus on binding ligand. The *C⁻* mutants have normal levels of the *Ah* receptor but are totally defective in nuclear translocation. The *D⁻* mutants have diminished levels of *Ah* receptor, which is also reduced in its ability to translocate to the nucleus.

Thus mutations in three complementation groups can affect functioning of the *Ah* receptor, in marked contrast to the situation with mutants of the apparently similar glucocorticoid receptor. Mutants analogous to our *B⁻* and *C⁻* classes have been isolated for this receptor (Gehring et al., 1977). However, the two classes belong to the same complementation group, which corresponds to the 86-kdalton ligand- (and DNA-) binding subunit of the glucocorticoid receptor (Miesfeld et al., 1984). It is conceivable that our *B⁻*, *C⁻*, and *D⁻* mutants all carry lesions in the same gene and show intragenic complementation. However, we think that it is much more likely that the *B*, *C*, and *D* complementation groups each correspond to a different gene, and thus three genes affect functioning of the receptor.

We found that the mutants are defective only in the enzymes investigated that are inducible by PAH and HAH. Thus, the mutants possess normal activities of cytochrome P-450 reductase, epoxide hydrolase, and ornithine decarboxylase (Duthu and Hankinson, 1963) but manifest a defect in induction of UDP-glucuronosyl transferase (the *D⁻* and dominant mutants were not tested; Robertson et al., 1987). Furthermore, the mutants also retain two liver-specific functions possessed by the parental Hepa-1 line, albumin secretion and transferrin secretion (Duthu and Hankinson, 1983); thus, the loss of AHH inducibility in the mutants does not reflect a change in the general state of differentiation of the cells. We also showed that all classes of mutant also retain normal levels of the glucocorticoid receptor and have undiminished ability to concentrate the glucocorticoid receptor-ligand complex in the nucleus (Hankinson and Bannister, 1988). Thus, the *B⁻*, *C⁻*, and *D⁻* mutations do not have a general effect on soluble steroid or steroid-like receptors.

Cloning of the Genes

We developed a "reverse selection" procedure that can be used to select for P-450IA1-inducible cells growing in the presence of a vastly greater number of noninducible cells (Van Gurp and Hankinson, 1983). We have used this procedure to isolate transfectants of each recessive class of AHH-deficient mutant, using rat or human DNA as donor material. The rat DNA-derived transfectants of an A^- mutant were all shown, by Southern blot analysis, to contain the rat P-450IA1 gene, providing additional evidence that the A gene is the P-450IA1 structural gene (Montisano and Hankinson, 1985). [Definitive evidence was later obtained by showing that two A^- mutants contain nucleotide substitution mutations in the P-450IA1 gene (Robertson et al., 1987).] Primary transfectants of a C^- mutant were obtained using human DNA, and secondary transfectants were obtained from two of the primaries. The secondaries contained a number of human sequences in common. An 18-kb *Bgl*II human fragment was isolated from one of the secondaries and used as a probe to look further into the C gene. The gene is at least 50 kb in size. We have also isolated cDNA for this gene (Hoffman et al., unpublished data), and it should be possible to clone the B and D genes in an analogous fashion. We have also successfully transfected the dominant gene into Hepa-1 cells (Watson and Hankinson, 1988) and propose to clone this gene by a marker rescue strategy.

Success in cloning the B, C, D, and dominant genes should lead to important insights into: (1) the structure, role, and mechanism of action of the Ah receptor; (2) the mechanism of interaction of the Ah receptor and the dominant repressor with the P-450IA1 gene; (3) the possible role of the Ah receptor in cell division and differentiation; and (4) the possible involvement of one or more of the genes in determining individual differences in susceptibility to cigarette-induced cancer in the human population.

ACKNOWLEDGMENTS

Work was supported by NCI grant 28868, DOE contract DE-SC03-87-ER60615, NCI Core Support Grant CA 16042, University of California CRCC Fellowship W-P880621 to R.M.B., a Predoctoral Fellowship from Associated Western Universities to E.C.H., a CICR Predoctoral Fellowship to H.R., and NIH Training Grant GM-07104 to A.J.W.

REFERENCES

Denison, MS, LM Vella, and AB Okey. 1986a. Hepatic Ah receptor for 2,3,7,8-tetrachlorodibenzo-p-dioxin: partial stabilization by molybdate. J Biol Chem 261:3987-3995.

Denison, MS, PA Harper, and AB Okey. 1986b. *Ah* receptor for 2,3,7,8-tetrachlorodibenzo-*p*-dioxin: codistribution of unoccupied receptor with cytosolic marker enzymes during fractionation of mouse liver, rat liver and cultured Hepa-1c1 cells. Eur J Biochem 155:223-229.

Duthu, GS and O Hankinson. 1983. The defects in all classes of aryl hydrocarbon hydroxylase-deficient mutant of mouse hepatoma line, Hepa-1, are restricted to activities catalyzed by cytochrome P-450. Cancer Lett 20:249-254.

Gehring, U, KR Yamamoto, and GM Tomkins. 1977. Complementation analysis of steroid hormone action. Res Steroids 7:43-48.

Gudas, JM and O Hankinson. 1986. Reversible inactivation of the *Ah* receptor associated with changes in intracellular ATP levels. J Cell Physiol 128:449-456.

Gudas, JM and O Hankinson. 1987. Regulation of cytochrome P-450c in differentiated and dedifferentiated rat hepatoma cells: Role of the *Ah* receptor. Somatic Cell Mol Genet 13:513-528.

Gudas, JM, SO Karenlampi and O Hankinson. 1986. Intracellular location of the *Ah* receptor. J Cell Physiol 128:441-448.

Hankinson, O. 1979. Single-step selection of clones of a mouse hepatoma line deficient in aryl hydrocarbon hydroxylase. Proc Natl Acad Sci USA 76:373-376.

Hankinson, O. 1981. Evidence that the benzo(a)pyrene-resistant, aryl hydrocarbon hydroxylase-deficient variants of the mouse hepatoma line, Hepa-1, are mutational in origin. Somatic Cell Genet 7:373-388.

Hankinson, O. 1983. Dominant and recessive aryl hydrocarbon hydroxylase-deficient mutants of mouse hepatoma line, Hepa-1, and assignment of recessive mutants to three complementation groups. Somatic Cell Genet 9:497-514.

Hankinson, O and RM Bannister. 1988. Genetic analysis of the *Ah* receptor and cytochrome P1-450 expression in the mouse hepatoma cell line, Hepa-1, pp. 39-46. In: *Microsomes and Drug Oxidations*, J Miners, D J Birkett, R Drew, and M McManus (eds.). Taylor and Francis, London, New York, and Philadelphia.

Hankinson, O, RD Andersen, BW Birren, F Sander, M Negishi, and DW Nebert. 1985. Mutations affecting the regulation of transcription of the cytochrome P1-450 gene in mouse Hepa-1 cell cultures. J Biol Chem 260:1790-1795.

Karenlampi, SO, C Legraverend, JM Gudas, N Carramanzana, and O Hankinson. 1988. A third genetic locus affecting the *Ah* (dioxin) receptor. J Biol Chem 263:10111-10117.

Kimura, S, HH Smith, O Hankinson, and DW Nebert. 1987. Analysis of two benzo[a]pyrene-resistant mutants of the mouse hepatoma Hepa-1 P_1-450 gene via cDNA expression in yeast. EMBO J 6:1929-1934.

Legraverend, C, R Hannah, H Eisen, O Owens, D Nebert, and O Hankinson. 1982. Regulatory gene product of the *Ah* locus: Characterization of receptor mutants among mouse hepatoma clones. J Biol Chem 257:6502-6507.

Miesfeld, R, S Okret, A-C Wikstrom, O Wrange, J-A Gustaffson, and KR Yamamoto. 1984. Characterization of a steroid hormone receptor gene and mRNA in wild-type and mutant cells. Nature 312:779-781.

Miller, AG, D Israel, and JP Whitlock Jr. 1983. Biochemical and genetic analysis of variant mouse hepatoma cells defective in the induction of benzo(a)pyrene-metabolizing enzyme activity. J Biol Chem 258:3523-3527.

Montisano, DF and O Hankinson. 1985. Transfection by genomic DNA of cytochrome P1-450 enzymatic activity and inducibility. Mol Cell Biol 5:698-704.

Nebert, DW and FJ Gonzalez. 1987. P450 genes: structure, evolution, and regulation. Annu Rev Biochem 56:945-993.

Poland, A. 1984. Reflections on the mechanism of action of halogenated aromatic hydrocarbons, pp. 109-117. In: *Banbury Report No. 18*, A Poland and RD Kimborough (eds.). Cold Spring Harbor Laboratory, Cold Spring Harbor, New York.

Poland, A and E Glover. 1987. Variation in the molecular mass of the *Ah* receptor among vertebrate species and strains of rats. Biochem Biophys Res Commun 146:1439-1449.

Robertson, JA, O Hankinson, and DW Nebert. 1987. Autoregulation plus positive and negative elements controlling transcription of genes in the [*Ah*] battery. Chem Scr 27A:83-87.

Van Gurp, JR and O Hankinson. 1983. Single-step phototoxic selection procedure for isolating cells that possess aryl hydrocarbon hydroxylase. Cancer Res 43:6031-6038.

Van Gurp, JR and O Hankinson. 1984. Isolation and characterization of revertants from four different classes of aryl hydrocarbon hydroxylase-deficient mutant of Hepa-1. Mol Cell Biol 4:1597-1604.

Watson, AJ and O Hankinson. 1988. DNA transfection of a gene repressing aryl hydrocarbon hydroxylase induction. Carcinogenesis 9:1581-1586.

Whitlock, JP, Jr and DR Galeazzi. 1984. 2,3,7,8-Tetrachlorodibenzo-*p*-dioxin receptors in wild type and variant mouse hepatoma cells. Nuclear location and strength of nuclear binding. J Biol Chem 259:980-985.

Whitlock, JP, HV Gelboin, and HG Coon. 1976. Variation in aryl hydrocarbon (benzo[a]pyrene) hydroxylase activity in heteroploid and predominantly diploid rat liver cells in culture. J Cell Biol 70:217-225.

EFFECTS OF TRIBUTYLTIN ON BIOMEMBRANES: ALTERATION OF FLOW CYTOMETRIC PARAMETERS AND INHIBITION OF Na$^+$, K$^+$-ATPase CRYSTALLIZATION

E. J. Massaro,[1] R. M. Zucker,[2] K. H. Elstein,[2] R. E. Easterling,[1] and H. P. Ting-Beall[3]

[1]Developmental Toxicology Division, U.S. Environmental Protection Agency, Health Effects Research Laboratory, Research Triangle Park, NC 27711

[2]NSI Technology Services Corp., Environmental Sciences Division, P.O. Box 12313, Research Triangle Park, NC 27709

[3]Department of Anatomy, Duke University Medical Center, Durham, NC 27710

Key words: *Tributyltin, membrane-active toxicant, flow cytometry, Na$^+$, K$^+$-ATPase*

ABSTRACT

The cell interacts with its enviroment via the plasma membrane and alteration of the composition/structure of this membrane can result in altered cell function. Therefore, the ability to detect subtle changes in the condition of the membrane may be of considerable value in predicting the response of cells to toxic insult. Tributyltin (TBT: tri-*n*-butyltin methoxide, 97% pure, #22,924-5, Aldrich, Milwaukee, WI) is a membrane-active toxicant. To gain insight into its mechanism of action, we have investigated its effect on (1) the murine erythroleukemic cell (MELC), employing fluorescent probes of membrane integrity/viability in conjunction with flow cytometry, and (2) *in situ* crystallization of Na$^+$, K$^+$-ATPase in porcine renal microsomal membrane preparations by electron microscopy.

MELC MEMBRANE INTEGRITY

The MELC (T3CL2, from Dr. Clyde Hutchison, University of North Carolina, Chapel Hill, NC) was selected for study primarily because of the large amount of literature on its biology and its ability to grow in suspension culture (for culture conditions, see Zucker et al., 1988a), minimizing potential membrane damage resulting from harvesting techniques.

Membrane integrity is an index of cell viability (Figure 1); the intact plasma membrane selectively excludes both acidic dyes (e.g., trypan blue) and basic dyes (e.g., propidium iodide: #P5264, Sigma, St. Louis, MO). Carboxyfluorescein diacetate (CFDA: #C-195, Molecular Probes, Eugene, OR), the neutral lipophilic, nonfluorescent precursor of the fluorescent vital stain carboxyfluorescein (CF), readily crosses the plasma membrane. In the cytoplasm, CFDA is converted by esterase-catalyzed hydrolysis to CF, a fluorescent anion that does not readily exit cells with an intact plasma membrane (Rotman and Papermaster, 1966; Watson, 1980; Goodall and Johnson, 1982; Shapiro, 1988).

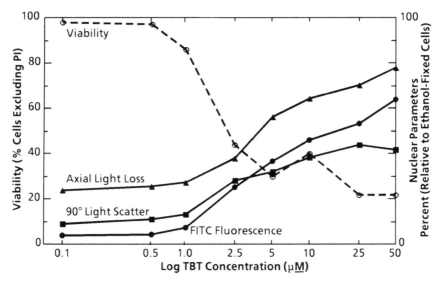

Figure 1. Cell viability and flow cytometric parameters of nuclei prepared by detergent (NP$_{40}$)-mediated lysis of murine erythroleukemic cells (MELC) exposed (4 hr) to tributyltin (TBT; 0.1-50 μM). As viability, measured by propidium iodide (PI) exclusion (O------O), decreases, resistance of the plasma membrane/cytoplasm complex to NP$_{40}$-mediated dissolution increases, resulting in increased axial light loss (▲——▲), 90° scatter (■——■), and fluorescein isothiocyanate (FITC) fluorescence (●——●) as a function of TBT concentration. Values are expressed as percentage of those obtained from ethanol-fixed cells treated with NP$_{40}$.

We have observed that mean cellular CF fluorescence ($\bar{x}F$) increases as a function of the product of TBT concentration (C) × duration of exposure (T), but only up to a value that we designate as the critical product value (CPV) (obtained, for example, by exposing 2×10^5 cells/ml growth medium to $1.0 \mu M$ TBT for 4 hr at 37°C). Above the CPV, $\bar{x}F$ decreases. The increase in $\bar{x}F$ in the range below the CPV may result from increased CFDA uptake, and/or CFDA hydrolysis (increased esterase activity), and/or decreased efflux of CF from the cell. Our evidence indicates a concentration-dependent increase in impedance of cellular CF efflux below the CPV. The mechanism of impedance is obscure and difficult to study because cellular CFDA uptake cannot be measured directly and the kinetics of CFDA hydrolysis are complicated by the apparent participation of more than one enzyme activity (Watson, 1980). In any case, the rate of CF efflux from control cells and from cells treated with 1.0 μM TBT for 4 hr is similar (Zucker et al., 1988a). However, the initial $\bar{x}F$ of TBT-treated cells is approximately 10 fold that of control cells. Therefore, if CF efflux is a function of diffusion (dependent on cellular CF concentration) and $\bar{x}F$ is proportional to mean cellular CF concentration, the TBT-treated cells exhibit increased resistance to CF efflux. Exceeding the CPV value (e.g., 1 μM TBT, 8 hr) results in a decrease in $\bar{x}F$. This decrease may be the result of increased leakage from membrane damage and/or decreased CFDA uptake and/or hydrolysis and/or CF fluorescence quenching. Other factors may also be involved.

Tosteson and Wieth (1979) demonstrated that TBT lowers the positive intrinsic dipole potential of phosphatidylethanolamine (PE) bilayers by approximately 70 mV (at a TBT concentration of 30 μM). A comparable decrease apparently would reduce the rate of diffusion of negatively charged molecules across the plasma membrane, which would be consistent with our observation of increased intracellular retention of the negatively charged fluorescent CF molecule as a function of TBT concentration below the CPV. However, employing the membrane-potential probe DiOC6 (dihexyloxacarbocyanine iodide: #D273, Molecular Probes), we observed no significant change in membrane potential below the CPV, a precipitous decrease above the CPV between 1.0 and 5.0 μM, and an increase above 5.0 μM (Zucker et al., in press). It would appear, therefore, that decreased transmembrane potential does not play a major role in CF retention in our system.

Exposure of MELC to TBT induced resistance to nonionic detergent (Nonidet P$_{40}$: #N6507, Sigma) mediated cytolysis (Zucker et al., 1988a). The resistance caused (see Figure 1) an increase in (1) the size (volume) of nuclei prepared by detergent treatment, which was manifested cytometrically as increased axial light loss; (2) fluorescein isothiocyanate (FITC: #7250, Sigma) fluorescence, resulting from the presence of FITC-binding residual proteinaceous cytoplasmic tags adherent to the nuclei; and (3) the flow cytometric parameter 90° light scatter, a measure of refractive index and protein content (Zucker et al., 1988b). These parameters increased as a function of TBT exposure.

PORCINE MICROSOMAL MEMBRANES

Alteration of membrane structure/function can be probed by monitoring vanadate-mediated crystallization of Na^+, K^+-ATPase in porcine microsomal membrane preparations (Zucker et al., 1988a). Crystallization requires appropriate Na^+, K^+-ATPase molecular structure and mobility within the membrane. Altering either parameter decreases the rate and extent of crystallization. We have observed that chemical (glutaraldehyde) or thermal protein denaturation inhibited Na^+, K^+-ATPase crystallization in the membrane preparations (Zucker et al., 1988a). Similarly, exposure to TBT (2.5 μM; Figure 2) inhibited crystallization. The electron microscopic appearance of glutaraldehyde-fixed or thermally denatured microsomes (data not shown) was essentially indistinguishable from that of TBT-treated microsomes, suggesting that TBT-induced protein denaturation is responsible for the inhibition of crystallization.

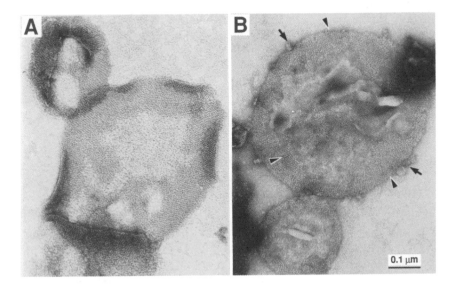

Figure 2. Effect of tributyltin (TBT) on Na^+, K^+-ATPase crystallization in microsomal membranes prepared from outer medulla of pig kidney. A. Microsomal membranes incubated for 2 hr at 20°C in the crystallization medium containing 5 mM MgCl$_2$, 1 mM NaVO$_3$ and 10 mM Tris-HCl, pH 7.5 (Zucker et al., 1988a). B. Microsomal membranes treated with 2.5 μM TBT for 30 min before induction of crystallization. *Arrowheads*, crystalline areas; *arrows*, surficial membrane blebbing. (Continued on facing page.)

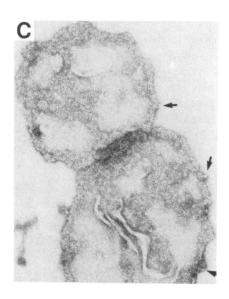

Figure 2 (continued). Effect of tributyltin (TBT) on Na$^+$, K$^+$-ATPase crystallization in microsomal membranes prepared from outer medulla of pig kidney. C. Microsomal membranes treated with 5 μM TBT for 30 min before induction of crystallization. *Arrows*, membrane blebbing. Crystallization is absent.

DISCUSSION

Carboxyfluorescein diacetate is a lipophilic nonfluorescent molecule that readily crosses the cell membrane. In the cytoplasm, it is hydrolyzed by nonspecific esterases to CF, a negatively charged fluorescent molecule that is retained incompletely by cells with an intact plasma membrane. Exposure of the MELC to TBT resulted in increased x̄F below the CPV. Above the CPV, x̄F was reduced, apparently as a consequence of perturbation of the structure of the plasma membrane-cytoplasm complex. For example, exposure of MELC to 2.5 μM TBT for 4 hr at 37°C produced resistance to detergent-mediated cytolysis and inhibition of vanadate-mediated crystallization of Na$^+$, K$^+$-ATPase molecules in porcine renal microsomal membrane preparations, a process requiring ATPase molecular structural integrity and mobility within the membrane. Taken together, the increased x̄F and resistance of the MELC to cytolysis, and inhibition of Na$^+$, K$^+$-ATPase crystallization in the microsomal membrane preparations, suggest fixation (protein denaturation, cross-linking, etc.) at the level of the plasma membrane cytoplasm complex as a mode of TBT's toxic action.

ACKNOWLEDGMENTS

The research described in this article has been reviewed by the Health Effects Research Laboratory, U.S. Environmental Protection Agency, and approved for publication. Approval does not signify that the contents necessarily reflect the views and policies of the Agency nor does mention of trade names or commercial products constitute endorsement or recommendation for use. This research was supported in part by NIH Grant GM-27804 to H. P. Ting-Beall.

REFERENCES

Goodall, H and MH Johnson. 1982. Use of carboxyfluorescein diacetate to study formation of permeable channels between mouse blastomeres. Nature 95:524-526.

Rotman, B and BW Papermaster. 1966. Membrane properties of living cells as studied by enzymatic hydrolysis of fluorogenic esters. Proc Natl Acad Sci USA 55:134-141.

Shapiro, H. M. 1988. *Practical Flow Cytometry*, 2nd Ed. Alan R Liss, New York, NY.

Tosteson, MT and JO Wieth. 1979. Tributyltin-mediated exchange diffusion of halides in lipid bilayers. J Gen Physiol 73:789-800.

Watson, JV. 1980. Enzyme kinetic studies in cell populations using fluorogenic substrates and flow cytometric techniques. Cytometry 1:143-151.

Zucker, RM, KH Elstein, RE Easterling, HP Ting-Beall, JW Allis, and EJ Massaro. 1988a. Effects of tributyltin on biomembranes: Alteration of flow cytometric parameters and inhibition of Na^+, K^+-ATPase two-dimensional crystallization. Toxicol Appl Pharmacol 96:393-403.

Zucker, RM, KH Elstein, RE Easterling, and EJ Massaro. 1988b. Flow cytometric discrimination of mitotic nuclei by right-angle light scatter. Cytometry 9:226-231.

Zucker, RM, KH Elstein, RE Easterling, and EJ Massaro. Flow cytometric comparison of the effects of trialkyltins on the murine erythroleukemic cell. Toxicology (in press).

DNA ADDUCT DISTRIBUTION IN THE RESPIRATORY TRACT OF RATS EXPOSED TO DIESEL EXHAUST

J. A. Bond,[1] R. K. Wolff,[2] J. R. Harkema,[1] J. L. Mauderly,[1] R. F. Henderson,[1] W. C. Griffith,[1] and R. O. McClellan[3]

[1]Lovelace Inhalation Toxicology Research Institute, P. O. Box 5890, Albuquerque, NM 87185

[2]Lilly Research Labs, Greenfield, IN 46140

[3]Chemical Industry Institute of Toxicology, Research Triangle Park, NC 27709

Key words: *DNA adducts, respiratory tract, rats, diesel exhaust*

ABSTRACT

Diesel exhaust, inhaled chronically at high concentrations, was previously found to be a pulmonary carcinogen in rats. The exhaust-induced tumors were located exclusively in the peripheral lung, although all respiratory tract tissues were exposed to the exhaust. The purpose of the study reported here was to determine whether there were differences in the level of DNA adducts among the regions of the respiratory tract that paralleled the site of tumors.

Groups of male F344/N rats were exposed for 7 hr/day, 5 days/wk for 12 wk, to diesel-engine exhaust at a soot concentration of 10 mg/m^3, or were sham-exposed to air. At necropsy, the maxilloturbinates, ethmoturbinates, trachea, left mainstem bronchus (airway generation 1), axial airway (airway generations 2 to 12), and peripheral lung tissue were dissected from the respiratory tract. The DNA was isolated from the dissected samples and analyzed for the presence of adducts, using the ^{32}P-postlabeling assay.

Chromatographic maps of DNA adducts demonstrated unique patterns of adducts for each region. The highest number of total DNA adducts was in peripheral lung tissue ($\sim$20 adducts per 10^9 bases). Approximately one-fourth to one-fifth as many DNA adducts were detected in the nasal tissues as in peripheral lung. There were less than 3 adducts per 10^9 bases in each region of the major conducting airways (i.e., trachea, bronchi, axial airways). In control rats, levels of DNA adducts ranged from 1 per 10^9 bases (mainstem bronchi, axial airway) to about 9 adducts per 10^9 bases (peripheral tissue).

The data from this study indicate that the highest levels of total DNA adducts and exhaust-induced adducts (i.e., exposed minus control adducts) were present in tissues where exhaust-induced tumors were located. This suggests that DNA adduct levels in discrete locations of the respiratory tract may be good measures of the "effective dose" of carcinogenic compounds.

The health effects of exposure to diesel exhaust have been a topic of intensive research during the last decade. Diesel exhaust consists of a mixture of gases, vapors, and soot particles of a respirable size (Cheng et al., 1984). Recent results from several studies (Mauderly et al., 1987; Stöber, 1986; Ishinishi et al., 1986; Brightwell et al., 1986) indicate that diesel exhaust, inhaled chronically at high concentrations, is a pulmonary carcinogen in laboratory rats. The carcinogenicity of inhaled diesel exhaust was shown to be both dose- and time related (Mauderly et al., 1987).

Several studies point to the potential role of the organic compounds associated with diesel exhaust soot as causative factors in the carcinogenic response of rodents (reviewed by McClellan, 1987). One proposed mechanism involves interaction of the organic chemicals with lung DNA as part of the initiation of carcinogenesis. The recent observation that organic chemicals associated with diesel soot can form DNA adducts in the lung (Wong et al., 1986) supports this hypothesis. However, while the studies of Wong et al. (1986) provide valuable information on whole-lung dosimetry, they did not provide information on the regional dosimetry of DNA adducts within the lung. The purpose of our studies, therefore, was to determine where in the respiratory tract DNA adducts occur after rats are exposed to diesel exhaust and to determine if the highest levels of DNA adducts were located in the region of the respiratory tract where exhaust-induced tumors have been found.

Male F344/N rats, 14-15 wk old at start of exposure, were used in these studies. The rats were born and raised in the Institute's barrier-maintained colony. Before exposure to diesel exhaust, rats were transferred from the animal housing quarters to inhalation exposure chambers (H2000, Hazleton Systems, Aberdeen, MD). Rats were housed in individual wire cages within the chambers and allowed to acclimate for 3 wk before initiation of exhaust exposure. After the 3-wk acclimation period, rats were exposed 7 hr/day, 5 days/wk for 12 wk to filtered air (controls) or to diluted diesel exhaust containing a nominal concentration of 10 mg particles/m^3. Food and water were available at all times except during the exposure period, when only water was available. Details of the exposure system used in these studies have been reported by Mokler et al. (1984).

Eighteen hours after the last exposure, two groups of 3-4 rats each were killed by CO_2 asphyxiation. Specific regions throughout the respiratory tract were sampled as described by Bond et al. (1988). These included two regions of the lateral wall of the left nasal airway (maxilloturbinates and ethmoturbinates), trachea, left mainstem extrapulmonary bronchus (airway generation 1), intrapulmonary axial airways (generations 2-12), and peripheral lung (i.e., alveolar tissue). After removal of the tissue samples, DNA was isolated by a modification (Gupta, 1984) of the Marmur procedure (Marmur, 1961). The DNA adducts in the tissue samples were quantitated by the ^{32}P-postlabeling method as described by Reddy and Randerath (1986). The nuclease P_1 procedure was used, and separation of DNA adducts by thin-layer chromatography was done as described by Bond et al. (1988).

Exposure to diesel exhaust did not cause overt signs of toxicity, and there were no significant exposure-related differences in body weight (data not shown). Lungs of rats exposed to diesel exhaust were darkly pigmented with black particles; control lungs were not. Lung burdens of soot in rats exposed to diesel exhaust for 12 wk were 3.50 ± 0.19 mg soot/lung (mean ± SE). The concentrations of key constituents of the exhaust atmospheres were summarized by Bond et al. (1988).

There appeared to be a unique pattern of DNA adducts for each of the different regions sampled (data not shown). Thus, although several DNA adducts were observed in each of the regions, the pattern of adducts differed from region to region. Table 1 summarizes the data for the level of total DNA adducts in different regions of the respiratory tract. The data shown in this table are the average of two groups (3-4 rats) for the maxillo-turbinates, ethmoturbinates, trachea, and peripheral lung, and one group (3-4 rats) for extrapulmonary mainstem bronchi and intrapulmonary axial airway. The highest level of DNA adducts was seen in the peripheral lung (~20 adducts per 10^9 bases). The level of adducts detected in nasal tissue was approximately one-fourth to one-fifth that detected in peripheral lung. Very few DNA adducts were measured in the major conducting airways. Thus, diesel exhaust exposure resulted in elevated levels of DNA adducts in both peripheral lung and nasal tissue (maxilloturbinates and ethmotur-binates), whereas there was no elevation of adducts above control levels in the major conducting airways (trachea, mainstem bronchi, and axial air-way). The level of exhaust-induced adducts was 1.5- to 3-fold greater in peripheral lung than in the nasal tissue.

Mauderly et al. (1987) reported the induction of lung tumors in rats exposed chronically to diesel exhaust. These exhaust-induced tumors, located in the peripheral lung, were derived from epithelial cells and consisted of both benign and malignant forms. The difference between the level of DNA adducts in the peripheral lung and the other regions of the respiratory tract probably resulted from several factors, including differences in deposition and clearance of the particles as well as differences in the metabolism and repair capacity of the various regions. The net effect of deposition and clearance may be to increase the "dose" of inhaled material to the peripheral lung as compared to other regions of the respiratory tract. Both the nasal and pulmonary tissues have considerably higher metabolic capacities than the tracheobronchial tissue, which would cause higher levels of reactive metabolites in these tissues. Therefore, the higher metabolic capability coupled with the large accumulation of particles in the peripheral lung may explain why this region of the respiratory tract has the highest level of DNA adducts. Further research is necessary to provide information on the cellular metabolic capability (i.e., metabolic activation, DNA repair) of the rat respiratory tract.

Table 1. Regional distribution of DNA adducts in the respiratory tract of rats exposed to diesel exhaust.[a]

Tissue	Total Adducts/10^9 Bases	Exposed Minus Control (Adducts/10^9 Bases)
Maxilloturbinates	3.8 ± 1.8	2.6
Ethmoturbinates	5.3 ± 1.2	5
Trachea	2.3 ± 2.2	0
Mainstem bronchi	1.3	0
Axial airway	1.1	0
Peripheral tissue	18 ± 10	8.4

[a]Values represent mean ± standard error, $n = 2$. Values with single numbers are from only one group of rats.

In summary, we have shown that the total level of DNA adducts was highest in the region of the respiratory tract where tumors formed after exposure to a carcinogenic concentration of diesel exhaust. This observation, while not proving causality between DNA adducts and tumors, lends support to the hypothesis that adduct formation and subsequent tumor formation are related. It will be important to understand the kinetics of formation and repair of *individual* adducts to elucidate the relationship of DNA adduct formation to carcinogenesis. These studies point to the importance of DNA adducts as measures of "effective dose" of inhaled carcinogens.

ACKNOWLEDGMENTS

This research was supported by the Office of Health and Environmental Research, U.S. Department of Energy, under Contract No. DE-AC04-76EV01013 in facilities fully accredited by the American Association for Accreditation of Laboratory Animal Care.

REFERENCES

Bond, JA, RK Wolff, JR Harkema, JL Mauderly, RF Henderson, WC Griffith, and RO McClellan. 1988. Distribution of DNA adducts in the respiratory tract of rats exposed to diesel exhaust. Toxicol Appl Pharmacol 96:336-346.

Brightwell, J, X Fouillet, A-L Cassano-Zopi, R Gatz, and F Duchosal. 1986. Neoplastic and functional changes in rodents after chronic inhalation of engine exhaust emissions, pp. 471-485. In: *Carcinogenicity and Mutagenicity of Diesel Engine Exhaust*, N Ishinishi, A Koizumi, R McClellan, and W Stöber (eds.). Elsevier, Amsterdam.

Cheng, YS, HC Yeh, JL Mauderly, and BV Mokler. 1984. Characterization of diesel exhaust in a chronic inhalation study. Am Ind Hyg Assoc J 45:547-555.

Gupta, RC. 1984. Nonrandom binding of the carcinogen N-hydroxyl-2-acetylaminofluorene to repetitive sequences of rat liver DNA *in vivo*. Proc Natl Acad Sci USA 81:6943-6947.

Ishinishi, N, A Koizumi, RO McClellan, and W Stöber (eds.). 1986. *Carcinogenicity and Mutagenicity of Diesel Engine Exhaust*, Elsevier, Amsterdam.

Marmur, JA. 1961. Procedure for the isolation of deoxyribonucleic acid from micro-organisms. J Mol Biol 3:208-218.

Mauderly, JL, RK Jones, WC Griffith, RF Henderson, and RO McClellan. 1987. Diesel exhaust is a pulmonary carcinogen in rats exposed chronically to inhalation. Fundam Appl Toxicol 9:208-221.

McClellan, RO. 1987. Health effects of exposure to diesel exhaust particules. Annu Rev Pharmacol Toxicol 27:279-300.

Mokler, BV, FA Archibeque, RL Beethe, CPJ Kelly, JA Lopez, JL Mauderly, and DL Stafford. 1984. Diesel exhaust exposure system for animal studies. Fundam Appl Toxicol 4:270-277.

Reddy, MV and K Randerath. 1986. Nuclease P$_1$-mediated enhancement of sensitivity of ^{32}P-postlabeling test for structurally diverse DNA adducts. Carcinogenesis 7:1543-1551.

Stöber, W. 1986. Experimental induction of tumors in hamsters, mice and rats after long-term inhalation of filtered and unfiltered diesel engine exhaust, pp. 421-439.

In: *Carcinogenicity and Mutagenicity of Diesel Engine Exhaust*, N Ishinishi, A Koizumi, R McClellan, and W Stöber (eds.). Elsevier, Amsterdam.

Wong, D, CE Mitchell, RK Wolff, JL Mauderly, and AM Jeffrey. 1986. Identification of DNA damage as a result of exposure of rats to diesel engine exhaust. Carcinogenesis 7:1595-1597.

QUESTIONS AND COMMENTS

Q: E. R. Blazek, Argonne National Laboratory, Argonne, IL
   Is cadmium a constitutent of diesel exhaust? This is of interest because certain metals, such as nickel (as $NiCO_3$), are carcinogenic in some model systems.

A: One study published by the National Institute for Occupational Safety and Health (M. M. Milson and R. D. Hull, *Trace Metals Analysis of Coal and Diesel Airborne Particulate*, Doc. PB 87-163226XAB, NIOSH, Cincinnati, OH, 1982) reports on the concentrations of 17 trace metals in samples of air removed from exposure chambers in which animals were exposed to diesel exhaust. Cadmium was one of the trace metals measured, and it was reported that levels of cadmium were less than 0.5 $\mu g/m^3$ air, which was the limit of quantitation.

Q: Has the diesel exhaust soot been studied by scanning electron microscopy? Not just mean size but *shape* (axial ratio) might be important, as has been shown in Syrian hamster transformation assays of apparent physical carcinogens such as asbestos.

A: A number of studies have described the physical characteristics of diesel exhaust particles (e.g., Cheng et al., Am. Ind. Hyg. Assoc. J. 45:547-555, 1984; Gray et al., J. Aerosol Sci. 16:211-216, 1985). Diesel exhaust particles have been characterized as chain aggregates of very small spherical primary particles in the size range 10-80 nm. Under the microscope they appear as chains of beads. The aggregates have a mass medium diameter of a few tenths of a micrometer. It is unlikely that diesel exhaust soot acts as a physical carcinogen in a manner suggested for fibers such as asbestos. We believe that the carcinogenic response of rodents to inhaled diesel exhaust stems from both the formation of lung DNA adducts by metabolites of soot-associated compounds and the possible role of the particulates that may be important in the promotion of the initiating event (i.e., DNA adduct formation).

Q: C. Leach, PNL, Richland, WA
   Were equal numbers of animals sacrificed at the 24- and 30-mo periods?

A: No, equal numbers of animals were not sacrificed at 24 and 30 mo. The sacrifices for histopathology at 6, 12, 18, and 24 mo included 10 rats (5 male, 5 female) per group (0, 0.35, 3.5, and 7 mg soot/m^3). All remaining rats were sacrificed at approximately 30 mo, including 5-10 males and 17-25 females per group (female rats live longer). The total numbers of rats sacrificed (male and female) are as follows:

Exposure Concentration (mg/m^3)	Time Until Sacrifice	
	24 mo	30 mo
0	10	22
0.35	10	31
3.5	10	35
7.0	10	24

Q: R. Renne, PNL, Richland, WA

Regarding the increased DNA adducts observed in the upper respiratory tract of diesel exhaust-exposed rats: Did you observe hyperplasia or neoplasia of nasal epithelium in the 30-mo bioassay of diesel exhaust?

A: As reported by **Mauderly** et al. (Fundam. Appl. Toxicol. 9:208-221, 1987), two other tumors of the respiratory tract were observed, both in the nasal cavity. A squamous carcinoma was found in the nasal cavity of a control female that died after 681 days of sham exposure. A well-differentiated chondrosarcoma was found in the nasal cavity of a high-level male that died after 781 days of exposure. The nasal tumors were not thought to be treatment related.

Q: R. Gantt, NCI

Are there any indications that adducts in the macrophage may affect the peripheral cells?

A: It is unlikely that the DNA adducts measured in macrophage DNA contributed to the level of DNA adducts measured in peripheral lung cells. I make this statement based on the observation that the pattern of DNA adducts seen in macrophage DNA is significantly different from the pattern of DNA adducts seen in the peripheral lung cells.

Multilevel Research in Relation to Epidemiology— Filling Information Gaps

STEPS TOWARD A WHOLE-SYSTEM VIEW OF RADIUM CARCINOGENESIS*

R. A. Schlenker

Biological, Environmental and Medical Research Division, Argonne National Laboratory, Argonne, IL 60439

Key words: *Bone-cancer induction, alpha particles, c-mos oncogene*

ABSTRACT ONLY

The shift of radiation health effects studies away from epidemiology and medicine toward the cellular and subcellular levels is based partly on the expectation that a new focus will ultimately improve the accuracy of cancer-risk estimation for humans at low exposure levels. To reach this goal, it will be necessary to integrate the new knowledge with existing epidemiological data to provide a predictive framework. A major step in this direction was made by the formulation of a quantitative model for the induction of bone cancer by Marshall and Gröer, linking hypothesized events at the cellular level to epidemiological data.

This model is reviewed as an example of an approach that creates a broader view of radium carcinogenesis than that provided by either epidemiological or cellular data. One element of the model is its parameterization in terms of the alpha-particle dose to the cells at risk rather than in terms of the indirect measures of the carcinogenic insult, such as average organ dose, which are popular in epidemiology.

In the arena of cellular dosimetry and its relationship to risk estimation, research by Lloyd on radium and the effects of alpha particles *in vitro* has been instrumental in showing: (1) that the presumed target cells for bone-cancer induction survive the intense radiation environment to which they are subjected in humans who develop bone cancer; (2) that alpha particles do not necessarily kill cells; and (3) that cell transformation is most likely to occur at cellular doses of several gray rather than hundreds of gray.

Lloyd's work and that of Schlenker have also shown that the relationship between cellular dose and the quantitative dose indices used in epidemiological analyses may be different in the dose range that produces demonstrable cancer than it is in the low-dose range. This suggests that extrapolation from high to low doses must be nonlinear along the dose axis as well as the normal extrapolation along the effects axis of the dose-response relationship.

*This research was sponsored by the U.S. DOE under Contract No. W-31-100-ENG-38.

Below the cellular level, Hardwick has found a frequent alteration in the *c-mos* oncogene in radium-exposed tissues that does not appear with nearly the same frequency in the tissues of unexposed persons. The data suggest a relationship to dose, but it is unclear whether the alterations are genetic or epigenetic. Whether such data can be incorporated within the framework of existing carcinogenesis models or will, instead, serve as a point of origin for new models awaits future developments. However, it seems clear that subcellular data must be linked to data on cancer frequency if they are to be useful for predicting low-dose radiation effects.

RADON RISKS IN ANIMALS WITH REFERENCE TO MAN

E. S. Gilbert and F. T. Cross

Pacific Northwest Laboratory, P.O. Box 999, Richland, WA 99352

Key words: *Animal experimental data, epidemiology, lung-cancer risks, radon*

ABSTRACT

Extensive studies have been conducted in dogs and rodents on the biological effects of inhaled radon daughters. Although estimates of lung-cancer risks in man have been obtained primarily from epidemiological studies of radon-exposed underground miners, animal experimental data provide important supplementary information.

Animal experiments have been designed specifically to assess the dependence of risks on radon-daughter cumulative exposure and of potential modifying effects, including exposure rate, unattached fraction, disequilibrium, and concomitant exposures to cigarette smoke. Data from human studies have been inadequate to answer all concerns regarding these factors. In addition, exposure to radon is one of the few areas in which risks in animals and man can be directly compared, and such comparisons are important for extrapolating from animals to man, especially when human data are inadequate.

Animal experimental data can contribute most effectively to understanding human risks when analyzed with statistical methods that consider time-related factors and competing risks and are comparable to analyses of epidemiological data. Recent analyses of underground uranium-miner data have modeled age-specific lung-cancer death rates as a function of exposure, and have evaluated the modifying effects of factors such as exposure rate, age at risk, and time from exposure.

In similar analyses of data on radon-exposed rats in experiments at Pacific Northwest Laboratory, the shape of the cumulative exposure-response function and the dependence of risks on exposure rate have been examined. Quantitative estimates of lifetime lung-cancer risks were roughly comparable to those obtained from epidemiological data, indicating that the rat provides a reasonable model for human lung-cancer risk.

INTRODUCTION

Human epidemiological data provide the most important information for assessing risks of radon exposure. Several groups of miners exposed to radon and radon progeny, including uranium miners in Colorado, Czechoslovakia, and Canada and metal miners in Sweden, have been carefully studied. These studies and their major findings were summarized in a recent report of the BEIR IV Committee (NAS, 1988).

Radon inhalation studies in animals provide important supplementary information to human data. Because the measurement of exposure characteristics is more precise in experimental than in epidemiological studies, animal studies may provide a more reliable assessment of the dependence of risks on radon-progeny cumulative exposure. Experimental data also provide information on the dependence of risks on radon-progeny exposure rate, unattached fraction, and disequilibrium, as well as on concomitant exposures to cigarette smoke. Cross (1988) provides a summary of radon studies in animals; Figures 1 and 2 show two examples from these studies, with results based on the percent of animals with lung tumors.

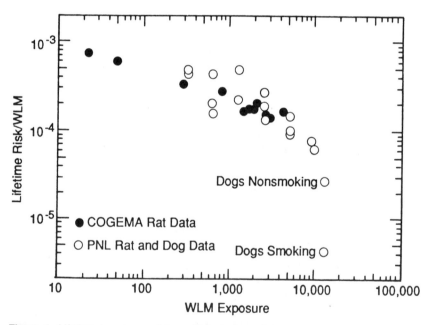

Figure 1. Lifetime lung-tumor risk coefficients for radon-progeny exposure (data unadjusted for life-shortening).

Figure 1 shows the lifetime risk of lung tumor per working level month (WLM) exposure for several experimental groups from the Pacific Northwest Laboratory (PNL) and Compagnie Générale des Matières Nucléaires

(COGEMA) radon studies. [Working level (WL) is defined as any combination of the short-lived progeny in 1 L air that will result in the ultimate emission of 1.3×10^5 MeV of potential α energy. Working level month is an exposure equivalent to 170 hr at a 1-WL concentration.] Figure 1 shows a downward trend in risk at high exposures, probably a result of lifespan-shortening from competing risks.

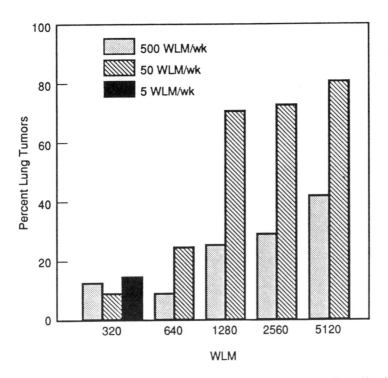

Figure 2. Percent of lung tumors in rats versus radon-progeny exposure rate and level.

Figure 2 shows results of PNL experiments addressing the effects of exposure rate. The graph compares the percentage of animals with lung tumors in each of several exposure-level groups with exposure received at rates of about 500, 50, and 5 WLM per week. With the exception of the lowest exposure-level group (320 WLM), higher percentages of tumors were seen in the lower exposure-rate groups.

STATISTICAL METHODS

Animal studies can be used most effectively to supplement epidemiological studies if data from both types of studies are analyzed using similar methods, and if the statistics used to summarize the data are comparable. Tumorigenesis data developed in the PNL radon studies are used here to illustrate this approach. The objective is to account for time-related factors and competing risks in a manner comparable to recent analyses in underground-miner epidemiological studies. Specifically, these methods are applied to data from PNL experiments designed to assess the effects of exposure rate; these data are summarized in Figure 2.

Recent analyses of miners exposed to radon and radon progeny include (1) those by Whittemore and McMillan (1983) and by Hornung and Meinhardt (1987), both based on Colorado Plateau uranium miners; (2) analyses by Thomas et al. (1985), based on published data from five studies (Colorado Plateau uranium miners, Czechoslovakian uranium miners, Newfoundland fluorspar miners, Swedish metal miners, and Ontario uranium miners); and (3) analyses by the BEIR IV Committee (NAS, 1988), based on combined data from four studies (Colorado Plateau uranium miners, Ontario uranium miners, Saskatchewan uranium miners, and Swedish metal miners). These analyses modeled the hazard, or age-specific lung-cancer death rates, as a function of cumulative WLM and also evaluated the modifying effects of factors such as exposure rate, age at first exposure, and time since exposure.

Specific findings of these analyses were that a linear exposure-response function fitted the data reasonably well, although some analyses suggested that a sublinear function or a function that allowed for cell-killing at higher exposures provided a slightly better fit. Risks were inversely related to exposure rate, and relative excess risks seemed to increase with increasing age at first exposure. Absolute risks increased with age at risk but not as rapidly as baseline risks; the relative excess risk declined with time since exposure. Most of these findings were interpreted tentatively because of data limitations in sample size, exposure assessments, and information on confounding factors.

Certain aspects of the data on radon-exposed rats require modification of the methods applied to human studies. First, baseline risks are more uncertain for laboratory rats than for humans. Human study populations frequently include large numbers of subjects with minimal exposure, and vital statistics provide additional information on baseline risks. The baseline lifetime risk of lung tumors in laboratory rats is estimated to be about one or two per thousand, and available data on control animals are not adequate for reliable estimation of the age-specific baseline risks needed for hazard modeling. For this reason, it is desirable to avoid expressing risks relative to the baseline, as is often done in epidemiological studies.

A second important difference between human and animal data is that substantial evidence indicates that lung tumors in rats are usually not the cause of death, but are, instead, found incidental to death from other causes (Cross, 1988; Chmelevsky et al., 1984; Gray et al., 1986). The correct approach to modeling is different if tumors are the cause of death (as has been assumed in analyses of data from epidemiological studies) than when tumors are incidental findings. Making the correct choice is especially important if competing risks depend on level of exposure and other factors of interest.

Details regarding the statistical methodology for analyses presented in this paper have been described elsewhere (Gilbert, in press). Analyses were based on the assumption that all tumors were incidental. However, alternative analyses, based on the assumption that all tumors were fatal, were also conducted and are discussed briefly. A Weibull function, or power function of age, was used to model the baseline risk and to provide for the possibility that radiation risks increase as animals age.

Specifically, the model emphasized is one in which the hazard for a given animal at age a^* is of the form

$$h(a^*) = (\alpha + 2)\, a^\alpha\, (\theta + \beta\, WLM_a) \qquad [1]$$

where a^* indicates the age of the animal in days $[a = (a^* - 60)/720$ is the age scaled to indicate the fraction of the average life span after 60 days; average survival time for control animals was about 780 days]; WLM_a denotes the cumulative exposure in WLM for the animal at age a; and α and β are parameters to be estimated. The parameter α is referred to as the "Weibull parameter," the parameter β is referred to as the "linear risk coefficient," and θ indicates the baseline risk. Both exposure and the Weibull function are lagged for 60 days, comparable to about 5 yr in a human life. The hazard, $h(a^*)$, is 0 for $a^* < 60$ days. With age scaled in the manner indicated, it can be shown that the linear risk coefficient β provides a reasonable estimate of the lifetime risk per WLM associated with lifetime exposure.

This model differs from those used in epidemiological analyses in that the Weibull function has been used for the baseline risk and the risk coefficient

β is not expressed relative to the baseline. However, important features of epidemiological analyses have been retained; the hazard is still being modeled, and the Weibull function allows the radiation-related risk to increase (or decrease) as animals age. The latter is an important feature of relative risk models employed in human studies.

RESULTS OF ANALYSES OF ANIMAL EXPERIMENTAL DATA

As noted, analyses presented here focus on recent PNL experiments in which male Wistar rats were exposed to radon progeny at three exposure rates (500, 50, and 5 WLM/wk) and several cumulative exposure levels. In all cases, exposure began about 90 days of age. These experiments have been described in detail by Cross (1987); the design is summarized in Table 1. Sacrificed animals (included in the 500- and 5-WLM/wk experiments) were excluded from analyses presented in this paper because of the potential for bias; sacrifice data were not available for the 50-WLM/wk experiments. Also, animals that survived less than 240 days were excluded because no lung tumors occurred before that time. Both malignant tumors and adenomas were included.

Table 1. Time (days) from initiation to scheduled completion of exposure (numbers of animals included in analyses[a] are given in parentheses).

Approximate Cumulative Exposure (WLM)[b]	Rate of Exposure (WLM/wk)[b]		
	500	50	5
0	0 (45)	0 (95)	0 (32)
320	3 (127)	43 (126)	438 (101)
640	8 (69)	86 (63)	
1,280	16 (38)	171 (32)	
2,560	36 (38)	354 (32)	
5,120	72 (41)	705 (32)	
10,240	138 (50)	—	

[a]Sacrificed animals and animals that survived less than 240 days were excluded.
[b]Actual exposures and exposure rates deviated slightly from tabulated values. For protracted exposures, not all animals lived to receive scheduled exposure.

The major reason for conducting these experiments was to assess the influence of radon-progeny exposure rate on lung-tumor risks. However, in varying exposure rate, variables such as age at exposure and time since exposure were necessarily varied as well, making it difficult to separate the modifying effects of these factors. Table 1 shows that, for higher cumulative exposure levels received at 50 WLM/wk as well as at 5 WLM/wk, the exposures continued through a substantial fraction of the life spans of the animals.

Figure 3 and Table 2 show results of incidental analyses fitting a model in which separate linear risk coefficients (β) were fitted to each of 12 exposure groups. As noted, these coefficients can be reasonably interpreted as estimates of lifetime risk per WLM. There is little indication of a decrease in the risk per WLM with increasing total exposure, even with cumulative exposures as large as 10,000 WLM. Similar analyses, based on the assumption that tumors were fatal, also showed little evidence of such a decrease. In general, the results indicated that risks for exposure at 50 WLM/wk were higher than for exposure at 500 WLM/wk, although this effect was not seen in the lowest cumulative exposure group (320 WLM).

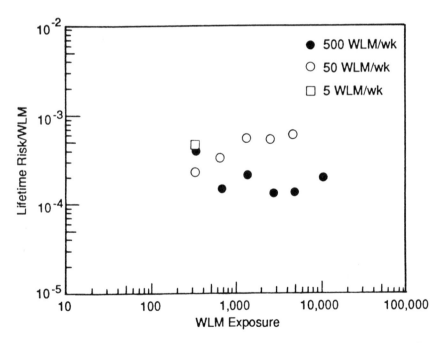

Figure 3. Linear lung-tumor risk coefficients (β) for radon-progeny exposure [see equation (1)]. Tumors are assumed incidental.

Table 2. Estimated linear lung-tumor risk coefficients[a] (95% confidence limits) for 12 exposure groups.[b]

Approximate Cumulative Exposure (WLM)	Rate of Exposure (WLM/wk)		
	500	50	5
320	401 (254, 635)	229 (136, 388)	459 (287, 735)
640	151 (71, 321)	329 (205, 528)	
1,280	219 (121, 398)	542 (342, 860)	
2,560	136 (77, 238)	522 (340, 840)	
5,120	140 (86, 227)	594 (337, 1,050)	
10,240	212 (129, 348)		

[a]Coefficients β from equation (1) are scaled to be interpreted as lifetime risk $\times$ 10^{-6}/WLM for lifetime exposure.
[b]Tumors are assumed incidental.

Shown in Table 3 are the results of incidental analyses fitting a single linear coefficient to combined data from all experimental groups and fitting separate linear coefficients for each of the three exposure rates. First, we consider the Weibull parameter, α. This parameter measures the increase in risk with age, with the value of zero corresponding to the absolute risk model in which the excess risk (per unit of time per unit of exposure) remains constant as the animals age. The Weibull parameter was estimated to be 2.0 and 1.4, respectively, for the two analyses in Table 3; in both cases, the estimates were significantly greater than zero. Thus, these analyses indicate that risks increased with age, and that the data were inconsistent with the absolute risk model.

Table 3. Parameter estimates with 95% confidence limits for linear Weibull models.

	Model A[a]	Model B[b]
α^c	2.00 (1.4, 2.6)	1.24 (0.5, 2.0)
β^d	294 (252, 342)	189 (146, 246) for 500 WLM/wk
		404 (330, 495) for 50 WLM/wk
		462 (289, 737) for 5 WLM/wk

[a]Coefficient β is assumed to be the same for all exposure-rate groups. (Tumors are assumed incidental.)
[b]Separate coefficients β were estimated for each exposure-rate group.
[c]Weibull parameter.
[d]Coefficients β from equation (1) are scaled to be interpreted as lifetime risk $\times$ 10^{-6}/WLM for lifetime exposure.

The estimated linear risk coefficient in adult nonsmoking male rats, based on the combined data, was about 300×10^{-6}/WLM. For the purpose of comparison with values obtained from human studies, it may be more appropriate to exclude the nonmalignant adenomas; if this is done, the risk estimate is reduced from 300 to about 250. This value may be compared with the value of 350×10^{-6}/WLM, the overall risk estimate given by the BEIR IV Committee (NAS, 1988), which is intended to apply to a population including both males and females and both smokers and nonsmokers. The value of 250×10^{-6}/WLM may also be compared, perhaps more appropriately, with the BEIR IV value of 140×10^{-6}/WLM for male nonsmokers. The value given by the NCRP model (NCRP, 1984) was 130×10^{-6}/WLM. Thus, estimates obtained from rats are roughly comparable to those obtained from human studies.

Results of the analyses in Table 3 indicate that the coefficients for protracted exposure were about double those at the higher exposure rate, and that consideration of exposure rate significantly improved the fit of the model ($p < 0.001$). The fit of the model with separate coefficients for the three exposure-rate groups has been examined by comparing the number of animals with tumors to the number predicted by the model. There was evidence of a poor fit at the cumulative 320-WLM level when the separate exposure-rate groups were examined. In this group, the risk per WLM was higher for the 500-WLM/wk group than for the 50-WLM/wk group, a reversal of the findings at the other exposure levels. The fit of the Weibull function was also examined by comparing observed and predicted tumors by categories defined by age. No evidence of lack of fit was found.

Analyses based on the assumption that tumors were fatal and in which separate linear risk coefficients were fitted for each of the exposure-rate groups resulted in a higher value for the Weibull parameter ($\alpha = 5.8$), but lower estimates for the risk coefficients; the estimates for the 500-, 50-, and 5-WLM/wk groups were 145, 172, and 220×10^{-6}/WLM, respectively. Thus, the evidence for an exposure-rate effect was not as great when tumors were assumed to be fatal, and the fitting of separate coefficients did not significantly improve the fit over that in a model in which a single coefficient was fitted ($p > 0.2$). Because most of the tumors were probably incidental, the results in Table 3 are probably more correct than those based on fatal analyses. However, because a few tumors probably did cause death, incidental analyses may have slightly underestimated the Weibull coefficient α and slightly overestimated the risk coefficient β.

Analyses of epidemiological data have addressed the modifying effects of factors such as age at risk and time since exposure, and have addressed evidence for reduced risks at older ages and with increasing time from exposure. Experimental data from rats can provide only limited information on these effects, because less information is available on the time of occurrence of tumors when tumors are incidental findings.

It has already been noted that the effects of exposure rate and time since exposure cannot be entirely separated in these experiments. Figure 4 shows the risk $\times$ 10^{-6}/WLM for the 12 exposure groups, plotted against the age when exposure was stopped in each experiment. The pattern is not entirely consistent, but the largest risks occurred in the groups where exposure was protracted to older ages. It is thus possible that the increased risk seen at lower exposure rates is partly explained by a dependence of risks on time since exposure or on time since cessation of exposure.

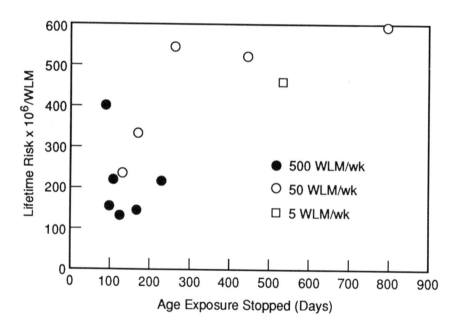

Figure 4. Linear lung-tumor risk coefficients (β) for radon-progeny exposure [see equation (1)] plotted by age at which exposure was stopped.

DISCUSSION AND SUMMARY

The attenuation of risks observed in simple analyses of experimental data at very high cumulative exposure levels (as shown in Figure 1) was not found when competing risks were accounted for either by assuming that all tumors were incidental or by assuming that all tumors were fatal. This result is similar to the conclusion drawn by Gray et al. (1986) from incidental analyses of data from experiments at the COGEMA laboratories.

Quantitative risk estimates were roughly comparable to those obtained from epidemiological data, although the estimates from rats were slightly high if the comparison was made with a nonsmoking human population. Although it was earlier thought that the ratio of the dose expressed in rad to exposure expressed in WLM was smaller for rats than for humans (NAS, 1988), a recent reevaluation of the rodent dosimetry data places the ratio for rats comparable to the value for humans (Cross, 1988). Thus, the estimated risks are roughly comparable for rats and humans regardless of whether they are expressed per WLM or per rad.

Risks observed at low exposure rates were generally higher than those observed at high exposure rates, consistent with recent results from epidemiological analyses. However, the reasons for these differences and the implications for risks resulting from exposure at very low levels are not fully understood. The strongest differences were at the higher cumulative exposure levels, with the intermediate exposure rate (50 WLM/wk) yielding higher risks than the highest exposure rate (500 WLM/wk). The pattern was reversed at the 320-WLM cumulative exposure level, but the differences in the groups at this level were not statistically significant.

Because the lower cumulative exposure-rate groups required the greatest protraction of exposure to attain a given cumulative exposure, it is possible that the exposure-rate effect was partly an effect of time since exposure or time since cessation of exposure, as suggested by modeling of data on human exposures. Evidence of such a decline was found in the BEIR IV analyses (NAS, 1988) and in analyses by Hornung and Meinhardt (1987). However, the decline seen in the epidemiological data could have resulted, in part, from changes in smoking habits over time; smoking data were available for only some of the human studies, and were inadequate to investigate changes with time.

Additional animal experiments could be designed to address questions that cannot be fully resolved with epidemiological data or current experimental data in laboratory animals. For example, groups exposed at high exposure rates but at older ages than those analyzed in this paper would help to clarify whether the observed elevated risks at low exposure rates resulted from exposure rate *per se* or from differences in time since exposure. Planned experiments in laboratory animals using females and/or with exposure initiated at very early ages would provide information on important subgroups, for which almost no human data exist. Overall, the rat seems to provide a reasonable model for human lung-cancer risks resulting from exposure to radon. Appropriately designed experiments could provide information on many issues that cannot be adequately addressed with available data from epidemiological studies.

ACKNOWLEDGMENT

This work was supported by the U.S. Department of Energy under Contract DE-AC06-76RLO 1830.

REFERENCES

Chmelevsky, D, AM Kellerer, J Lafuma, and J Chameaud. 1984. Maximum likelihood estimation of the prevalence of nonlethal neoplasms—An application to radon-daughter inhalation studies. Radiat Res 98:519-535.

Cross, FT. 1987. Inhalation hazards to uranium miners, pp. 37-40. In: *Pacific Northwest Laboratory Annual Report for 1986 to the DOE Office of Energy Research, Part 1*. PNL-6100, Pacific Northwest Laboratory, Richland, WA.

Cross, FT. 1988. *Radon Inhalation Studies in Animals: A Radon Health Effects Literature Review*. Report to the U.S. Department of Energy Office of Health and Environmental Research. Pacific Northwest Laboratory, Richland, WA.

Gilbert, ES. 1989. Lung cancer risk models from experimental animals. In: *Radon*. National Council on Radiation Protection and Measurements, Proceedings of Twenty-Fourth Annual Meeting, March 1988. Nuclear Regulatory Commission, Washington, DC (in press).

Gray, RG, J Lafuma, SE Parish, and R Peto. 1986. Lung tumors and radon inhalation in over 2000 rats: Approximate linearity across a wide range of doses and potentiation by tobacco smoke, pp. 455-470. In: *Lifespan Radiation Effects Studies in Animals: What Can They Tell Us?*, Proceedings of the Twenty-Second Hanford Life Sciences Symposium. CONF-830951, NTIS, Springfield, VA.

NAS (National Academy of Sciences). **1988**. *Health Risks of Radon and Other Internally Deposited Alpha-Emitters*. National Academy Press, Washington, DC.

NCRP (National Council on Radiation Protection and Measurements). **1984**. *Evaluation of Occupational and Environmental Exposures to Radon and Radon Daughters in the United States*. NCRP Report No. 78, NCRP, Bethesda, MD.

Hornung, RW and TJ Meinhardt. **1987**. Quantitative risk assessment of lung cancer in U.S. uranium miners. Health Phys 50:417-430.

Thomas, DC, KG McNeill, and C Dougherty. **1985**. Estimates of lifetime lung cancer risks resulting from Rn progeny exposures. Health Phys 5:825-846.

Whittemore, AS and A McMillan. **1983**. Lung cancer mortality among U.S. uranium miners: A reappraisal. J Natl Cancer Inst 1:489-499.

EXPRESSION OF EPIDERMAL GROWTH-FACTOR RECEPTOR AND BOMBESIN IN ARCHIVED PARAFFIN-BLOCK URANIUM-MINER LUNG TUMORS

F. C. Leung[1] and G. Saccomanno[2]

[1]Pacific Northwest Laboratory, P. O. Box 999, Richland, WA 99352

[2]St. Mary's Hospital, Grand Junction, CO 81501

Key words: *GFR, uranium-miner lung tumors, non-small-cell carcinoma, bombesin*

ABSTRACT

The expression of epidermal growth-factor receptor (EGFR) and bombesin was examined in two lung tumors from uranium miners who were also smokers. We applied the immunocytochemical assay in archived paraffin-block serial sections (>30 yr old) with a specific monoclonal antibody generated against human EGFR and with a specific polyclonal antibody generated against bombesin. Strong positive staining for bombesin, with marginal positive staining for EGFR, were observed in one lung tumor; in the other tumor, there was strong positive staining for EGFR but none for bombesin. These data demonstrate that archived paraffin-block uranium-miner lung-tumor samples are suitable for use in the immunocytochemical assay for cellular biochemical analysis of GF and GFR. The data also suggest that the abnormal expression of EGFR and bombesin may be involved in oncogenesis of the lung in uranium miners who smoke.

INTRODUCTION

Recent studies have shown abnormally high levels of expression of EGFR in human non-small-cell carcinoma of the lung (non-SCCL) and of bombesin in small-cell carcinoma (SCCL) of the lung. Sherwin et al. (1981) reported that EGFR binding increased in five of six non-SCCL cell lines examined and that there was no detectable EGFR binding in eight of eight SCCL cell lines examined. Using a monoclonal antibody to EGFR and indirect immunoperoxidase staining techniques, Cerny et al. (1986) reported that 80% of 48 non-SCCL tissue samples examined stained positively and that all 15 SCCL samples were negative. The abnormally high expression of EGFR found in non-SCCL were confirmed by Berger et al. (1987), Gamou et al. (1987), and Sobol et al. (1987). More specifically, the abnormally high expression of EGFR has been associated more often with squamous cell carcinoma than other types of lung tumors (Berger et al., 1987; Sobol et al., 1987). Moody et al. (1983, 1985) demonstrated that 94% of SCCL lines synthesize bombesin and have bombesin receptors, and that non-SCCL cell lines do not. Abe et al. (1984) reported that gastrin-releasing peptide immunoactivities were highest in SCCL and in carcinoid lung tumors.

Previous studies of EGFR and bombesin expression in human lung tumors have not addressed the etiology of the disease, e.g., in smokers versus non-smokers, and in radiation-induced versus spontaneous lung tumors. Occupational exposure of underground uranium miners to high levels of radon daughters has been correlated with a significantly increased incidence of pulmonary lung cancer in that group (NCRP, 1984). The uranium-miner data represent the largest and most detailed comparison now available of human radon exposures with the pathology of precancerous lesions and pulmonary lung cancers (Saccomanno et al., 1988; Samet, 1989). Most miners are smokers, and cigarette smoking plays a significant role in causing lung cancer in humans. Saccomanno et al. (1988) showed a synergistic and/or additive effect of these two carcinogens in uranium-miner lung tumors.

This paper describes the feasibility of using archived uranium-miner lung tumors for studying the biochemical cellular changes of GF and GFR by immunocytochemical assay.

MATERIALS AND METHODS

Tissue Samples

Two lung-tumor samples were collected, in 1965 (65-144743-3) and 1967 (67-5155-3), from uranium miners who were smokers. The specimens were fixed in 10% neutral buffered formalin and embedded in paraffin blocks.

Immunocytochemical Assays

The immunocytochemical assay procedure for measuring the expression of EGFR and bombesin is described in Leung et al. (this volume). Briefly, the Vectastain ABC (peroxidase) system was used to detect EGFR and bombesin in serial 5-μm-thick paraffin sections. A monoclonal antibody against human EGFR (clone no. 29.1, mouse IgG1) was obtained from Sigma (St. Louis, MO), and the polyclonal antibody against bombesin was obtained from ICN ImmunoBiologicals (Lisle, IL). The EGFR AB-1 was diluted and used at 1:50; the bombesin was diluted and used at 1:1000-2000. One lung tumor specimen (67-5155-3) was also examined for the expression of transforming growth factor-α (TGF-α). TGF-α polyclonal antibody was obtained from Biotop (Seattle, WA) and was used at 1:1000-2000. The appropriate Vectastain ABC kits were used, based on the species of the primary antibody, and appropriate (isotype) normal animal sera were used as a blocking reagent for both the specific and nonspecific sections. The nonspecific section was taken from the tissue section immediately adjacent to the specific section. It was treated with exactly the same reagents as the specific section except that normal serum was substituted for primary antibody. Positive tissue samples for immunocytochemistry were also examined in each assay: human placenta for EGFR and TGF-α, rat duodenum for bombesin. Normal rat lung and tumor-free dog lung tissues were also examined in each assay. Immunohistochemistry slide samples were evaluated as positive or negative.

RESULTS

Strong positive specific staining of bombesin was observed in sections of sample 67-5155-3, and weak positive staining of EGFR was observed in an adjacent section of the same tumor. Staining for bombesin and EGFR was homogeneous, and most tumor cells displayed strong staining for bombesin (Figure 1A and 1B) and weak staining for EGFR (Figure 2A and 2B). There was no positive staining for the expression of TGF-α in sample 67-5155-3 (Figure 3A and 3B). There was no positive staining for bombesin in sample 65-144743 (Figure 4A and 4B), but strong positive staining for EGFR (Figure 5A and 5B) was observed in an adjacent section. The positive staining for EGFR in sample 65-144743 was intense but not homogeneous (Figure 5A). There were no obvious morphological differences between EGFR-positive and EGFR-negative SCCL carcinoma in sample 65-144743.

DISCUSSION

We have applied immunocytochemical assays to examine the expression of EGFR, TGF-α, and bombesin in archived lung tumors from uranium miners that have been embedded in paraffin blocks for more than 30 yr. The abnormal expression of bombesin found in sample 67-5155-3 agrees with the findings of Moody et al. (1983, 1985) that SCCL in humans expresses a high level of bombesin. The positive staining for EGFR in both tumors and of bombesin in sample 67-5155-3 suggests abnormally high expression of both EGFR and bombesin in these lung tumors, which were obtained from uranium miners who were smokers. The intense positive staining for bombesin in sample 67-5155-3 and for EGFR in sample 65-144743-3 gives credence to the negative staining for other GF and GFR in each tumor. The heterogeneous expression of EGFR in sample 65-144743 is of particular interest because Berger et al. (1987), Gamou et al. (1987), and Sobol et al. (1987) found no abnormal expression of EGFR in SCCL. The biological and clinical significance of this differential expression of EGFR in SCCL is unknown. It would be interesting to determine whether SCCL that stained positive for EGFR share biological and clinical features with non-SCCL that stained positive for EGFR.

Because of the limited sample number, it is hard to establish the physiological significance of the differential expression of GF and GFR in two samples of SCCL tumors obtained from uranium miners, both of whom smoked and were exposed to radioactive radon gas. One might hypothesize that the differential expression of EGFR, TGF-α, and bombesin in these two tumors may reflect the quality and quantity of the chemical and radioactive insult from radon gas and cigarette smoke. Neither Sobol et al. (1987) or Cerny et al. (1986) reported abnormal expression of EGFR in SCCL in their studies; however, the etiology of their lung tumors was not given. The expression of EGFR that we observed in sample 65-144743 SCCL warrants further investigation to establish its biological and clinical significance.

It is important to point out that immunocytochemical assay methods are not quantitative and do not definitely rule out a very weak expression of GF or GFR in the section that stained negatively. However, the assay indicates a relative difference in the expression of GF and GFR between positive- and negative-staining tumors and also between positive-staining tumors and negative-staining normal lung tissue.

In conclusion, our findings demonstrate that the archived paraffin-block lung tumor samples from uranium miners are suitable for immunocytochemical analysis for the expression of GF and GFR. Further investigations will be required to elucidate the biological significance of the expression of EGFR and bombesin by lung carcinomas. Investigation is also needed to determine whether the aberrant expression of EGFR and bombesin is an important factor in pulmonary oncogenesis and the relationship of this expression to the specific insults, for example, chemical versus radiation.

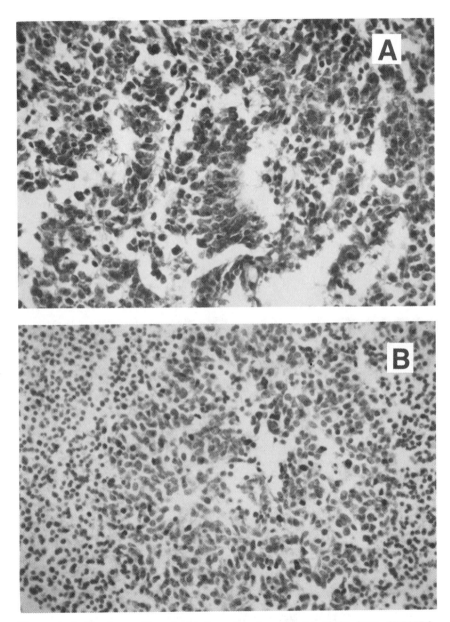

Figure 1. Archived, paraffin-embedded small cell carcinoma of the lung, 67-5155-3, obtained from a uranium miner and immunocytochemically stained for bombesin; A, specific staining with a polyclonal antibody; B, nonspecific staining with normal serum.

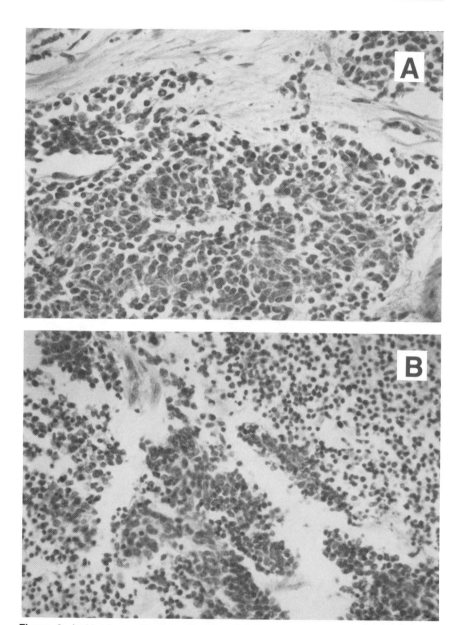

Figure 2. Archived, paraffin-embedded small cell carcinoma of the lung, 67-5155-3, obtained from a uranium miner and immunocytochemically stained for epidermal growth-factor receptor; A, specific staining with a monoclonal antibody; B, nonspecific staining with normal mouse isotype IgG.

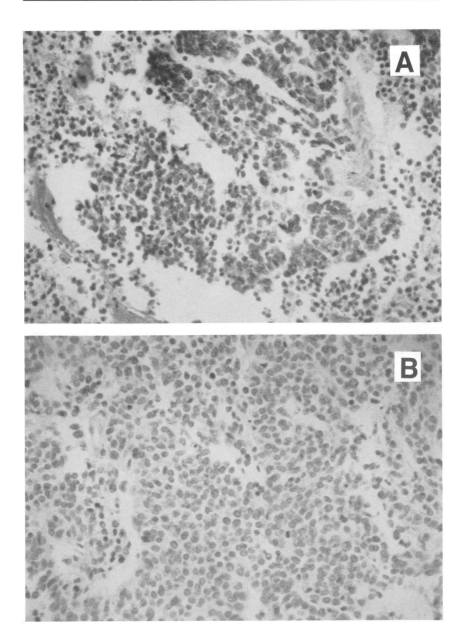

Figure 3. Archived, paraffin-embedded small cell carcinoma of the lung, 67-5155-3, obtained from a uranium miner and immunocytochemically stained for transforming growth factor-α; A, specific staining with a polyclonal antibody; B, nonspecific staining with normal serum.

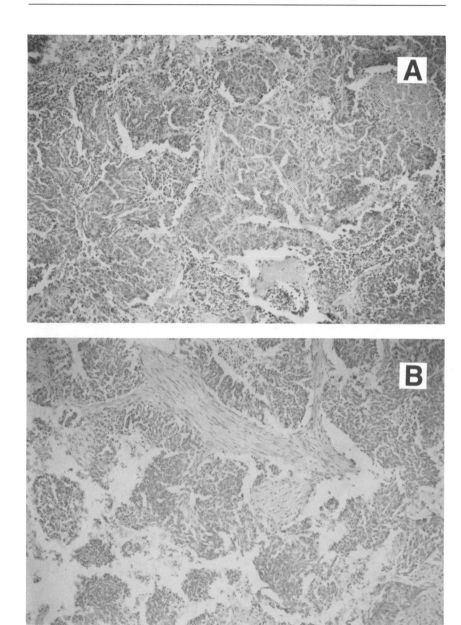

Figure 4. Archived, paraffin-embedded small cell carcinoma of the lung, 65-144743, obtained from a uranium miner and immunocytochemically stained for bombesin; A, specific staining with a polyclonal antibody; B, nonspecific staining with normal serum.

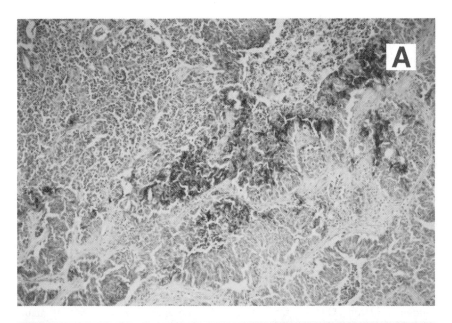

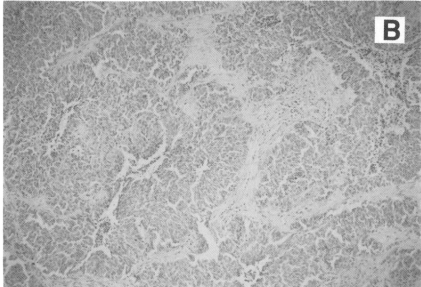

Figure 5. Archived, paraffin-embedded small cell carcinoma of the lung, 65-144743, obtained from a uranium miner and immunocytochemically stained for epidermal growth-factor receptor; A, specific staining with a monoclonal antibody; B, nonspecific staining with normal mouse isotype IgG.

ACKNOWLEDGMENTS

This work was supported by the U.S. Department of Energy under Contract DE-AC06-76RLO 1830. We thank Ms. Ruth Michaels and Ms. Lisa Smith, Mr. Jim Coleman, and Mr. Bob Boettcher for their technical assistance. We also thank Ms. D. Felton and Ms. Susan Kreml for expert editing and Ms. H. B. Crow for wordprocessing assistance.

REFERENCES

Abe, K, T Kameya, K Yamaguchi, K Kikuchi, I Adachi, M Tanaka, S Kimura, T Kodama, Y Shimosato, and S Ishikawa. 1984. Hormone-producing lung cancers, pp. 549-595. In: *The Endocrine Lung in Health and Disease*, KL Becker and AF Gazdar (eds.). WB Saunders, Philadelphia, PA.

Berger, MS, WJ Gullick, C Greenfield, S Evans, BJ Addis, and MD Waterfield. 1987. Epidermal growth factor receptors in lung tumors. J Pathol 152:297-307.

Cerny, T, DM Barnes, P Hasleton, PV Barber, K Healy, W Gullick, and N Thatcher. 1986. Expression of epidermal growth factor receptors (EGFR) in human lung tumors. Br J Cancer 54:265-269.

Gamou, S, J Hunts, H Harigai, S Hirohashi, Y Shimosato, I Pastan, and N Shimizu. 1987. Molecular evidence for the lack of epidermal growth factor receptor gene expression in small cell lung carcinoma cells. Cancer Res 47:2668-2673.

Moody, T, V Bertness, and D Carney. 1983. Bombesin-like peptides and receptors in human tumor cell lines. Peptides 4:683-686.

Moody, TW, DN Carney, F Cuttitta, K Quattrocchi, and JD Minna. 1985. Current concepts: I. High affinity receptors for bombesin/GRP-like peptides on human small cell lung cancer. Life Sci 37:105-113.

National Council on Radiation Protection and Measurements (NCRP). 1984. Evaluation of Occupational and Environmental Exposures to Radon and Radon Daughters in the United States. NCRP, Bethesda, MD.

Saccomanno, G, GC Huth, O Auerback, and M Kuschner. 1988. Relationship of radioactive radon daughters and cigarette smoking in the genesis of lung cancer in uranium miners. Cancer 62:1402-1408

Samet, JM. 1989. Radon and lung cancer. J Natl Cancer Inst 81:745-757.

Sherwin, SA, JE Minna, AF Gazdar, and GJ Todaro. 1981. Expression of epidermal and nerve growth factor receptors and soft agar growth factor production by human lung cancer cells. Cancer Res 41:3538-3542.

Sobol, RE, RW Astarita, C Hofeditz, H Masui, R Fairshter, I Royston, and J Mendelsohn. 1987. Epidermal growth factor receptor expression in human lung carcinomas defined by a monoclonal antibody. J Natl Cancer Inst 79:403-405.

GENETIC PREDISPOSITION TO CANCER AND ENHANCED CHROMATID ABERRATIONS IN HUMAN CELLS X-IRRADIATED IN G$_2$ PHASE

R. Gantt,[1] K. K. Sanford,[2] R. Parshad,[3] and R. E. Tarone[4]

[1]Radiation Effects Branch, National Cancer Institute, Bethesda, MD 20892

[2]Laboratory of Cellular and Molecular Biology, National Cancer Institute, Bethesda, MD 20892

[3]Department of Pathology, Howard University College of Medicine, Washington, DC 20059

[4]Biostatistics Branch, National Cancer Institute, Bethesda, MD 20892

Key words: *DNA repair, cancer predisposition, chromosome aberrations*

ABSTRACT

Compared to normal cells, malignant or nontumorous cells from individuals genetically predisposed to cancer have increased chromatid aberrations at 2 to 3 hr after 1 Gy of x-irradiation in the G$_2$ phase of the cell cycle. This response is a genetic trait observed in cells from individuals with a variety of clinical syndromes or conditions predisposing to cancer, including ataxia telangiectasia, Bloom's syndrome, Fanconi's anemia, xeroderma pigmentosum (XP), familial polyposis, Gardner's syndrome, hereditary cutaneous malignant melanoma, dysplastic nevus syndrome, Wilms' tumor, and retinoblastoma. This trait was acquired by human keratinocytes before their neoplastic transformation in culture and could provide the basis of a test for genetic susceptibility to cancer.

The enhanced chromatid aberrations (gaps and breaks) do not appear to be caused by increased sensitivity to damage because initial aberration frequencies in normal and cancer-prone cells were equivalent. Nor do differential rates of progression through the G$_2$ phase account for the enhanced aberrations, because these rates were similar.

Evidence for a deficiency in processing the DNA damage includes the following: (1) XP group A cells, virtually devoid of DNA-repair strand incision activity, are an exception and manifest the normal chromatid aberration phenotype. This observation suggests that DNA strand incision is required for chromatid gaps and breaks. (2) Treatment of normal cells with the repair polymerase inhibitor β-cytosine arabinoside (5×10^{-5} M) after x-irradiation increases the level of aberrations to that of the cancer-prone cells but has little effect on the latter. (3) Frequencies of chromatid aberrations decrease precipitously with time after irradiation in normal cells but remain high or even increase in cancer-prone or cancer cells, suggesting incomplete ligation during the repair process. (4) Comparison of DNA from normal and cancer-prone cells by alkaline elution indicates that either cancer-prone cells repair breaks more slowly or acquire breaks more rapidly than normal cells. (5) Catalase protects both normal and cancer-prone cells from x-ray-induced chromatid aberrations, which indicates that they are the result of secondary and indirect enzymatic DNA strand breaks rather than of direct breaks.

An unbalanced or deficient DNA-repair process could lead to genetic instability, which is the *sine qua non* of the cancer cell. This instability could increase the probability of losing genetic heterozygosity or of defective homozygosity at cancer-predisposing loci and thereby increase the process of malignant transformation and tumor progression.

INTRODUCTION

The association between malignancy and chromosomal aberrations or aneuploidy has been known for decades. Our long-standing interest in "spontaneous" transformation in cultured rodent cells led to the idea that genetic instability alone, manifested as chromosomal alterations, is the key to "spontaneous" transformation (Sanford et al., 1978, 1979). Specific nonrandom chromosomal aberrations were not an essential precondition for malignant transformation in these studies. This paper briefly describes an analogous human genetic instability found in individuals at high risk for cancer.

DNA DAMAGE, CHROMOSOMAL ABERRATIONS, AND PREDISPOSITION TO CANCER

When fibroblasts or stimulated blood lymphocytes from individuals at high risk for cancer or malignant cells are irradiated (1 Gy of x ray) in the G_2 phase, the frequencies of chromatid gaps and breaks are significantly higher than in cells from normal individuals. Figure 1 shows test results from 103 individuals, 1 to 96 years old; 39 of these, of whom 2 tested high, were clinically normal; 28 had cancer-prone genetic disorders and, except for 2 xeroderma pigmentosum (XP) group A individuals, all tested high, as did skin fibroblasts from 36 hereditary or familial cancer patients. The genetic disorders tested included ataxia telangiectasia (AT), Fanconi's anemia, Bloom's syndrome, Gardner's syndrome, familial polyposis, and XP. The hereditary or familial cancers tested include breast cancer, retinoblastoma, Wilms' tumor, and hereditary cutaneous malignant melanoma (HCMM) (with its precursor lesion, the dysplastic nevus). The DNA-damaging agent can be either x rays or visible fluorescent light (Parshad et al., 1985a; Sanford et al., 1986a). X-ray-sensitive AT is also sensitive to visible light and, unexpectedly, ultraviolet- (UV-) light-sensitive XP is also sensitive to x rays (except XP-A cells). Cells from an additional five individuals who were 3 months old or less (one fetus, three 3-day-old foreskins, and one 3-month-old infant) all tested high, perhaps reflecting developmental processes that do not require additional genomic stability in the protected *in utero* environment.

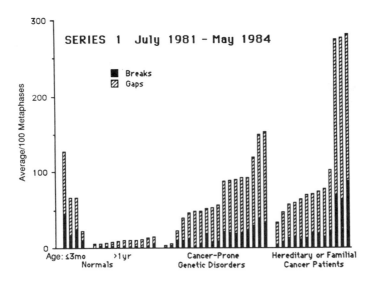

Figure 1. Comparison of chromatid damage in skin fibroblasts from normal donors, those with cancer-prone genetic disorders, and those with familial or hereditary cancer; cells were fixed 2 hr after G$_2$-phase x-irradiation (1 Gy). *Series 1*: The genetic disorders represented were (left to right; numbers in parentheses indicate numbers of individuals if more than 1, throughout figure): xeroderma pigmentosum (XP)-A (2), XP variant, Gardner's syndrome, Fanconi's anemia, XP-E, Gardner's syndrome, Bloom's syndrome, XP-E, familial polyposis, ataxia telangiectasia (AT) heterozygote (3), XP-C, AT heterozygote (2), AT (2). Cancer patients had (left to right): hereditary cutaneous malignant melanoma (HCMM) (3), osteosarcoma, medulloblastoma, acute myeloid leukemia (AML), liposarcoma, basal cell carcinoma syndrome, HCMM, breast cancer, HCMM (2), and dysplastic nevus syndrome (DNS). Sources of normal cells 3 months old or less were (left to right): fetal skin, 3-day foreskin (3). (Continued on following page.)

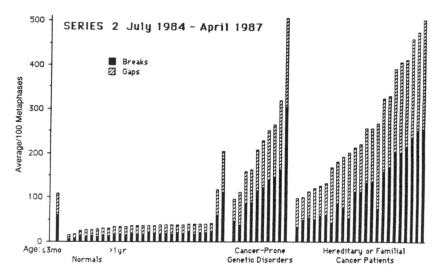

Figure 1 (continued). Comparison of chromatid damage in skin fibroblasts from normal donors, those with cancer-prone genetic disorders, and those with familial or hereditary cancer; cells were fixed 2 hr after G_2-phase x-irradiation (1 Gy). *Series 2*: Cancer-prone genetic disorders were (left to right): AT heterozygote, XP-C, AT heterozygote (5), AT, AT heterozygote, AT. First individual in cancer patient group (left to right) was from a high-incidence breast cancer family; the other patients had: retinoblastoma, Wilms' tumor, retinoblastoma, DNS, Wilms' tumor, HCMM (2), retinoblastoma, DNS (4), HCMM, DNS, HCMM, retinoblastoma (3), HCMM, retinoblastoma (3). Normal donor (far left) was 3 months old.

Important considerations regarding the experimental protocol include the necessity to renew the culture medium and add colcemid 30 min after irradiation; first, to allow cells in metaphase at the time of irradiation to complete mitosis and be excluded from analysis, and second, to allow both normal and cancer-prone cells to repair direct strand breaks. Metaphase cells collected between 0.5 and 2 hr after irradiation show the differential response. During this period cells are particularly susceptible to environmental factors that can affect chromatid aberrations, including pH, temperature, cell density, culture medium or serum, microbial contamination, and visible light exposure. With adequate control of these factors, this method could provide the basis of a test for detecting individuals genetically predisposed to cancer.

ENHANCED CHROMATID ABERRATIONS MANIFEST A GENETIC TRAIT

Three experimental approaches demonstrated the genetic character of enhanced chromatid aberrations after DNA damage in G_2 phase and its strong association with susceptibility to cancer. The first approach, somatic cell hybridization, showed that when HeLa cells were hybridized with normal skin fibroblasts, the immediate progeny manifested the small number of chromatid aberrations and the nontumorigenicity of a normal cell (Sanford et al., 1986b). Thus, the aberration enhancement behaved as a recessive trait in these hybrids.

The second approach, injection of pristane in susceptible BALB/cAnPt mice, resulted in plasmacytoma induction in a large fraction of the animals, although few or no tumors were induced in resistant DBA/2NPt mice; F_1 hybrids between these two strains resulted in resistant progeny. After x-irradiation of stimulated lymphocytes, chromatid aberrations in cells from BALB/cAnPt were enhanced twofold over those from either DBA/2NPt or the F_1 progeny (Sanford et al., 1986a), directly demonstrating the recessive genetic character of enhanced chromatid aberrations in this case.

Finally, the strong association with genetic susceptibility to human cutaneous melanoma observed in 25 members of 9 melanoma-prone families, 12 spouses, and 11 other unrelated normal individuals clearly indicated the genetic basis of enhanced G_2 chromatid aberrations (Sanford et al., 1987). Cells from obligate carriers of the recessive conditions AT and XP also showed enhanced G_2 chromatid aberrations, although to a lesser extent than cells from their homozygous counterparts (Parshad et al., 1985b; Sanford et al., 1988; Shiloh et al., 1986). In addition, a clinically normal obligate carrier of the HCMM gene and two individuals who later developed clinical symptoms showed enhanced G_2 aberrations (Sanford et al., 1987). It thus appears feasible to identify the heterozygous gene carriers in families from at least these three cancer-predisposing conditions. It also seems that enhancement of aberrations after G_2 irradiation may behave as a dominant trait in some cases.

EVIDENCE THAT DEFICIENT DNA REPAIR RESULTS IN ENHANCED CHROMATID ABERRATIONS

There are three plausible explanations for the enhanced chromatid aberrations. First, transit time through the G_2 phase of the cell cycle may be faster for the cells that manifest enhanced aberrations, resulting in less time available for repair. However, transit time was found to be the same for those lines tested (Parshad et al., 1983, 1984, 1985a). Second, cells that manifest enhanced aberrations may be more susceptible to DNA damage than normal cells. This is unlikely because the initial numbers of chromatid aberrations observed in normal and susceptible cells are essentially the same (Gantt et al., 1987, Figure 7; Parshad et al., 1983, Figure 1; 1984, Figure 3; 1985a, Figure 2; Sanford et al., 1986c, Figure 1).

The third plausible explanation, that deficient or unbalanced repair of DNA results in enhancement of chromatid aberrations after damage in the G_2 phase, seems likely for the following reasons: (1) Kinetic experiments clearly show the rapid decrease of chromatid aberrations with time in normal cells compared with that in cancer-prone or malignant cells (Gantt et al., 1987; Parshad et al., 1983, 1984, 1985a; Sanford et al., 1986c). (2) Direct measure of DNA strand breaks by the membrane alkaline elution technique indicates that the newly synthesized DNA from tumor- or cancer-prone cells either repairs breaks more slowly or acquires more breaks than that of normal cells (Gantt et al., 1986); breaks can accumulate during incomplete or deficient repair processes. The kinetic difference between normal and tumor- or cancer-prone cells in DNA-strand-break repair reaches a maximum within 2 hr, and this maximum corresponds to the kinetic difference in chromatid aberration incidence following x-irradiation (Parshad et al., 1983, 1984, 1985a). (3) The presence of catalase in culture medium at the time of x-irradiation eliminates or greatly reduces both the low chromatid aberration frequencies in normal cells and those greatly enhanced in malignant cells (Parshad et al., 1980, 1982). This indicates that these chromatid aberrations are largely a result of indirect or secondary DNA damage, not the initial direct strand breaks. (4) The presence of β-cytosine arabinoside (ara-C) during the repair period after irradiation greatly increases the chromatid aberrations in normal cells to levels approaching that of tumor cells. However, the ara-C does not significantly affect the aberrations in the tumor cells (Parshad et al., 1982, 1983, 1984; Preston, 1982; Sanford et al., 1985). This indicates that a repair mechanism present in normal cells and inhibited by ara-C is deficient in the tumor cells. (5) XP-A cells are an exception to the general association of cancer proneness and enhanced chromatid aberrations after DNA damage in the G_2 phase. Also, chromatid aberrations in XP-A cells are not affected by ara-C in the medium during the repair period (Parshad et al., 1983; Sanford et al., 1985). Because the repair defect in XP-A cells is known to be the virtual lack of DNA strand incision in the nucleotide excision repair process, this indicates that enzymatic DNA strand incision activity is required to manifest the chromatid aberrations. It also indicates that the aberrations observed are not complicated by residual S-phase DNA synthesis during G_2, because XP-A is normal in that regard and shows no increase in aberrations. (6) One genetic disorder associated with enhanced chromatid aberration and a high risk for cancer, Bloom's syndrome, has been reported to be deficient in DNA ligase activity (Chan et al., 1987; Willis and Lindahl, 1987).

A MODEL FOR MALIGNANT TRANSFORMATION AND TUMOR PROGRESSION

Our results and recent findings on hereditary neoplasms (Ali et al., 1987; Cavenee et al., 1983; Naylor et al., 1987; Okamoto et al., 1988; Orkin et al., 1984) suggest that two classes of gene defects or deficiencies are involved in the process of malignant transformation and progression. Class I genes are associated with the specific cell and tissue type predisposed to undergo transformation. Among deficient genes in this class are those currently referred to as the retinoblastoma gene(s), the genes for familial polyposis, Gardner's syndrome, HCMM, Wilms' tumor, etc. Class II genes are more general, in that they are associated with many diverse cancer types. When these genes are deficient, they impart a genetic instability to the predisposed cell that results from breakdown of a precise system for monitoring and repairing DNA damage during the G_2 phase before distribution of chromosomes to daughter cells, thus increasing the probability of mutation. After the complete loss of function for the normal class I gene, the process of transformation, promotion, and tumor progression persists, driven by continued proliferation in the presence of genetic instability. Genetic instability is dependent on cell cycling, since the repair deficiency is manifest only when DNA damage is sustained during G_2. Thus, rapid cycling resulting from activation of genes that control cell proliferation (such as oncogenes) would increase the rate of malignant change. The absence of genetic instability would greatly reduce, or possibly preclude acquiring in a single cell, the necessary genetic change(s) for cancer.

Some important implications of this model are as follows: (1) Defective class II genes resulting in enhanced chromatid aberrations in malignant cells after damage to DNA in G_2 phase explain genetic instability, the *sine qua non* of the cancer cell. (2) The conclusion by Matsunaga (1978) that expression of the retinoblastoma gene is affected significantly by inherited genes at other loci is consistent with the presence of defective class II genes. It should be possible to test whether the class II genes are involved in loss of retinoblastoma gene expression with appropriate family studies. (3) Cells with the G_2 lesion from defective class II genes have the properties of "initiated" cells, which explains the temporal and dose characteristics associated with the multistep model of tumor initiation, promotion, and progression. (4) Oncogenes participate in the transformation and progression process by providing a proliferative stimulus. Proliferation of a genetically unstable cell population (cells with defective class II genes) in the presence of low levels of DNA damage provides the driving force for malignant transformation and tumor progression. (5) Association of defective class II genes and consequent genetic instability with genetic heterozygosity greatly increases the chance that normal gene function will be lost in cell progeny, resulting in defective homozygosity and uncovering of recessive genes. This process could have important implications for health in areas other than cancer, including various chronic diseases, degenerative neurological disorders, immunological deficiencies, and aging.

REFERENCES

Ali, IU, R Lidereau, C Theillet, and R Callahan. 1987. Reduction to homozygosity of genes on chromosome II in human breast neoplasia. Science 238:185-188.

Cavenee, WK, TP Dryja, RA Phillips, WF Benedict, R Godbout, BL Gallie, AL Murphree, LC Strong, and RL White. 1983. Expression of recessive alleles by chromosomal mechanisms in retinoblastoma. Nature 305:779-784.

Chan, JYH, FF Becker, J German, and JH Ray. 1987. Altered DNA ligase I activity in Bloom's syndrome cells. Nature 325:357-359.

Gantt, R, R Parshad, FM Price, and KK Sanford. 1986. Biochemical evidence for deficient DNA repair leading to enhanced G_2 chromatid radiosensitivity and susceptibility to cancer. Radiat Res 108:117-126.

Gantt, R, KK Sanford, R Parshad, FM Price, WD Peterson, Jr., and JS Rhim. 1987. Enhanced G_2 chromatid radiosensitivity, an early stage in the neoplastic transformation of human epidermal keratinocytes in culture. Cancer Res 47:1390-1397.

Matsunaga, E. 1978. Hereditary retinoblastoma: Delayed mutation or host resistance? Am J Hum Genet 30:406-424.

Naylor, SL, BE Johnson, JD Minna, and AY Sakaguchi. 1987. Loss of heterozygosity of chromosome 3p markers in small-cell lung cancer. Nature 329:451-454.

Okamoto, M, M Sasaki, K Sugio, C Sato, T Iwama, T Ikeuchi, A Tonomura, T Sasazuki, and M Miyaki. 1988. Loss of constitutional heterozygosity in colon carcinoma from patients with familial polyposis coli. Nature 331:273-277.

Orkin, SH, DS Goldman, and SE Sallan. 1984. Development of homozygosity for chromosome 11p markers in Wilms' tumor. Nature 309:172-174.

Parshad, R, KK Sanford, and GM Jones. 1983. Chromatid damage after G_2 phase x-irradiation of cells from cancer-prone individuals implicates deficiency in DNA repair. Proc Natl Acad Sci USA 80:5612-5616.

Parshad, R, KK Sanford, and GM Jones. 1985a. Chromatid damage induced by fluorescent light during G_2 phase in normal and Gardner syndrome fibroblasts: Interpretation in terms of deficient DNA repair. Mutat Res 151:57-63.

Parshad, R, KK Sanford, GM Jones, and RE Tarone. 1985b. G_2 chromosomal radiosensitivity of ataxia telangiectasia heterozygotes. Cancer Genet Cytogenet 14:163-168.

Parshad, R, R Gantt, KK Sanford, and GM Jones. 1984. Chromosomal radiosensitivity of human tumor cells during the G_2 cell cycle period. Cancer Res 44:5577-5582.

Parshad, R, R Gantt, KK Sanford, GM Jones, and RE Tarone. 1982. Repair of chromosome damage induced by x-irradiation during G_2 phase in a line of normal human fibroblasts and its malignant derivative. J Natl Cancer Inst 69:404-414.

Parshad, R, WG Taylor, KK Sanford, RF Camalier, R Gantt, and RE Tarone. 1980. Fluorescent light-induced chromosome damage in human IMR-90 fibroblasts. Mutat Res 73:115-124.

Preston, RJ. 1982. The use of inhibitors of DNA repair in the study of the mechanism of induction of chromosome aberrations. Cytogenet Cell Genet 33:20-26.

Sanford, KK, R Parshad, and R Gantt. 1978. Light and oxygen effects on chromosomes, DNA and neoplastic transformation of cells in culture, pp. 117-148. In: *Nutritional Requirements of Cultured Cells*, H Katsuta (ed.). University Park Press, Baltimore, MD.

Sanford, KK, R Parshad, and R Gantt. 1985. Enhanced G_2 chromosomal radiosensitivity, susceptibility to cancer and neoplastic transformation, pp. 811-820. In: *Progress in Leucocyte Biology: Genetic Control of Host Resistance to Infection and Malignancy*, E Skamene (ed.). Alan R Liss, New York, NY.

Sanford, KK, R Parshad, and R Gantt. 1986a. Responses of human cells in culture to hydrogen peroxide and related free radicals generated by visible light, pp. 373-394. In: *Free Radicals, Aging, and Degenerative Diseases*, J Johnson (ed.). Alan R Liss, New York, NY.

Sanford, KK, R Parshad, EJ Stanbridge, JK Frost, GM Jones, JE Wilkinson, and RE Tarone. 1986b. Chromosomal radiosensitivity during the G_2 cell cycle period and cytopathology of human normal × tumor cell hybrids. Cancer Res 46:2045-2049.

Sanford, KK, R Parshad, M Potter, GM Jones, RP Nordan, SE Brust, and FM Price. 1986c. Chromosomal radiosensitivity during G_2 phase and susceptibility to plasmacytoma induction in mice. Curr Top Microbiol Immunol 132:202-208.

Sanford, KK, R Parshad, MH Greene, RE Tarone, MA Tucker, and GM Jones. 1987. Hypersensitivity to G_2 chromatid radiation damage in familial dysplastic naevus syndrome. Lancet ii:1111-1116.

Sanford, KK, R Parshad, GM Jones, S Handleman, C Garrison, and F Price. 1979. Role of photosensitization and oxygen in chromosome stability and "spontaneous" malignant tranformation in culture. J Natl Cancer Inst 63:1245-1255.

Sanford, KK, R Parshad, KH Kraemer, RE Tarone, and GM Jones. 1988. Carrier detection in XP. Clin Res 36:691a.

Shiloh, Y, R Parshad, KK Sanford, and GM Jones. 1986. Carrier detection in ataxia telangiectasia. Lancet i:689-690.

Willis, AE and T Lindahl. 1987. DNA ligase I deficiency in Bloom's syndrome. Nature 325:355-357.

QUESTIONS AND COMMENTS

Q: T. Seed, Argonne National Laboratory, Chicago, IL
Do the spontaneous rates of chromosome breaks/gaps in cells of cancer-prone individuals correlate with subsequent measures of chromosomal repair in these cells?

A: No, the spontaneous rates do not generally correlate, although certain conditions such as AT and Bloom's syndrome do have increased spontaneous rates.

S: M. Smerdon, WSU, Pullman, WA
It is possible that the gaps you see represent regions of chromatin that are "opened up" for the repair of the initial lesions and are not regions of damage per se. These regions, if they persist, may then be "hot spots" for chromosomal aberrations. Your araC data support this notion because araC is known to block excision repair at the repair synthesis step, and this would cause the gaps to persist. Finally, the XP(A) results may indicate that these cells are deficient in a preincision process involving opening up of chromatin.

R: We think there are various genetic lesions an individual can have which would lead to enhanced chromatid aberrations. Your suggestion is a plausible and interesting one.

INTERINDIVIDUAL VARIATION WITH RESPECT TO DNA REPAIR IN HUMAN CELLS

R. C. Leonard, [1,3] J. C. Leonard, [1,4] M. A. Bender, [1] J. Wieland, [1,5] and R. B. Setlow[2]

[1]Medical Department, Brookhaven National Laboratory, Upton, NY 11973

[2]Biology Department, Brookhaven National Laboratory, Upton, NY 11973

[3]Consultants in Epidemiology and Occupational Health, Washington, DC 20007

[4]Wilson Genetics Center, George Washington University, Washington, DC 20037

[5]Department of Obstetrics, State University of New York, Stony Brook, NY 11794

Key words: *DNA repair, variability, cytogenetics, mutagenic assays*

ABSTRACT

Ecogenetics is the study of genetically determined differences among individuals in terms of their susceptibility to the actions of physical, chemical, and biological agents in the environment. An individual's most basic level of response to these environmental agents may well be the ability to repair physical and chemical damage to DNA. We have surveyed DNA-repair measurements in a healthy working human population to determine the extent of their variability in DNA repair, and to identify individuals who are at the extremes of the distributions for DNA repair. In addition, we are measuring the interindividual variation over time, as well as the correlations among measurements of different systems of repair.

We have measured cytogenetic responses [sister chromatid exchanges (SCE) and micronuclei formation] and DNA excision repair (unscheduled DNA synthesis and removal of O^6-methylguanine) in human peripheral lymphocytes exposed to ultraviolet light, x rays, mitomycin C, and N-methyl-N-nitro-nitrosoguanidine (MNNG). Our efforts to identify specific factors (e.g., age, gender, race, and cigarette-smoking) that contribute to the variances of these measurements show that the SCE response to MNNG is positively correlated with age when treatment occurs during cell division but not when MNNG is added before blast transformation. Cigarette-smoking affects both SCE formation and the number of micronuclei produced after x-irradiation. We have not established a statistically significant correlation between O^6-methylguanine transferase activity and the number of SCE following treatment with MNNG.

Ecogenetics is the study of genetically determined differences among individuals in their susceptibility to the actions of physical, chemical, and biological agents in the environment. An individual's most basic level of response to these environmental agents may be the ability to repair physical and chemical damage to DNA. We have surveyed DNA-repair measurements in a healthy working population to determine the extent of the population variability in these end points and to assess the value of these screening protocols in identifying individuals who are at the extremes of the distributions. We are also measuring intraindividual variation over time and the correlations between measurements of different repair systems. We have chosen to use, as end points, cytogenetic responses [sister chromatid exchanges (SCE) and micronucleus formation] and DNA excision repair [unscheduled DNA synthesis and removal of O^6 guanine methylation] in human peripheral lymphocytes exposed to 254-nm ultraviolet light, x rays, the bifunctional alkylating agent mitomycin C, or the monofunctional alkylating agent N-methyl-N-nitro-nitrosoguanidine (MNNG). These four test mutagens produce spectra of DNA lesions eliciting different types of DNA repair.

We use autoradiography of G_1 lymphocytes labeled with ^{3}H-thymidine to determine, by grain counting, variability in the amount of ultraviolet-induced repair synthesis among cells within individual samples. Levels of O^6-methylguanine methyl transferase activity were determined in lymphocyte extracts (Waldstein et al., 1982).

Cultures are exposed to MNNG ($3\ \mu M$) before or 24 hr after phytohemagglutinin (PHA) stimulation; the frequencies of sister chromatid exchanges induced by each treatment, as well as the background frequency, are measured. Each of these assays is conducted with separated lymphocytes. Ionizing radiation sensitivity is measured by the frequency of occurrence of micronuclei in whole blood cultures exposed to 3 Gy of 250-Kvp x rays before PHA stimulation and harvested after 72 hr. Because micronucleus frequency depends on the number of *in vitro* cell divisions after exposure, a parallel group of cultures are grown with 5-bromodeoxyuridine and stained by the Hoechst 33258-Giemsa method, so that we can assess the number of first-, second-, third-division, and subsequent metaphases. Whole blood cultures also are used to measure the frequencies of SCE produced by 4-hr exposure to mitomycin C before PHA stimulation.

Our analyses of the various end points are as yet incomplete, and should be regarded as preliminary because population sampling is continuing. The preliminary results for some end points, however, are of interest. Induction of SCE by MNNG currently yields a mean SCE frequency ($\pm$ SEM) for untreated controls of 10.1 ± 0.28; frequency for the G_0-treated cultures is 13.1 ± 0.49, and that for the G_1-phase cultures is 19.4 ± 0.60. In examining the effect of current cigarette smoking on the level of MNNG-induced SCE, we are still at some disadvantage because of the few cigarette smokers (8) in our current sample. Comparison of mean SCE of smokers and nonsmokers shows a statistically significant increase in the smokers only in the cycling-phase data ($p < 0.01$). Interestingly, the white blood count (WBC) of the smokers is also significantly increased ($p = 0.05$). When stepwise multiple regression is used to examine the effects of age, WBC, sex, and smoking status, the variables that make a significant contribution to r^2 are smoking and WBC. Further examination of WBC data shows that although there is no correlation between WBC and the control level of SCE, there is a significant correlation between WBC and MNNG-induced SCE during G_0 phase ($r = 0.34$; $p = 0.03$). This correlation of WBC and mean SCE increases to a highly significant level for cells treated with MNNG during cycling phase ($r = 0.64$; $p < 0.001$).

We had hoped to establish a correlation between the level of MNNG-induced SCE and the level of the O^6 acceptor protein. The O^6 acceptor protein was measured in both PHA-stimulated and unstimulated lymphocyte cultures. We have SCE counts and O^6 acceptor protein levels for 38 persons, but as yet have found no significant correlation between the G_0-phase SCE and the unstimulated culture O^6 acceptor levels, nor do we see any correlation between the cycling phase, MNNG-induced SCE, and the level of the O^6 acceptor in PHA-stimulated cultures.

We have also examined the effect of age, sex, race, cigarette smoking, and WBC on the level of mitomycin C- (150 ng/ml) induced SCE but have found no significant effect. We have mitomycin C data for only four smokers, so the lack of significance of cigarette smoking may be caused by the small sample size. Unlike the MNNG-induced SCE, SCE induction by mitomycin C appears to be unaffected by WBC.

A synergistic effect of caffeine and mitomycin C on the induction of SCE was reported by Ishii and Bender (1978). In mitomycin C-treated cultures we find a large increase in SCE frequency if cells are incubated in caffeine (200 μg/ml) (35.4 compared to 26.8/cell), but this difference may be accounted for by the increase in frequency in control cultures incubated in caffeine (18.5 compared to 10.5). Thus, in contrast to the case reported by Ishii and Bender, in these cases there seems to be only an additive effect and no interaction between mitomycin C and caffeine.

One major goal of this investigation is to measure the extent of the population variability in these end points of DNA damage/repair and to determine whether these measurements can be used in screening protocols to identify particularly susceptible subsets of the population. Radiation effects on chromosomal structure can be measured with considerable accuracy by examining chromosomal aberrations. Scoring this end point, however, requires considerable time and technical expertise, and therefore this end point is expensive to use in mass screening protocols. Micronuclei, usually acentric chromosomal fragments that fail to be incorporated in either daughter nucleus during mitosis, can be used as a convenient assay of chromosome breakage. Counting micronuclei is relatively simple and, because it can be automated, comparatively inexpensive. The micronucleus assay is less than ideal for our purposes because of the variability of progression through the cell cycle by human lymphocytes, even though the ease with which they can be obtained is important for large sampling schemes. Our goal has been to remove the effects of differential cell cycle delay between persons and thus to establish the range of variation in sensitivity to irradiation as measured by micronucleus formation in a population sample.

We used multivariate regression and simple linear regression with parameters that measure aspects of progression through the cell cycle to adjust total micronuclei in irradiated cultures. The first type of analysis regressed total micronuclei with the difference in the replicative index (Schneider and Lewis, 1981) of the control and irradiated cultures. The second approach used a weighted replicative index that gave proportionally more weight to the percentages of third and fourth divisions. In the third approach, multivariate regression was used with the mitotic index and the percent second divisions in the irradiated culture to adjust total micronuclei for the percent of cells actually dividing and the percent of cells that would express micronuclei.

Table 1 shows results for the three adjustment methods. These results indicate that the distribution of micronuclei produced in human peripheral blood lymphocytes by irradiation with 3 Gy of x rays can be made more consistent within a population when measures of cell cycle delay are used to adjust the total number of micronuclei. The variance is reduced the most by simple linear regression with the replicative index (without extra weighting of the individual cell generation numbers). The mitotic index shows a negative coefficient when regressed with micronucleus frequency; the reason is unclear, although it could be related to the loss of micronuclei in third and later divisions. Distributions resulting from the adjusted values of micronucleus frequency should make it easier to distinguish individuals who may be either more sensitive or less sensitive to radiation than the general population. Experiments on repeat samples are currently attempting to establish the validity of the adjusted micronucleus count as a stable marker for an individual's radiation sensitivity.

Table 1. Mean micronucleus frequency induced by 3 Gy of x rays in unstimulated whole blood cultures adjusted in various ways for the frequency of cells in other than second postirradiation cell cycle (see text).[a]

		Adjusted By:		
	Unadjusted	Replicative Index $(y = 124.6 + 50.4x)^*$	Weighted Index $(y = 123.0 + 49.8x)^{**}$	Mitotic Index $(y = 163.7 - 1.8x)^{***}$
Mean	135.0	131.4	131.1	121.6
SD	55.0	12.9	15.9	25.8

[a] Values are mean estimate $\pm$ SD for micronuclei induced by 3 Gy of x rays and adjusted in the indicated ways.
   $^*x$ = replicative index = % first division + (% second divisions $\times$ 2) + (% third divisions $\times$ 3) + (% fourth divisions $\times$ 4)/100.
 $^{**}x$ = weighted replicative index = % first divisions + (% second divisions $\times$ 2) + (% third divisions $\times$ 4) + (% fourth divisions $\times$ 16)/100.
$^{***}x$ = mitotic index (contribution of % second division to r^2 was significant).

ACKNOWLEDGMENTS

This research was supported by the Office of Health and Environment Research of the U.S. Department of Energy.

REFERENCES

Ishii, Y and MA Bender. 1978. Caffeine inhibition of prereplication repair of mitomycin C-induced DNA damage in human peripheral lymphocytes. Mutat Res 51:419-425.

ALLOANTIGENIC CHALLENGE AND ACQUIRED IMMUNODEFICIENCY SYNDROME (AIDS)

C. Hoff

Pacific Northwest Laboratory, P. O. Box 999, Richland, WA 99352

Key words: *AIDS, HLA alloantigens, suppression, pregnancy*

ABSTRACT

Early in pregnancy, women are exposed to paternally derived, foreign (allo) fetal histocompatibility antigens (HLA). This alloantigenic challenge results in the production of maternal anti-HLA IgG antibodies that bind to fetal HLA alloantigens on the placenta. These HLA + IgG immune complexes are noncytotoxic and apparently shield the fetus from a maternal lymphocytotoxic attack. Some of these immune complexes also enter the maternal circulation and directly affect maternal immunosuppression. Because only regional lymph nodes are involved, immunosuppression is localized in the endometrium. It is believed these events promote fetal survival by blocking maternal immune reactions against stage-specific, alloantigenic growth factors produced by the fetoplacental unit.

The major route of human immune deficiency virus (HIV) infection is exposure to HIV-contaminated blood, blood products, semen, or body fluids in which HLA antigens are present. Exposure to HLA alloantigens by transfusion of blood or blood products or by insemination during anal intercourse results in systemic alloantigenic challenge.

Evidence is presented from human and laboratory animal studies that HLA alloantigenic challenge via the routes just described results in systemic immunosuppression. Conceivably, this could increase the risk of HIV infection after exposure and enhance progression to AIDS once infection has occurred. Some research strategies to test this hypothesis are discussed.

The major routes of transmission of the human immunodeficiency virus (HIV) are through intravenous (parenteral) and rectal exposure to contaminated body fluids and across the maternofetal interface. Most cases of parenteral/anal infection occur in individuals *chronically* exposed to foreign body fluids. It has been assumed that increased exposure to foreign body fluids increases the risk of encountering and thus becoming infected with HIV. However, chronic exposure to foreign body fluids also increases exposure to foreign (allo-) antigens of the major histocompatibility complex (MHC), and MHC alloantigenic challenge can lead to immunosuppression.

Chronic exposure to MHC alloantigenic challenge is hypothesized to increase the risk of infection after HIV exposure and may increase the rate of progression to manifest acquired immunodeficiency syndrome (AIDS) after HIV infection. Support for this hypothesis is based on clinical investigations of HIV-infected individuals and studies of the immunological effects of chronic MHC alloantigenic challenge resulting from pregnancy, transfusion of blood or blood products, and anal sexual intercourse. Evidence from studies of reproductive immunology is presented first because the model of maternal response to fetal MHC alloantigenic challenge is among those well documented.

In humans, the MHC is called the human leukocyte A (HLA) complex. Expression of the HLA antigens is controlled by gene loci in close linkage on chromosome 6 (Klein and Figueroa, 1986). Because of a high degree of HLA polymorphism, nearly all fetuses have one or more paternally derived HLA antigens that are alloantigenic to the mother. Although the fetus is an allograft to the mother, it is not rejected by her immune system. In fact, the the greater the fetal alloantigenicity, the better the pregnancy outcome in terms of reduced rates of maternal preeclampsia and fetal morbidity and of enhanced fetal growth. Figure 1 (Hoff et al., 1989) explains this paradox.

Maternal exposure to fetal MHC antigens is a normal event during pregnancy (Ahrons, 1971; Billington, 1987). Fetal MHC antigens that are alloantigenic to the mother trigger antigen-specific cell-mediated and humoral responses (Voisin, 1983). Anti-MHC antibodies of the gamma globulin class (IgG) are produced by the mother and some bind to fetal MHC alloantigens, forming immune complexes (Davies, 1985). Some of the immune complexes and free IgG eventually attach to trophoblast receptors, providing a temporary shield against a maternal lymphocytotoxic attack directed toward the fetoplacental unit (Johnson et al., 1976). *In vitro*, the free immune complexes and maternal IgG block maternal-paternal mixed lymphocyte reactions (MLR) (Albrechtsen et al., 1977; Jonker and De Rooyer-Doyer, 1980). These immune complexes and IgG may also stimulate the proliferation of antigen-specific suppressor T cells by the mother (Voisin, 1983, 1987), inhibiting further cell-mediated activity against fetal MHC alloantigens. Over time, antiidiotypic antibodies are formed by the mother against the various epitopes on her own anti-MHC IgG (Suciu-Foca et al., 1983; Singal et al., 1984). These antiidiotypic antibodies stimulate the proliferation of suppressor cells (T and non-T/non-B) with nonspecific activity, resulting in general suppression of the cell-mediated arm of the mother's immune system (Chaouat and Lankar, 1988).

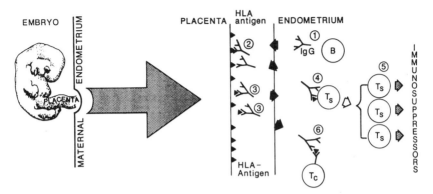

Figure 1. Model of the effects of fetal alloantigenic challenge on the maternal immune system. 1. Fetal alloantigens enter maternal circulation and stimulate production of anti-HLA IgG antibodies. 2. Some anti-HLA antibodies cross maternofetal interface and bind to fetal HLA antigens on placenta; these *immune complexes* (fetal allo-HLA antigen + maternal antibody) help provide protection from maternal cell-mediated cytotoxic response against fetoplacental unit. 3. Free immune complexes in the maternal circulation stimulate the proliferation of specific suppressor T cells. 4. These cells produce substances that down-regulate a cell-mediated response directed against fetal alloantigens; immune complexes may also stimulate the proliferation of nonspecific suppressor cells that down-regulate cell-mediated responses against other alloantigens. 6. In addition, immune complexes interfere with a maternal cell-mediated attack against a broad class of fetoplacental alloantigens by binding to T-cell receptors and blocking their cytotoxic activity. This response to HLA alloantigens may provide protection to the fetus by blocking potential maternal cytotoxic response against alloantigenic, stage-specific growth factors produced by fetoplacental unit during development.

The maternal response to MHC alloantigenic challenge tends to be localized, occurring in the lymph nodes draining the uterus and at the maternofetal interface (Billington, 1987). Nonetheless, a mild systemic effect can be observed among some pregnant women that includes reduced levels of helper T cells, elevated levels of suppressor T cells and blocking antibodies/immune complexes, increased susceptibility to infection (Brabin, 1985), and extended allograft rejection times (Ward et al., 1978). These findings may explain why the transfusion of sera from such women prolongs renal allograft survival (Riggo et al., 1978) and why these sera have tumor-enhancing activity (Voisin and Chaouat, 1974). Although the localized maternal immune response to fetal MHC alloantigenic challenge tends to be advantageous to the fetus, convincing evidence exists that parenteral and anal exposure to MHC alloantigenic challenge can result in systemic lymph node and splenic involvement leading to general systemic immunosuppression.

Patients receiving frequent heterologous blood transfusions often develop elevated levels of suppressor T cells and pregnancy-like IgG that block antibodies/immune complexes and show *in vitro* impairment of cell-mediated responses to mitogenic and antigenic stimuli (Sengar et al., 1973; Burlingham, 1988). The presence of these IgG in transfused renal transplant recipients is associated with enhanced renal allograft survival (MacLeod et al., 1983). Many HIV-negative hemophiliacs receiving Factor VIII (which contains HLA alloantigenic fragments) also show the same signs of immunosuppression as observed in transfused patients (Lee et al., 1984; Kreiss et al., 1986; Sullivan et al., 1986).

The HLA antigens present in semen can be transported across the rectal mucosa into the general circulation, and rectal abrasions can augment this transport (Mavligit et al., 1984). HIV-negative human recipients in anal sexual intercourse have inverted T4/T8 ratios and subnormal graft-versus-host reactions (Mavligit et al., 1984). HIV-negative homosexual males often have elevated levels of both suppressor T8 cells (Schwartz et al., 1985; Weber et al., 1986) and non-T/non-B cells bearing the Leu 7 marker (Hester et al., unpublished data). Because the same cell populations are elevated among HIV-infected individuals who are immunosuppressed (Gupta, 1986; Stites et al., 1986), these HIV-negative homosexuals may be partially immunosuppressed, increasing their susceptibility to HIV infection (Seyda and Krueger, 1987).

Evidence exists that chronic HLA alloantigenic challenge can lead to immunosuppression, impairing the immune system ability to detect and neutralize virus and augmenting the immunosuppressive action of HIV. In addition, *in vitro* HLA alloantigenic challenge has been shown to enhance *both* entry of HIV into uninfected T4 cells (Lewis et al., 1988) and HIV expansion from infected cells (Margolick et al., 1987). Sera from HIV-infected patients contain an antibody component that enhances HIV entry into uninfected target cells *in vitro* (Robinson et al., 1988); it has been assumed that the enhancing antibody is anti-HIV. Because exposure to HIV is associated with HLA alloantigenic challenge, it is possible that this component also contains anti-HLA and antiidiotypic antibodies having suppressive and enhancing activity.

An argument has been made that chronic alloantigenic challenge increases the risk for AIDS. Before HIV was identified as the etiological agent of AIDS, alloantigen challenge was considered a possible contributing factor (Shearer, 1983; Sonnabend et al., 1983; Hsia et al., 1984). However, this idea lost favor as HIV came to dominate the attention of AIDS researchers. This hypothesis merits reexamination.

REFERENCES

Ahrons, S. 1971. HLA-A antibodies: Influence on the human fetus. Tissue Antigens 1:121-136.

Albrechsten, D, BG Solheim, and E Thorsby. 1977. Antiserum inhibition of the mixed lymphocyte culture (MLC) interaction. Inhibitory effect of antibodies reactive with HLA-D associated determinants. Cell Immunol 28:258-273.

Billington, WD. 1987. Immunological aspects of implantation and fetal survival: The central role of the trophoblast, pp. 209-232. In: Recent Advances in Mammalian Development. Current Topics in Development of Biology, Vol. 23, C McLaren and G Siracusa (eds.). Academic Press, New York.

Brabin, BJ. 1985. Epidemiology of infection in pregnancy. Rev Infect Dis 7:570-603.

Burlingham, WJ. 1988. What is known about blocking factors in renal allograft recipients. Am J Reprod Immunol Microbiol 16:15-20.

Chaouat, G and D Lankar. 1988. Vaccination against spontaneous abortion in mice by preimmunization with an anti-idiotypic antibody. Am J Reprod Immunol Microbiol 16:146-150.

Davies, M. 1985. Antigenic analysis of immune complexes formed in normal human pregnancy. Clin Exp Immunol 61:406-415.

Gupta, S. 1986. Abnormality of Leu2$^+$7$^+$ cells in acquired immune deficiency syndrome (AIDS), AIDS-related complex, and asymptomatic homosexuals. J Clin Immunol 6:502-509.

Hoff, C, RM Garruto, and NM Durham. 1989. Human adaptability and medical genetics, pp. 69-81. In: Human Population Biology, MA Little and JD Haas (eds.). Oxford University Press, New York.

Hsia, H, DM Doran, RK Shockley, PC Galle, CL Lutcher, and LD Hodge. 1984. Hypothesis: Unregulated production of virus and/or sperm specific antiidotypic antibodies as a cause of AIDS. Lancet i:1212-1214.

Johnson, PM, WP Faulk, and AC Wang. 1976. Immunological studies of human placentae: Subclass and fragment specificity of binding of aggregated IgG by placental endothelial cells. Immunology 31:659-664.

Jonker, M and L De Rooyer-Doyer. 1980. Possible mechanisms by which alloantisera inhibit in the MLC test. Tissue Antigens 15:1-10.

Klein, J and F Figueroa. 1986. Evolution of the major histocompatibility complex. Crit Rev Immunol 6:275-278.

Kreiss, JK, LW Kitchen, HE Prince, CK Kasper, AL Goldstein, PH Naylor, O Preble, JA Stewart, and M Essex. 1986. Human T cell leukemia virus type III antibody and acquired immune deficiency syndrome in hemophiliac subjects. Results of a prospective study. Am J Med 80:345-350.

Lee, CA, PBA Kernoff, P Karayiannis, J Waters, and HC Thomas. 1984. Abnormal T-lymphocyte subsets in hemophilia: Relation to HLA proteins in plasma products. N Engl J Med 310:1058.

Lewis, DE, B Yoffe, CG Bosworth, FB Hollinger, and RR Rich. 1988. Human immunodeficiency virus-induced pathology favored by cellular transmission and activation. FASEB J 2:251-255.

MacLeod, AM, RJ Mason, KN Stewart, DA Power, WG Shewan, N Edward, and RGD Catto. 1983. Fc-receptor-blocking antibodies develop after blood transfusions and correlate with good graft outcome. Transplant Proc 15:1019-1021.

Margolick, JB, DJ Volkman, TM Folks, and AS Fauci. 1987. Amplification of HTLV-III/LAV infection by antigen-induced activation of T cells and direct suppression by virus of lymphocyte blastogenic responses. J Immunol 138:1719-1723.

Mavligit, GM, M Talpaz, FT Hsia, W Wong, B Lichtiger, PWA Mansell, and DM Mumford. 1984. Chronic immune stimulation by sperm alloantigens. Support for the hypothesis that spermatozoa induce immune dysregulation in homosexual males. JAMA 2512:237-241.

Riggio, RR, SD Saal, JS Cheigh, SJ Kim, WT Stubenbord, KH Stenzel, and AL Runin. 1978. Improved survival-rates in pre-sensitised recipients of kidney transplants by immunosuppression with maternal-source gamma-globulin. Lancet i:233-235.

Robinson, WE, Jr., DC Montefiori, and WM Mitchell. 1988. Antibody-dependent enhancement of human immunodeficiency virus type 1 injection. Lancet i:790-795.

Schwartz, K, BR Visscher, R Detels, J Taylor, P Nishanji, and JL Fahey. 1985. Immunological changes in lymphadenopathy virus positive and negative symptomless male homosexuals: Two years after observation. Lancet ii:831-832.

Sengar, DPS, G Opelz, and PT Terasaki. 1973. Suppression of mixed lymphocyte response by plasma from hemodialysis patients. Transplant Proc 5:641-647.

Seyda, M and GRF Krueger. 1987. Complex infectious copathogenesis of AIDS in HIV-positive individuals. Clin Immunol Newsl 8:81-86.

Shearer, GM. 1983. Allogeneneic leukocytes as a possible factor in induction of AIDS in homosexual men. N Engl J Med 308:223-224.

Singal, DP, L Butler, SK Liao, and S Joseph. 1984. The fetus as an allograft. Evidence for antiidiotypic antibodies induced by pregnancy. J Reprod Immunol 6:145-151.

Sonnabend, J, SS Witkin, and DT Purtilo. 1983. Acquired immunodeficiency syndrome, opportunistic infections, and malignancies in male homosexuals: A hypothesis of etiologic factors in pathogenesis. JAMA 249:2370-2374.

Stites, DP, CH Casavant, TM McHugh, AR Moss, SL Beal, JL Ziegler, AM Saunders, and NL Warner. 1986. Flow cytometric analysis of lymphocyte phenotypes using monoclonal antibodies and simultaneous dual immunofluorescence. Clin Immunol Immunopathol 38:161-177.

Suciu-Foca, N, E Reed, C Rohowsky, P Kung, and DW King. 1983. Anti-idiotypic antibodies to anti-HLA receptors induced by pregnancy. Proc Natl Acad Sci USA 80:830-834.

Sullivan, JL, FE Brewster, DB Brettler, AD Forsberg, SH Cheeseman, KS Byron, SM Baker, DL Willitts, RA Lew, and PH Levine. 1986. Hemophiliac immunodeficiency: Influence of exposure to factor VIII concentrate, LAV/HTLV-III, and herpesvirus. J Pediatr 108:504-510.

Voisin, GA. 1983. Immunological interventions of the placenta in maternal immunological tolerance to the fetus, pp. 179-204. In: *Immunology of Reproduction*. TG Wegman and TJ Gill (eds.). Oxford University Press, New York.

Voisin, GA. 1987. Regulatory facilitation reaction and active tolerance: A non-Euclidian view of the immune reaction authenticated by immunology of reproduction. Immunol Lett 16:283-290.

Voisin, GA and G Chaouat. 1974. Demonstration, nature and properties of maternal antibody fixed on placenta and directed against paternal antigens. J Reprod Fertil (Suppl) 21:89-103.

Ward, FE, NR Mendell, HF Seigler, JM MacQueen, and DB Amos. 1978. Factors which have a significant effect on survival of human skin grafts. Transplantation 26:194-198.

Weber, JN, J Wadsworth, LA Rogers, O Moshtael, K Scott, T McManus, E Berrie, DJ Jeffries, JRW Harris, and AJ Pinching. 1986. Three-year prospective study of HTLV-III/LAV infection in homosexual men. Lancet i:1179-1182.

IMPLICATIONS OF RECENT FINDINGS IN CARCINOGENESIS FOR ASSESSMENT OF LOW-EXPOSURE CANCER RISK

J. D. Wilson

Monsanto Company, St. Louis, MO 63167

Key Words: *Carcinogenesis, cancer risk, genotoxicity*

ABSTRACT

Results of carcinogenesis research during the last two decades require that we alter assessment of cancer risk. Significant observations contradicting all the key elements of the circa-1970 theory—on which present risk assessment methodology is based—have appeared over these years. In 1981, a new theory incorporated concepts from cancer genetics, epidemiology, and mutagenesis. The theory rationalizes many observations from experiment and experience, and predictions from the theory have been verified experimentally. For genotoxic carcinogens in exposure regimes in which mitotic rate is not increased, the added hazard is proportional to cumulative dose. However, when mitotic rate is increased, the two effects act synergistically and the apparent dose response climbs very rapidly. For nongenotoxic agents, hazard is a function of both dose and duration of exposure, and is not proportional to cumulative exposure.

Methods used today for estimating low-exposure hazard were developed in the mid-1970s, deriving from the theory as it was understood about 1970. Given the enormous amount of excellent research in the past 20 yr into cancer and its origins, it would be very surprising if those results did not signal the need for change, and they do. This paper explores the modern theory and its implications for cancer risk assessment.

Crump's model for the dependence of tumor incidence (yield) on dose (Guess and Crump, 1977; Crump et al., 1977) is derived from the epidemiological age-specific incidence model of Armitage and Doll (1954), adding the assumption that effect is directly proportional to dose. That assumption is justified by the observation (Miller and Miller, 1977) that most carcinogens recognized before 1970 were chemical "electrophiles," or could be metabolically transformed to such species. These electrophiles were postulated to speed the transit of normal cells through the "stages" of the Armitage-Doll "multistage" model by reaction with cellular DNA. From chemistry it is known that the rate of reaction of electrophiles with "bases" comparable to those of DNA is directly proportional to the electrophile's concentration, which is in turn proportional to dose in animal studies. The mathematical formula developed by Crump is a polynomial in dose, with the low-exposure hazard assumed to be dominated by the linear term; thus, the phrase "linearized multistage" model. The U.S. Environmental Protection Agency (EPA) today uses this procedure as the preferred method for estimating low-exposure hazard, justifying the choice by its derivation from the 1954 theory.

Ironically, by the time of the Guess and Crump publication, the Armitage-Doll multistage model was already recognized as inadequate to its initial task—describing the age-specific incidence of human cancer by the epidemiological community (Moolgavkar, 1977). Observations contradicting other assumptions essential to the validity of the multistage theory were accumulating and have since overwhelmed that theory. A new theory, partly based on the old concept but incorporating more recent developments from epidemiology and classical and molecular genetics, was developed. First articulated and given mathematical form by Moolgavkar and Knudson (1981), and independently in different form soon thereafter by Greenfield et al. (1984), this theory accords cell division a central role in the development of cancer.

This new theory can be summarized by four statements:

- Cancer begins when a cell suffers two critical irreversible genetic changes (mutations).
- Mutations occur when DNA lesions remain unrepaired at mitosis.
- A substantial background flux of DNA damage results from cosmic rays, oxidation, natural mutagens in food, and irreducible errors of DNA transcription.
- Once formed, a cancer cell can undergo further mutations and phenotypic changes that confer survival advantages on the daughter clone.

This theory provides a framework for relating a remarkable variety of observations (Moolgavkar, 1986; Knudson, 1987; Thorslund et al., 1987; Wilson, in press). In particular, it explains: (1) why a substantial number of "carcinogens" are not "electrophiles" and do not induce mutations and why the predictability of carcinogenic activity by mutagenic tests is poor; (2) why "nongenotoxic" "promoters" nevertheless increase the tumor yield (a small amount) when tested in the absence of "initiators;" (3) why powerful mutagenic carcinogens [e.g., dimethylbenzanthracene, (DMBA)] can induce tumors with a single exposure, even though rapidly detoxified and cleared from the body; (4) why chronic wounding or irritation (e.g., of the urinary bladder epithelium) leads to cancer; and (5) why relatively few rat liver "enyzme-altered foci" or skin or colon polyps become cancerous. None of these observations is really comprehensible in terms of the Armitage-Doll framework, even as it had evolved by the early 1970s.

In addition, in their 1981 paper, Moolgavkar and Knudson predicted that following an "initiation-promotion" protocol with a second "initiation" step (giving the so-called I-P-I protocol) would greatly increase the number of tumors and shorten the time to their appearance. [Potter, also in 1981, made the same prediction on somewhat different but compatible grounds; it was verified a short time later (Hennings et al., 1983)]. Cohen and Ellwein predicted that simultaneous dosing of an initiator and a mitogenic agent would increase tumor yield, as would wounding and subsequent or simultaneous treatment with a mitogen; they quantitatively verified those predictions in the rat bladder (Ellwein and Cohen, in press).

In the context of this theory, the terms "initiation" and "promotion" evolve somewhat from their phenomenological definitions. "Initiation" refers to the transformation of a normal cell to a mutant-"initiated" cell, one that has suffered one of the two critical irreversible genetic changes, and "promotion" refers to an increase in the net birth rate of initiated cells, causing "clonal expansion." Initiation is rare, occurring naturally at the background mutation frequency of about 10^{-6} per genetic locus per mitotic event. The probability that initiation will occur is increased by treatment with radiation or chemical mutagens. The second critical mutation also can occur naturally or be increased by treatment.

IMPLICATIONS

1. Low-exposure hazard is proportional to cumulative exposure only for genotoxic agents in treatment regimes in which no mitotic rate increase occurs. Thus, the linear multistage (LMS) procedure is not generally valid. In the approximate formula for age-specific incidence given by Moolgavkar (Moolgavkar and Venzon, 1979; Moolgavkar and Knudson, 1981; Moolgavkar, 1986), the probabilities of mutation appear as multipliers of the mitotic events integrated over duration of exposure. Holding that factor constant and assuming that the added probability of either mutation (or both) is directly proportional to dose yields an equation identical to Crump's, if the number of "stages" (in Crump's terms) is kept to two. That is, the tumor incidence (at low incidence) has approximately a linear-quadratic dose dependence. At very low exposures, the linear term will dominate.

However, if treatment increases the mitotic rate of either normal or initiated cells (or both), that identity disappears. [It also disappears at high incidence, but the Crump approximation is not then valid anyway (Moolgavkar, 1986)]. Now the duration of exposure becomes very important, because the mutagenic and mitogenic stimuli act synergistically, causing the apparent dose response to rise dramatically (Ellwein and Cohen, in press). This effect can also be seen as a dependence of incidence on dose rate, which Littlefield and Gaylor (1986) observed in the bladder cancers from the ED01 study. Thus, the LMS procedure is valid only under a very limited set of conditions that are seldom found. We know of three verified examples: 2-AAF in the mouse liver (Littlefield and Gaylor, 1985), "FANFT" in the rat bladder (Hasegawa et al., 1986), and benzo[a]pyrene in the rat forestomach (Zeise and Crouch, 1985).

2. Because nongenotoxic carcinogens act by increasing the mitotic rate of cells in the target organ, this increase should be used as the basis for hazard assessment.

Mitotic rate can be affected by many mechanisms, probably more than we now know. Nevertheless, the activity leading to increased tumor yield is in the cell dynamics. Thus, the dose response for increasing mitotic rate should be the basis for hazard assessment.

It may be neither appropriate nor possible to estimate risk from exposure to nongenotoxic carcinogens. Ellwein and Cohen (in press) have shown that the incidence depends on both dose and duration of exposure, and that incidence is not simply proportional to duration. Because continuous, uniform exposure over a lifetime almost never occurs, the actual exposure needs to be known for risk to be estimated. However, Ellwein and Cohen have also shown, at least for the substance they studied, that the dose-response curve rises very rapidly. This suggests that a "negligible risk" level of exposure can be defined, but more work is needed.

3. The conventional lifetime bioassay does not yield information adequate for dose-response assessment. Protocols should be modified to identify effects of mitotic rate increase.

At present, lifetime bioassays are almost never begun until the substance has been tested for genotoxic activity, yet the results from those experiments are not taken into account in the design of the lifetime test. Risk assessors need to know something about carcinogenicity in the absence of mitogenicity to properly assess low-exposure risk. Thus, bioassays conducted on genotoxins should include extra animals for periodic mitotic rate elevation measurements. Adding a low-dose group, perhaps at MTD/20, might give an indication of genotoxic hazard.

For compounds not testing "positive" in genotoxic assays, a different situation obtains. It is not clear now what information is really needed. Are powerful promoters, such as phorbol esters, the main concern? This, too, needs to be investigated.

4. Activation of *ras* and other oncogenes may or may not be a critical step toward cancer. This field needs to develop further before implications for risk assessment can be drawn.

In retinoblastoma and, perhaps, other tumors, deactivation of both copies of the critical *rb* gene is required for the tumor to begin (Friend et al., 1986; Kimchi et al., 1988). It is tempting to speculate that this double deactivation provides the link between molecular genetics—with its plethora of oncogenes and anti-oncogenes—and epidemiology and classical cancer genetics, whence comes the evidence that just two critical mutations are the critical path between normal cells and cancer. This part of molecular biology is exploding now; by the time this is published, the answer may be known (or perhaps not). In either case, those of us involved in risk assessment will wait impatiently until we can put the molecular genetic information to profitable use.

REFERENCES

Armitage, P and R Doll. 1954. The age distribution of cancer and a multi-stage theory of carcinogenesis. Br J Cancer 8:1-12.

Crump, KS, HA Guess, and KL Deal. 1977. Confidence intervals and test of hypotheses concerning dose response relations inferred from animal carcinogenicity data. Biometrics 33:437-451.

Ellwein, LB and SM Cohen. 1988. A cellular dynamics model of experimental bladder cancer: Analysis of the effect of sodium saccharin in the rat. Risk Anal 8:215-221.

Ellwein, LB and SM Cohen. Comparative analyses of the timing and magnitude of genotoxic and nongenotoxic cellular effects in urinary bladder carcinogenesis. In: *Biologically Based Models for Cancer Risk Assessment*, CC Travis (ed.). Pergamon Press, New York (in press).

Friend, SH, R Bernards, S Rogelj, RA Weinberg, JA Rapaport, DM Albert, and TP Dryja. 1986. A human DNA segment with properties of the gene that predisposes to retinoblastoma and osteosarcoma. Nature 323:643-646.

Greenfield, RE, LB Ellwein, and SM Cohen. 1984. A general probabilistic model of carcinogenesis: Analysis of experimental bladder cancer. Carcinogenesis 5:437-445.

Guess, HA and KS Crump. 1977. Best-estimate low-dose extrapolation of carcinogenicity data. Environ Health Perspect 22:149-152.

Hasegawa, R, SM Cohen, M St. John, M Cano, and LB Ellwein. 1986. Effect of dose on the induction of urothelial proliferation by N-[4-(5-nitro-2-furyl)-2-thiazolyl] formamide and its relationship to bladder carcinogenesis in the rat. Carcinogenesis 7:633-636.

Hennings, H, R Shores, ML Wenk, EF Spangler, R Tarone, and SH Yuspa. 1983. Malignant conversion of mouse skin tumours is increased by tumour initiators and unaffected by tumour promoters. Nature 304:67-69.

Kimchi, A, XF Wang, RA Weinberg, S Chiefetz, and J Massague. 1988. Absence of TGF-beta receptors and growth inhibitory responses in retinoblastoma cells. Science 240:196-199.

Knudson, AG. 1987. A two-mutation model for human cancer. Adv Viral Oncol 7:1-17.

Littlefield, NA and DJ Gaylor. 1985. Influence of total dose and dose rate carcinogenicity studies. J Toxicol Environ Health 15:545-550.

Miller, JA and EC Miller. 1977. Ultimate chemical carcinogens as reactive mutagenic electrophiles, pp. 605-627. In: Origins of Human Cancer, HH Hiatt, JD Watson, and JA Winstein (eds.). Cold Spring Harbor Laboratory, Cold Spring Harbor, New York.

Moolgavkar, SH. 1977. The multistage theory of carcinogenesis (letter). Int J Cancer 19:730.

Moolgavkar, SH. 1986. Carcinogenesis modeling: From molecular biology to epidemiology. Annu Rev Public Health 7:151-169.

Moolgavkar, SH and AG Knudson. 1981. Mutation and cancer: A model for human cancer. J Natl Cancer Inst 66:1037-1052.

Moolgavkar, SH and DJ Venzon. 1979. Two-event models for carcinogenesis: Incidence curves for childhood and adult tumors. Math Biosci 47:55-77.

Potter, VR. 1981. A new protocol and its rationale for the study of initiation and promotion of carcinogenesis in rat liver. Carcinogenesis 2:1375-1379.

Thorslund, TW, CC Brown, and G Charnley. 1987. Biologically motivated cancer risk models. Risk Anal 7:109-119.

Wilson, JD. Assessment of low-exposure risk from carcinogens: Implications of the Knudson-Moolgavkar two-critical mutation theory. In: Biologically Based Models for Risk Assessment, CC Travis (ed.). Pergamon Press, New York (in press).

Zeise, L and EAC Crouch. 1985. Experimental variation in the carcinogenic potency of benzo[a]pyrene. Unpublished manuscript. Energy and Environmental Policy Center, Harvard University, Cambridge, MA.

QUESTIONS AND COMMENTS

C: F. T. Cross, PNL, Richland, WA

Data from approximately 1800 rats previously exposed to radon, radon daughters, and uranium or dust were recently analyzed by Suresh Moolgavkar of the Fred Hutchinson Cancer Research Center, Seattle, WA, for parameters in the two-mutation recessive oncogenesis model. Preliminary main conclusions reached are that radon and daughters strongly affect the first mutation rate, have a significant effect on the kinetics of intermediate cells (dust exposure-mediated?), and have a lesser effect on the second mutation rate.

A MATHEMATICAL DOSE-RESPONSE MODEL: A STOCHASTIC APPROACH TO CELL SURVIVAL

C. Rossi

Dipartimento di Matematica, II Università di Roma, Via Orazio Raimondo, 00173 Rome, Italy

Key words: *Cell survival curves, dose-analysis response*

ABSTRACT ONLY

The study of cell survival curves is an important tool for quantifying the effects of radiotherapy, chemotherapy, or both, and to optimize protocols used in tumor disease therapy.

Several mathematical models have been proposed to obtain suitable parameters for dose-response analysis. In this paper we propose, on the basis of genetic considerations, a comprehensive model to describe cell-survival curves (e.g., from exposure to ionizing radiation, chemotherapeutic agents, etc.) by parameters related to dose.

Some years ago a model was proposed by de Finetti and Rossi to deal with the onset of degenerative diseases as the final event of a genetic decay process. The genetic basis of the model was suggested by articles that appeared in the literature. Analogous considerations that can be applied to the dose-response problem form the basis of our model.

The basic parameters of the mathematical model are the redundance parameter (multitarget model); the repair parameter, the probability that damage in a cell can be repaired; and the environmental parameter, which takes into account the effects of the therapy as a function of dose. For simplicity, a model with a repair parameter = 1 will be considered in depth, but the general expression for the survival function will also be derived and reported. The estimation problems related to the model will then be handled by the maximum likelihood estimation approach.

Data collected by the Istituto Tumori "Regina Elena," of Rome, are analyzed, using the proposed model. Results will be reported in tabular and graphic forms.

In addition, two other models (the multitarget, single-hit model and the linear-quadratic model) that have been widely reported in the literature are considered, using the same set of data, with the aim of making some comparisons.

Detection of DNA Adducts
and Other Measures of Primary Cell Damage

MAPPING UV PHOTOPRODUCTS IN NUCLEOSOME DNA

M. J. Smerdon, J. M. Gale, and K. A. Nissen

Biochemistry/Biophysics Program, Washington State University, Pullman, WA 99164-4660

Key words: *Ultraviolet, chromatin, T4 polymerase*

ABSTRACT

The strong absorption of ultraviolet (UV) light near 260 nm by DNA bases leads to a number of stable photoproducts in the DNA molecule. The major lesion produced is the *cis-syn* cyclobutane pyrimidine dimer (PD). These photoproducts are classic examples of mutagenic and carcinogenic DNA lesions. The next most prevalent photoproduct, which occurs, on average, at ∼10% the frequency of PD, is the pyrimidine-pyrimidone (6-4) adduct. These lesions have also been implicated in forming mutagenic "hot spots" in DNA.

We have mapped the distribution of these photoproducts at the single nucleotide level in nucleosome core DNA from UV-irradiated mononucleosomes, chromatin fibers, and human cells in culture, using the $3' \rightarrow 5'$ exonuclease activity of T4 DNA polymerase. This enzyme is quantitatively blocked at the $3'$ side of both types of photoproducts. The results show that the quantum yield of PD is strongly modulated with a 10.3 ($\pm$ 0.1) base periodicity throughout nucleosome core DNA. The maxima in this distribution map to positions where the DNA strand is farthest from the core histone surface. Furthermore, the individual intensities of this distribution are modulated in a unique and characteristic manner. This manner reflects core histone-DNA interactions and, possibly, local DNA structure, giving rise to a "photo-footprint" of core histone binding.

In marked contrast, the distribution of pyrimidine-pyrimidone (6-4) photoproducts is much more random throughout nucleosome core DNA. Thus, protein-DNA interactions in chromatin can modulate the formation of stable UV photoproducts in DNA, as well as having differential effects on the distribution of UV photoproducts. This work represents one approach to studying the effect of chromatin structure on DNA damage in human cells.

INTRODUCTION

The strong absorption of ultraviolet (UV) light near 260 nm by DNA bases leads to a number of stable photoproducts in the DNA molecule (Wang, 1976). The major lesion produced is the *cis-syn* cyclobutane pyrimidine dimer (PD). These photoproducts are classic examples of mutagenic and carcinogenic DNA lesions (Harm, 1980). The next most prevalent photoproduct, occurring at ~10% the frequency of PD on average, is the pyrimidine-pyrimidone (6-4) adduct. These lesions have also been implicated in forming mutagenic "hot spots" in DNA (Tang et al., 1986).

The "target" for UV photoproduct formation in intact cells is DNA folded into the compact structure of chromatin (for recent reviews on chromatin structure, see Pederson et al., 1986; Adolph, 1988). Thus, it is important to understand the influence of this packaging on the distribution of UV photoproducts in the genome, especially because the location of these lesions may be significant in determining their removal by repair enzymes (Leadon and Hanawalt, 1984; Lan and Smerdon, 1985; Bohr et al., 1985). Several studies have indicated that at both the total genome level (Cohn and Lieberman, 1984; Leadon and Hanawalt, 1984; Bohr et al., 1985) and the chromatin domain level (Leadon and Hanawalt, 1984; Bohr et al., 1985), PD form randomly, indicating that there is no significant bias between large domains of chromatin. Studies have also been performed at the nucleosome level of chromatin, focusing on the distribution of PD between nucleosome core DNA and linker DNA (Williams and Friedberg, 1979; Niggli and Cerutti, 1982). Once again, the results indicated that chromatin structure has little effect on the formation of PD in cellular DNA after irradiation with UV light.

We have recently developed a sensitive assay to measure the UV photoproduct yield *within* nucleosome core regions at the single nucleotide level (Gale et al., 1987). This assay uses the observations of Hazeltine and coworkers (Doetsch et al., 1985; Chan et al., 1985) that the $3' \rightarrow 5'$ exonuclease activity of T4 DNA polymerase is quantitatively blocked at the $3'$ side of both PD and pyrimidine-pyrimidone (6-4) dimers. Our results showed that the packaging of DNA by core histones dramatically influences the distribution of PD. This distribution shows a striking 10.3 ($\pm$ 0.1) base periodicity in which regions of enhanced PD formation map to positions along the DNA strands that are farthest from the core histone surface (Gale et al., 1987). A detailed analysis of this pattern demonstrates that certain characteristics correlate well with known structural features of isolated nucleosome core particles and indicates that these features are preserved in intact chromatin (Gale and Smerdon, 1988). Thus, the photochemistry of PD formation in DNA is influenced by the folding of DNA into the nucleosome unit.

One explanation for these results is that the binding of core histones to DNA physically restrains the formation of PD. Indeed, formation of PD requires a significant change in the orientation of adjacent pyrimidines from the normal B conformation and local deformation of the DNA helix (Pearlman et al., 1985; Husain et al., 1988). The binding of histones may therefore restrict movement in the DNA backbone, making PD formation in that region less favorable. This effect could be further enhanced by energy transfer in the DNA (Georghiou and Saim, 1986), after absorption of photons in more constrained locations, to less physically constrained regions (i.e., where the DNA backbone is farthest from the histone surface). Thus, regions where PD formation is less constrained may act as "energy sinks" for uniformly absorbed UV radiation.

More recently, we have measured the distribution of pyrimidine-pyrimidone (6-4) dimers by removing PD with *Escherichia coli* UV photolyase (Sancar and Sancar, 1988) before the T4 polymerase-exonuclease digestion step (J. M. Gale and M. J. Smerdon, in preparation). In marked contrast to the periodic distribution of PD, the distribution of pyrimidine-pyrimidone (6-4) photoproducts is much more random throughout nucleosome core DNA. This marked difference between the two different classes of stable UV photoproducts may reflect the difference in helix distortion required for formation of these adducts (Franklin et al., 1985; Pearlman et al., 1985). Thus, protein-DNA interactions in chromatin can modulate the formation of stable UV photoproducts in DNA, as well as have differential effects on different types of UV photoproducts.

ACKNOWLEDGMENTS

This work was supported by NIH grants ES02614 and ES03720, and by NIH Research Career Development Award ES00110 (MJS).

REFERENCES

Adolph, KW. 1988. *Chromosomes and Chromatin*, Vol. I. CRC Press, Boca Raton, FL.

Bohr, VA, CA Smith, DS Okumoto, and PC Hanawalt. 1985. DNA repair in an active gene: Removal of pyrimidine dimers from the DHFR gene of CHO cells is much more efficient than in the genome overall. Cell 40:359-369.

Chan, GL, PW Doetsch, and WA Hazeltine. 1985. Cyclobutane pyrimidine dimers and (6-4) photoproducts block polymerization by DNA polymerase. I. Biochemistry 24:5723-5728.

Cohn, SM, and MW Lieberman. 1984. The use of antibodies to 5-bromo-2'-deoxyuridine for the isolation of DNA sequences containing excision repair sites. J Biol Chem 259:12456-12462.

Doetsch, PW, GL Chan, and WA Hazeltine. **1985**. T4 DNA polymerase (3'-5') exonuclease, an enzyme for the detection and quantitation of stable DNA lesions: The ultraviolet light example. Nucleic Acids Res 13:3285-3304.

Franklin, WA, PW Doetsch, and WA Hazeltine. **1985**. Structural determination of the ultraviolet light-induced thymine-cytosine pyrimidine-pyrimidone (6-4) photoproduct. Nucleic Acids Res 13:5317-5325.

Gale, JM and MJ Smerdon. **1988**. UV photofootprint of nucleosome core DNA in intact chromatin having different structural states. J Mol Biol 204:949-958.

Gale, JM, KA Nissen, and MJ Smerdon. **1987**. UV-induced formation of pyrimidine dimers in nucleosome core DNA is strongly modulated with a period of 10.3 bases. Proc Natl Acad Sci USA 84:6644-6648.

Georghiou, S and AM Saim. **1986**. Excited state properties of DNA methylated at the N-7 position of guanine and its free fluorophore at room temperature. Photochem Photobiol 44:733-740.

Harm, W. **1980**. *Biological Effects of Ultraviolet Radiation*. Cambridge University Press, London.

Husain, I, J Griffith, and A Sancar. **1988**. Thymine dimers bend DNA. Proc Natl Acad Sci USA 85:2558-2562.

Lan, SY and MJ Smerdon. **1985**. A nonuniform distribution of excision repair synthesis in nucleosome DNA. Biochemistry 24:7771-7783.

Leadon, SA and PC Hanawalt. **1984**. Ultraviolet irradiation of monkey cells enhances the repair of DNA adducts in alpha DNA. Carcinogenesis 5:1505-1510.

Niggli, HJ and PA Cerutti. **1982**. Nucleosomal distribution of thymine photodimers following far- and near-ultraviolet irradiation. Biochem Biophys Res Commun 105:1215-1223.

Pearlman, DA, SR Holbrook, DH Pirkle, and SH Kim. **1985**. Molecular models for DNA damaged by photoreaction. Science 227:1304-1308.

Pederson, DA, F Thoma, and RT Simpson. **1986**. Core particle, fiber, and transcriptionally active chromatin structure. Annu Rev Cell Biol 2:117-147.

Sancar, A and GW Sancar. **1988**. DNA repair enzymes. Annu Rev Biochem 57:29-67.

Tang, M-S, J Hrncir, D Mitchell, J Ross, and J Clarkson. **1986**. The relative cytotoxicity and mutagenicity of cyclobutane pyrimidine dimers and <6-4> photoproducts in *Escherichia coli* cells. Mutat Res 161:9-17.

Wang, SY. **1976**. *Photochemistry and Photobiology of Nucleic Acids*. Academic Press, New York.

Williams, JI and EC Friedberg. **1979**. Deoxyribonucleic acid excision repair in chromatin after ultraviolet irradiation of human fibroblasts in culture. Biochemistry 18:3965-3972.

QUESTIONS AND COMMENTS

Q: Springer, PNL, Richland, WA
   When you digest with T4 polymerase (3'→5' exonuclease activity) is there variability, i.e., does the enzyme always stop next to the dimer?

A: We do not see variability. However, we do not know if the enzyme *always* terminates digestion immediately 3' to PD and (6-4) dimers, or whether it stops one or two bases 3' to these lesions in some fragments. This is why it is best to use restriction fragments that have been UV irradiated and digested with T4 polymerase as markers on gels.

FEMTOMOLE DETECTION OF PAH-ADDUCTED DNA BY ORGANIC SECONDARY ION MASS SPECTROMETRY

D. F. Barofsky, J. G. Pavlovich, and D. A. Griffin

Department of Agricultural Chemistry, Oregon State University, Corvallis, OR 97331

Key words: *PAH/DNA-adduct, organic SIMS, field-desorption mass spectrometry (FDMS), dosimetry*

ABSTRACT

Among the most promising procedures for monitoring human exposure to environmental polycyclic aromatic hydrocarbons (PAH) are protocols that employ mass spectrometry. The view that it is possible to use field desorption (FD) and organic secondary ionization to make quantitative mass spectrometric measurements of DNA adducts at levels found *in vivo* is supported by the fact that less-than-nanogram amounts of certain nonvolatile biological molecules have been detected by these two techniques (Desiderio et al., 1983; Wood, 1982).

We have just begun an investigation in which the general goal is to establish an experimental basis for developing mass spectrometric methods to detect and identify dosimetric indicators of human exposure to PAH. Our specific analytical objective is to evolve one or more methods capable of detecting ≤ 0.2 fmol (≤ 0.1 pg) of individual PAH-adducted nucleosides without unduly sacrificing the mass spectrometry's qualitative specificity. Our experimental program includes the following unique components: (1) a pulsed version of an FD ion source coupled to a time-of-flight (TOF) mass analyzer; (2) a liquid metal ion (LMI) column to produce finely focused primary beams for secondary ionization mass spectrometry (SIMS); (3) a small-diameter wire to serve as sample holder for SIMS and combined FD/SIMS; and (4) a combination of certain features of the FD and secondary ionization methods to enhance ionization efficiency and to control fragmentation of sample molecules.

It is generally acknowledged that FD mass spectrometry possesses a relatively high sensitivity for nucleosides. In general, the precision and accuracy of FD data compare well with those of more common ionization techniques such as electron impact or chemical ionization (Schulten and Lehmann, 1980). FD/TOF mass analysis of organic compounds would be novel and might mitigate or eliminate some of the major problems associated with the analysis of organic compounds by this form of mass spectrometry. For example, the high transmission of a TOF mass analyzer would greatly increase the efficiency of ion collection, and its nonscanning, integrating feature would reduce the effects of pronounced fluctuations in FD ion currents.

Our conviction that it might be possible to detect subpicogram quantities of PAH-adducted nucleosides with some specialized form of SIMS is based on the facility with which particle-induced desorption mass spectra are produced from many compounds of this sort (Mitchum et al., 1985; Dino et al., 1985), on the high sensitivity (∿femtomole) that has been demonstrated for other compounds (Day et al., 1980; Chait and Field, 1984), and on our pioneering use of focusing LMI columns as primary sources for SIMS of organic molecules (Barofsky et al., 1982, 1983a,b). LMI columns produce intense, finely focused beams of a wide variety of metal ions. Using an LMI column and a wire as the sample probe, it is possible to analyze small sample amounts in the liquid-assisted form of organic SIMS. For example, we have employed this technique to produce fully resolved molecular ion profiles with good signal-to-noise ratios from 10 to 50 pmol of oligopeptides, oligonucleotides, and oligosaccharides weighing between 2000 and 4000 daltons (Barofsky et al., unpublished data) and from 0.5 to 10 pmol of oligopeptides and oligosaccharides weighing less than 1000 daltons (Jiang et al., 1988). With respect to this study, we have already succeeded in recording a full spectrum of less than 20 pmol of a synthesized PAH-guanosine adduct (Pavlovich et al., unpublished data). In addition to having a favorable geometry for use in conjunction with a liquid metal primary ion source, small-diameter wire sample holders permit investigation of the effects of heating and electric-field strength on secondary ionization and fragmentation of sample molecules, facilitate loading of exceedingly small samples, and might facilitate an interface to microbore liquid chromatography.

Wire sample holders can also be used to reduce sample waste in the TOF mode of SIMS. For example, a 1-nl droplet of a 1-fmol/μl solution (a reasonable concentration for a substance eluting from a microbore liquid chromatography column) deposited on a 30-μm length of a 10-μm-diameter wire ($\sim 10^{-5}$ cm^2) would provide a detectable surface coverage of about 0.001 monolayer. Additionally, the geometry of a wire is naturally compatible with the operation of the pulsed secondary ionization necessary for TOF mass analysis. For a given sweep rate of the primary beam, the wire itself (instead of a slit) would serve to define the starting interval for the secondary ions. This could lead to faster sweep rates and, consequently, improved mass resolution.

As a rule, little fragmentation of sample molecules results from either FD or secondary ionization processes, and there is a consequent shortage of qualitative information in mass spectra produced by these methods. Auxiliary methods, such as chemical degradation or tandem mass spectrometry, have been employed to induce fragmentation at will, but these techniques are not practical for the exceedingly small amounts of sample that will be used in this study. Our approach to this problem, which has not been previously investigated, will be to combine certain features of the FD and secondary ionization methods and create a field-enhanced secondary ionization process. It is possible that the small desorption energy for ionic emission from field-induced surface states can be supplied by bombardment with fast ions. We think that a field-promoted secondary ionization process could have greater sensitivity than that available from either FD or secondary ionization individually. The ion signal from a given amount of sample might be stronger than in the case of pure FD because it would be generated by controlled ionic bombardment rather than resulting from an uncontrolled spontaneous process. The ionic yield might be greater than in the case of pure secondary ionization, either the static or liquid-assisted variety, because a larger number of molecules would be predisposed to desorb as ions and because the desorption zones around individual impact points would be broadened because of the reduction in desorption energy.

In normal FD, ion emission occurs at a lower temperature than does thermal cracking of the sample; hence, very little evidence of thermal degradation is observed in FD mass spectra. If, however, a polar sample were heated in the absence of a high electric field, the sample's temperature can be increased to the point of cracking. By subsequently lowering the temperature and returning to the conditions for either secondary ionization or field-promoted secondary ionization, it should be possible to cause emission of the thermal fragment ions. If we observe this phenomenon, we can use it to induce fragmentation of sample molecules at will and thus to exercise some degree of control over the structural information contained in mass spectra.

Our study certainly has innovative and, therefore, speculative components. We believe, however, that the likelihood is good that this investigation will lead to femtomole detection of PAH-adducted DNA by organic secondary ion mass spectrometry and, consequently, to procedures for monitoring human exposure to environmental PAH.

REFERENCES

Barofsky, DF, U Giessmann, LW Swanson, and AE Bell. 1982. Use of a liquid metal point source for secondary ion mass spectrometry of organic compounds, pp. 425-432. In: *Proceedings of the 29th International Field Emission Symposium*, H-O Andrén and H Nordén (eds.). Almqvist & Wiksell, Stockholm.

Barofsky, D, U Giessmann, LW Swanson, and AE Bell. 1983a. Molecular SIMS with a liquid metal field ion point source. J Mass Spectrom Ion Phys 46:495-497.

Barofsky, DF, U Giessmann, AE Bell, and LW Swanson. 1983b. Molecular secondary ion mass spectrometry with a liquid metal ion primary source. Anal Chem 55:1318-1323.

Chait, BT and FH Field. 1984. A highly sensitive pulsed ion bombardment time-of-flight mass spectrometer, pp. 237-238. In: *32nd Annual Conference on Mass Spectrometry and Allied Topics*, American Society for Mass Spectrometry, San Antonio, TX.

Day, RJ, SE Unger, and RG Cooks. 1980. Molecular secondary ion mass spectrometry. Anal Chem 52:557A-572A.

Desiderio, DM, I Katakuse, and M Kai. 1983. Measurement of leucine enkephalin in caudate nucleus tissue with fast atom bombardment-collision activated dissociation-linked field scanning mass spectrometry. Biomed Mass Spectrom 10:426-429.

Dino, JJ, GD Marbury, and RK Boyd. 1985. Tandem mass spectrometry of oligonucleotides and in vitro adducts of benzo[a]pyrene diol-epoxide with nucleosides, p. 518. In: *33rd Annual Conference on Mass Spectrometry and Allied Topics*, American Society for Mass Spectrometry, San Diego, CA.

Jiang, LF, E Barofsky, and DF Barofsky. 1988. Liquid assisted SIMS with a liquid metal ion microprobe, pp. 683-686. In: *Secondary Ion Mass Spectrometry*, A Benninghoven, AM Huber, HW Werner (eds.). Wiley, New York, NY.

Mitchum, RK, JP Freeman, FA Beland, and FF Kadlubar. 1985. Mass spectrometric identification of DNA adducts formed by carcinogenic aromatic amines, pp. 547-580. In: *Mass Spectrometry in the Health and Life Sciences*. AL Burlingame, N Castagnoli, Jr. (eds). Elsevier, Amsterdam.

Schulten, HR and WD Lehmann. 1980. Field desorption mass spectrometry. Trends Biochem Sci 5:142-146.

Wood, GW. 1982. Field desorption mass spectrometry: Applications. Mass Spectrom Rev 1:63-102.

QUESTIONS AND COMMENTS

Q: Smerdon, Washington State University, Pullman, WA
    What is the level of detection you would predict for glycosylation of proteins using this method?

A: Barofsky

No SIMS or FD mass spectrum has been produced from an intact glycoprotein to date. Glycoasparagines are amenable to fast atom or fast ion bombardment but not at the same sensitivity as nucleosides. I think glycoasparagines might be analyzed at picomole levels using our method.

ANALYSIS OF CLASSICAL AND NONCLASSICAL ADDUCTS*

R. M. Bean, B. L. Thomas, D. A. Dankovic, D. B. Mann, G. A. Ross, and D. L. Springer

Pacific Northwest Laboratory, P.O. Box 999, Richland, WA 99352

Key words: *DNA adducts, GC/MS, carcinogenesis, PAH, BaP, fluorescence*

ABSTRACT

Metabolites of cancer-causing organic compounds are known to form covalent bonds with cellular DNA. The formation of these DNA adducts is currently thought to be a critical step in the chain of events leading to carcinogenic response. Because many DNA adducts remain intact for relatively long periods of time, analysis of DNA for the adducts can serve as an integrated dosimetric measurement of recent environmental exposure to carcinogens.

The structure of adducts formed from polycyclic aromatic hydrocarbon metabolites has received much study, and the principal structures have been characterized for many carcinogenic compounds. However, when adducts are formed from radiolabeled hydrocarbons and DNA, both *in vitro* and *in vivo*, not all the radiolabel incorporated into the DNA can be accounted for. While the role of these so-called "nonclassical" adducts in carcinogenesis is not known, the characterization of these adduct species would add significantly to understanding adduct formation processes.

We have been studying methods of direct analysis of adducts, using a variety of isolation, separation, and detection techniques. Several analytical approaches are discussed, including derivatization gas chromatography/selected ion monitored mass spectrometry, liquid chromatography, and capillary electrophoresis. The potential for specific detection by laser fluorescence, chemiluminescence, and electrospray mass spectrometry is discussed.

In addition, we discuss some of the newly developed analytical methods that have been applied to a study of the nonclassical fraction of DNA adducted with benzo[a]pyrene. Release of quinones from the nonclassical fraction by acid hydrolysis has provided evidence that at least some of the material is formed through a mechanism other than the well-accepted diolepoxide route. The nature of the quinone precursor is under investigation.

*This work was supported by the U.S. DOE under Contract No. DE-AC06-76RLO 1830.

INTRODUCTION

Metabolites of carcinogenic organic compounds can bond with deoxyribonucleic acid (DNA) to form DNA adducts. These species are retained for relatively long periods of time in the body and are thought to be associated with the formation of cancer. Analysis of DNA for adducts may therefore provide an estimate of individual exposure to carcinogens. Methods currently being used for analysis of DNA adducts have been reviewed by Wogan and Gorelick (1985). In general, the currently available methods suffer from either a lack of sufficient sensitivity for environmental screening or from a lack of qualitative specificity. Although data on humans are sparse, allowing for initial rapid decay after environmental exposure, we may expect adduct levels of 0.1-0.01 ng per milligram of DNA. Research at Pacific Northwest Laboratory (PNL) is directed toward developing methods for the analysis of DNA adducts that will permit identification and quantitation of adducted polycyclic aromatic hydrocarbon (PAH) metabolites at environmental levels. Included within this objective are the preparation and characterization of DNA adducts to be used as analytical standards.

Several approaches to the analysis of DNA adducts are being undertaken. A primary analytical approach is to isolate the bound metabolites by cleaving the covalent bonds that attach them to the purine or pyrimidine bases of DNA, then to treat the isolated metabolites with reagents that will increase their separability and their sensitivity to gas chromatography/mass spectrometry (GC/MS) detection. However, analysis of the metabolites while still bound to the nucleic acid base (as adducted nucleosides or nucleotides) would provide more specific information about the nature of the adduction process and its relation to carcinogenesis. Thus, separation and detection methods that do not require cleavage of the metabolite from the DNA bases are also being explored. These methods involve liquid chromatography and capillary electrophoresis, using fluorescence, chemiluminescence, or electrospray MS detection.

PREPARATION OF ANALYTICAL STANDARDS

One limitation inherent in the direct analysis of adducts has been the lack of analytical standards. In initial experiments, we prepared nucleotide adducts of benzo[a]pyrene (BaP) in nanogram quantities with calf thymus DNA, using microsomal preparations to allow the adduction process. The microsomal method produced experimental artifacts and did not produce adducts in the microgram quantities required for analytical study. A method using intact rat hepatocytes, developed in our Biology and Chemistry Department, appears to be satisfactory for obtaining the required quantities of various PAH adducts (Dankovic et al., 1989). The products from this *in vitro* method seem to approximate very closely the adduct distributions found from *in vivo* studies of adducts. Thus, for the first time, research quantities of many different adducts can be prepared from adducting hydrocarbons and pure DNA. To date, about 5 µg adducted BaP, 1.5 µg adducted fluoranthene, 200 ng dibenz[a,h]anthracene, and 110 ng 7,12-dimethylbenz[a]anthracene have been made available for study. Using the hepatocyte system, the rate of metabolism of each hydrocarbon is different; hence, the incubation conditions require preliminary experiments before microgram-scale experiments can be successfully conducted.

GC/MS OF DERIVATIZED METABOLITES

On treatment with hydrochloric acid, the adducting moiety from PAH adducts is liberated as a tetrahydrotetrahydroxy compound (tetrol) that is subject to derivatization by a number of agents before analysis by GC/MS. BaP tetrol forms a tetramethyl ether as well as a tetraacetate that is detectable by selected ion monitoring (SIM) MS at the picogram level (Bean et al., 1987). A principal research problem is to prepare these derivatives reliably, in good yield, and at the concentrations required, with background noise sufficiently low for unambiguous identification. Although we have extended the sensitivity of the permethylation method to 10 pg of tetrol (Bean et al., 1987), we have not yet been able to do so reliably and without unacceptable accompanying chemical noise. During a study of the mass spectral properties of derivatives of BaP metabolites (Chess et al., 1988), we found that the methyl ether derivatives of several PAH tetrols produced a unique spectrum resulting from a reverse Diels-Alder (RDA) cleavage. This cleavage is not observed with PAH acetate or with trifluoroacetate derivatives, which fragment by other mechanisms. We have found that the trimethylsilyl derivative of BaP tetrol also undergoes the RDA cleavage to yield a fragment ion of 404 atomic mass units (amu) that has very little interference in the single-ion chromatogram. The derivative is more readily and reliably prepared than the corresponding methyl ethers, and unoptimized detection levels are approaching the 1-pg level.

DETECTION OF INTACT ADDUCT BY CHEMILUMINESCENCE

Chemiluminescence is a powerful and specific detection method that has been recently applied to the analysis of a number of PAH compounds

(Sigvardson and Birks, 1983). Amino-PAH compounds are particularly sensitive to this detection technique, with detection limits one to two orders of magnitude lower than fluorescence detection (Sigvardson et al., 1984). The structures of DNA adducts formed from PAH compounds comprise both a fluorescent hydrocarbon moiety and an aromatic amine linkage. Thus, preliminary studies were conducted to determine if these compounds are amenable to specific detection by chemiluminescence. The chemiluminescence response we are investigating depends on electronic excitation of the analyte by the reaction between an aryl oxalate and hydrogen peroxide. A variety of oxalates can be used for the reaction, each giving different light intensities and durations that are pH dependent.

Although in principle the reaction is simple, from a practical standpoint the process is more difficult because of the need for compatibility between separation column eluent and postcolumn reagents and solvents, the mechanical arrangements for reagent metering, and the short elapsed time required between postcolumn mixing and detection. For these experiments, bis-(2,4,6-trichlorophenyl) oxalate was used with hydrogen peroxide to initiate chemiluminescence response from a synthetic BaP-guanosine adduct and the response was compared with fluorescence detection. The results of these preliminary experiments, conducted without a separation column, indicate that the adduct does exhibit a strong chemiluminescence response that is comparable in intensity with fluorescence under the conditions used. It is very likely that the chemiluminescence response can be increased substantially by increasing oxalate concentration, choosing a more responsive oxalate, and optimizing solvent, pH, and postcolumn mixing conditions. Further chemiluminescence studies are planned.

SEPARATION OF ADDUCTS BY CAPILLARY ZONE ELECTROPHORESIS

Electrophoretic separation of high molecular weight compounds in silica capillaries filled with buffer solutions has several advantages that lend themselves well to the analysis of adducts. Separation of adducts by capillary zone electrophoresis (CZE) separation efficiencies can be high for molecules with higher molecular weights, because mobility depends mainly on charge. Further, electroosmotic flow is relatively frictionless, resulting in essentially "plug" flow for the separated analyte. PAH-adducted nucleotides and nucleosides are sufficiently polar to give good electrophoretic mobility with excellent separation efficiency. Good separations can also be obtained at both high and low pH. In our studies, detection was by laser fluorescence; although detection wavelength was not optimized, it appears that about 100 attomoles (amol) can be detected under the conditions used. We have found that the use of a mixed solvent/buffer system as the mobile phase is critical to good performance. If water alone is used, several peaks appear, presumably because of hydrolysis under the strongly acid or basic conditions of the separation. A principal problem with CZE is the small sample capacity. The column must be very small in diameter to avoid overheating; thus, only about 10 nl of sample can be applied to the column, giving an overall detection level of 10 pg/ml using fluorescence detection.

The next step in this technology is to interface the CZE system with a mass spectrometer. Normal mass spectrometric analysis is not sensitive enough to detect femtogram quantities of analyte. An electrospray interface, pioneered at PNL (Olivares et al., 1987), can detect femtogram quantities of certain polypeptide analytes. Research is being conducted to interface CZE with a new triple-quadrupole atmospheric-inlet mass spectrometer recently acquired for this and other biochemical studies. Another refinement of the CZE approach to adduct analysis will be an investigation of the CZE and mass spectrometric properties of the BaP-nucleotide adduct (containing a phosphate moiety).

INVESTIGATION OF NONCLASSICAL DNA ADDUCTS

We are trying to identify forms of hydrocarbon adducts that do not exhibit the behavior of "classical" adducts formed through normal diolepoxide addition to DNA bases. A number of researchers, for example, Shen et al. (1980) and Ashurst and Cohen (1982), have reported that when radiolabeled BaP adducts are isolated by the conventional method, one-third to one-half of the radiolabeled nucleoside material is not recovered as the classical adduct. We have examined this "nonclassical" adduct material by treating it with 0.12 N HCl to release it from the residual DNA structure. This process was followed by solid reverse-phase adsorption of the hydrolyzed product.

Reverse-phase chromatography of this material revealed that, in addition to tetrols, 10%-33% of the nonclassical material had retention times consistent with BaP-3,6-quinone and BaP-6,12-quinone. We have confirmed the presence of these quinones with mass spectrometry. Quinones are not found in the nonclassical fraction unless the acid hydrolysis step is performed, leading us to believe that the appearance of quinones after acid treatment results from cleavage of covalent bonds to the DNA structure. Formation of nonclassical structures may be a consequence of a competing adduct-formation mechanism, as suggested by Cavielieri and Rogan (1985). The project will continue to confirm these results and to investigate the nature of the quinone-precursor structure.

ACKNOWLEDGMENT

Work was supported by the U. S. Department of Energy, Office of Health and Environmental Research, under Contract DE-AC06-76RLO 1830.

REFERENCES

Ashurst, SW and GM Cohen. 1982. The formation of benzo[a]pyrene-dioxyribonu-cleoside adducts in vivo and in vitro. Carcinogenesis 3:267-273.

Bean, RM, EK Chess, BL Thomas, DL Springer, DB Mann, and DJ Hendren. 1987. Abstracts, Eleventh International Symposium on Polynuclear Aromatic Hydrocar-bons, Gaithersburg, MD, September 23-25, 1987. (Available from National Insti-tute of Standards and Technology, Gaithersburg, MD).

Cavielieri, EL and EG Rogan. 1985. Polycyclic Hydrocarbons and Carcinogenesis, pp. 289-305. ACS Symposium Series 283, RG Harvey (ed.). American Chemical Society, Washington, DC.

Chess, EK, BL Thomas, DJ Hendren, and RM Bean. 1988. Biomed Environ Mass Spectrom 15:485-493.

Dankovic, DA, DL Springer, DB Mann, BL Thomas, LG Smith, and RM Bean. 1989. Preparation of microgram quantities of BaP-DNA adducts using isolated rat hepatocytes in vitro. Carcinogenesis 10:789-791.

Olivares, JA, NT Nguyen, CR Yonker, and RD Smith. 1987. On-line mass spectro-metric detection for capillary zone electrophoresis. Anal Chem 59:1230-1232.

Shen, AL, WE Fahl, and CR Jefcoate. 1980. Metabolism of benzo[a]pyrene by isolated hepatocytes and factors affecting covalent binding of benzo[a]pyrene metabolites to DNA in hepatocyte and microsomal systems. Arch Biochem Biophys 204:511-523.

Sigvardson, KW and JW Birks. 1983. Peroxylate chemiluminescence detection of polycyclic aromatic hydrocarbons in liquid chromatography. Anal Chem 55:432-435.

Sigvardson, KW, JM Kennish, and JW Birks. 1984. Peroxylate chemiluminescence detection of polycyclic aromatic amines in liquid chromatography. Anal Chem 56:1096-1102.

Wogan, GN and NJ Gorelick. 1985. Chemical and biochemical dosimetry to genotoxic chemicals. Environ Health Perspect 62:5-18.

MAPPING OF BaP ADDUCTS TO THE 5S rRNA GENE CARRIED ON A PLASMID TARGET

D. B. Mann, G. L. Stiegler, and D. L. Springer

Biology and Chemistry Department, Pacific Northwest Laboratory, P.O. Box 999, Richland, WA 99352

Key words: *BaP adducts, 5S rRNA gene, adduct mapping*

ABSTRACT

Even though formation of adducts to DNA is believed to be the initial event in tumor development following exposure to polycyclic aromatic hydrocarbons (PAH) and other carcinogens, the mechanism for DNA damage from these adducts has not been identified. It has been postulated that the controlling event in tumor initiation is the activation of oncogenes as a result of mutation or an error in control mechanisms. For several genes it has been shown that the activity or inactivity of the gene may be correlated with changes in its chromatin structure.

Because of this, we have been using simple *in vitro* systems to determine the influence of bulky adducts on chromatin structure. For this we prepared the pXP-14 plasmid containing the 5S rRNA gene and the SP-6 promoter. This plasmid was incubated with ($\pm$)r-7,t-8-dihydroxy-t-9,10-epoxy-7,8,9,10-tetrahydrobenzo[a]pyrene (*anti*-BPDE); we found that binding was linear with doses of 5 to 125 μM BPDE, with the highest concentration resulting in an average of one adduct per 500 bp.

Digestion of the plasmid with the restriction enzymes *Hin*fI/*Pst*I, *Sal*I/*Hin*fI, *Sal*I/*Eco*RI and *Eco*RI/*Sal*I resulted in isolation of double-stranded DNA fragments that contain the 5S rRNA gene and the SP-6 promoter region. The ^{32}P-5′-end-labeled, transcribed and nontranscribed strands of the fragment containing the 5S rRNA gene will be incubated with T4 polymerase, which has 3′-5′ exonuclease activity and digests the DNA until it reaches a base with a bulky adduct attached. Using this approach, we will locate adduction sites on the 5S rRNA gene and the promoter region. Results from this work will contribute to our understanding of the influence of bulky adducts on nucleosome positioning.

Although the initial event in the induction of tumors by chemical carcinogens is the formation of carcinogen-DNA adducts, the mechanism by which the cell then progresses into a tumor is not yet known. Investigation of this progression must begin with an understanding of how individual genes are turned on and off. One indicator of the activity or inactivity of genes appears to be the structural formation of the gene's chromatin. Transcriptionally active genes have been shown to have a more open chromatin structure than those that are inactive. At a very basic level, this structure is controlled by the positioning of the nucleosomes and other control proteins within a gene. The induction of one such system was shown to be accompanied by the loss or alteration of a single nucleosome (Richard-Foy and Hager, 1987). It has been shown for the β-major globin gene that the nucleosomes are in a phased array on specific sites in L cells in which the gene is inactive; however, in Friend cells in which the gene is expressed, there is a 300-base-pair (bp) nucleosome free region at the 5' end of the gene (Benezra et al., 1986). Although this mechanism needs further evaluation, these results suggest that the positioning of certain nucleosomes is critical to gene expression.

The positions of the nucleosomes within a gene are determined to a large extent by the sequence-specific nature of the DNA binding. It has been shown that certain sequences have preferred orientations with respect to the core histones, and other sequences, most notably long nonalternating sequences of poly[(dA)-(dT)] or poly[(dG)-(dC)], as well as Z DNA, tend to be excluded from the nucleosome (Drew and Calladine, 1987; Garner and Felsenfeld, 1987). The left-handed Z DNA, which is substantially stiffer than the right-handed B DNA, has a more irregular zigzag pattern to the phosphodiester backbone in contrast to the smoother helical coil of the B DNA. This irregularity in the phosphodiester backbone presents a further hindrance to the interaction of DNA with the core histones. Chemical interactions with the DNA, such as the adduction of benzo[a]pyrene (BaP), have been shown to alter the equilibrium between the B and Z DNA forms. Chen (1985) demonstrated that BaP adduction causes a destabilization of the B DNA, favoring a transition to Z DNA at a point several base pairs from the adduct. This implies that the adduct, in addition to its direct effect, may also influence nucleosome positioning at some distance from the site of adduction.

Because of this, we are looking at the influence of bulky chemical adducts on the positioning of nucleosomes within a gene. We are using the pXP-14 plasmid (Figure 1), which is 3250 bp long and contains the 5S rRNA gene and the SP6 promoter. This model system is ideal for this type of study because the 5S rRNA gene, which is about 120 bp long, forms a single nucleosome located at a tightly fixed position along the DNA, with the midpoint of the nucleosome located at the beginning (5' end) of the transcribed gene. Thus, any alterations in the positioning of the nucleosome should be visible.

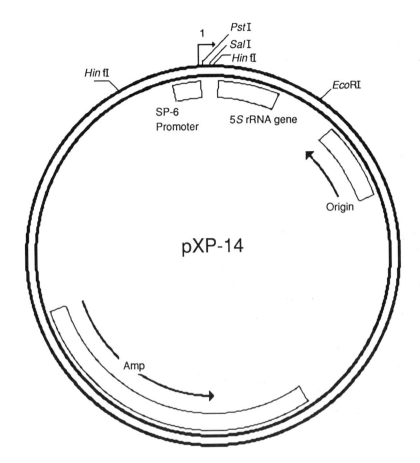

Figure 1. Map of plasmid pXP-14 shows locations of ampicillin-resistance gene, origin of replication, SP-6 promoter region, 5S rRNA gene, and cleavage sites of restriction enzymes used to isolate SP-6 promoter and 5S rRNA gene.

We have adducted the pXP-14 plasmid with (±)r-7,t-8-dihydroxy-t-9,10-epoxy-7,8,9,10-tetrahydrobenzo[a]pyrene [*anti*-BaP diol epoxide (BPDE)] at levels that result in an average of 6.7 adducts per plasmid. This corresponded to an adduction level of one BPDE per two copies of the fragment containing the 5S rRNA gene. The plasmid was then digested with restriction enzymes, dephosphorylated, and 5'-end-labeled with [32]P.

Using other restriction enzymes, the fragments were digested for a second time to remove the ^{32}P from one of the strands. This resulted in fragments containing either the 5S rRNA gene or the SP6 promoter with a ^{32}P on the

5' end of either the transcribed or the nontranscribed strand (Figure 2). Each of these 5'-end-labeled fragments was digested with the T4 polymerase, which contains a 3'-5' exonuclease activity in the absence of free nucleotide triphosphates. This resulted in a population of fragments with a BPDE adduct on the 3' end and a ^{32}P label on the 5' end. These fragments were separated on a denaturing polyacrylamide gel with a Maxam-Gilbert sequence for the same strand (Figure 3). This approach provided a map of the adduct locations within each strand of the 5S rRNA gene and the SP6 promoter. Preliminary data indicated that there were preferred binding sites for the BPDE within the DNA, with certain deoxyguanosines being more heavily adducted than others. Using this approach in conjunction with footprinting techniques will allow us to determine the effects of chemical adducts on nucleosome position.

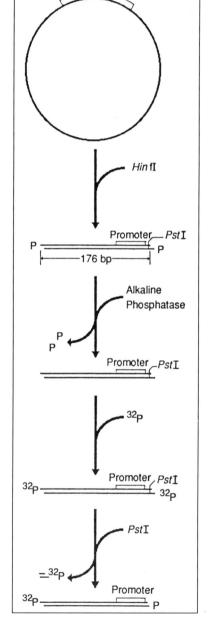

Figure 2. Diagram shows isolation of fragment containing SP-6 promoter region from pXP-14 plasmid. In this case, nontranscribed strand was ^{32}P labeled on 5' end.

Figure 3. Diagram shows mapping of benzo[a]pyrene (BaP) adducts. Locations of adducts within fragments are determined by comparing sizes of adducted fragments to sequence of same fragment.

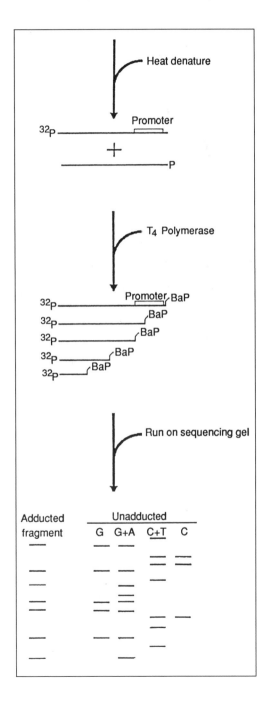

REFERENCES

Benezra, R, CR Cantor, and R Axel. **1986**. Nucleosomes are phased along the mouse β-major globin gene in erythroid and nonerythroid cells. Cell 44:697-704.

Chen, FM. **1985**. Covalent binding of (+)- and (-)-trans-7,8-dihydroxy anti-9,10-epoxy-7,8,9,10-tetrahydrobenzo[a]pyrene of B and Z DNAs. Biochemistry 24: 6219-6227.

Drew, HR and CR Calladine. **1987**. Sequence-specific positioning of core histones on an 860 base-pair DNA. J Mol Biol 195:143-173.

Garner, MM and G Felsenfeld. **1987**. Effect of Z-DNA on nucleosome placement. J Mol Biol 196:581-590.

Richard-Foy, H and GL Hager. **1987**. Sequence-specific positioning of nucleosomes over the steroid-inducible MMTV promoter. EMBO J 6:2321-2328.

QUESTIONS AND COMMENTS

Q: Smerdon, Washington State University, Pullman, WA
Once you've completed the adduct mapping studies, will you examine the blockage of SP6 polymerase at the different sites?

A: Mann
Yes, we expect to look at that following our studies to determine the effects of the adducts on nucleosome positioning.

IMMUNOQUANTITATION AND CHARACTERIZATION OF THE XENOBIOTIC METABOLIZING CYTOCHROME P-450 ISOZYMES FROM RAINBOW TROUT

C. L. Miranda,[1] J.-L. Wang,[1] M. C. Henderson,[1] D. E. Williams,[2] and D. R. Buhler[1]

[1]Department of Agricultural Chemistry, Marine/Freshwater Biomedical Center, Oregon State University, Corvallis, OR 97331

[2]Department of Food Science and Technology, Marine/Freshwater Biomedical Center, Oregon State University, Corvallis, OR 97331

Key words: *Cytochrome P-450, xenobiotic-metabolizing enzymes, rainbow trout*

ABSTRACT

The role of constitutive cytochrome P-450 isozymes (designated LMC1 to LMC5) in the metabolism of xenobiotics and endogenous compounds by trout liver microsomes was examined, using polyclonal antibodies raised in rabbits against trout P-450. Anti-LMC2 IgG markedly inhibited the microsomal hydroxylation of testosterone and the bioactivation of aflatoxin B_1, as measured by covalent binding of reactive metabolites to DNA. In contrast, anti-LMC5 IgG inhibited the activities of microsomal progesterone hydroxylase, estradiol 2-hydroxylase, benzphetamine N-demethylase, and benzo[a]pyrene hydroxylase. Anti-LMC1 IgG had a slight inhibitory effect on lauric acid hydroxylase activity. Anti-LMC3 IgG and anti-LMC4 IgG had no effect on any of the microsomal enzyme activities measured in this study.

To gain understanding of the regulation of P-450 isozyme activities, the concentrations of the individual isozymes (except LMC4) in trout liver microsomes were determined by the Western blot technique. The LMC2 was the most abundant isozyme in juvenile males (15 mo old) and juvenile females (15 mo old), whereas LMC5 was most abundant in 7-wk-old fry. Quantities of both LMC2 and LMC5 were substantially less in juvenile females than in juvenile males of the same age (15 mo). However, juvenile females had higher levels of LMC1 and LMC3 than sexually mature females. Treatment with β-naphthoflavone (BNF) reduced the concentration of LMC2 in juvenile males but not in juvenile females. Females injected intraperitoneally with BNF (100 mg/kg body weight) 2 wk before spawning produced fry with lowered concentrations of LMC2. However, the concentrations of LMC1 and LMC3 were higher in the fry of BNF-treated females than in controls of similar age (7 wk after hatching). These results suggest that constitutive P-450 isozymes in trout liver differ in their ability to metabolize xenobiotics and endogenous substrates and that these isozymes are subjected to developmental, sexual, and chemical regulation.

Cytochrome P-450 (P-450) is a key component of the mixed-function oxidase system that plays an important role in the metabolic transformation of xenobiotics and endogenous compounds. The different forms or isozymes of P-450 vary with species, age, and sex of animal, and with exposure to xenobiotics. At least five hepatic P-450 isozymes have been isolated from β-naphthoflavone- (BNF-) treated rainbow trout *(Salmo gairdneri)* in our laboratory (Williams and Buhler, 1984). The isozyme LM4, which is the inducible form, has high benzo[a]pyrene (BaP) hydroxylase activity; another isozyme, LM2, is very effective in activating aflatoxin B_1 (AFB$_1$), a potent carcinogen.

We recently purified five P-450 isozymes from untreated rainbow trout (Miranda et al., 1989). The isozymes are designated LMC1, LMC2, LMC3, LMC4, and LMC5, with molecular weights of 50, 54, 56, 58, and 59, respectively. In a reconstituted system, these forms vary in their ability to catalyze the metabolism of xenobiotics and steroids. LMC2 is most active toward AFB$_1$ whereas LMC1 is most active toward lauric acid. LMC5 has the highest activity toward progesterone; LMC3 and LMC4 have no activity toward the substrates used. Presented here is a summary of recent findings from immunoinhibition studies conducted to define the contribution of the constitutive trout P-450 isozymes to the hepatic microsomal metabolism of xenobiotics and endogenous compounds. In addition, we examined the levels of P-450 isozymes in trout as a function of age, sex, and chemical treatment.

INHIBITION OF MICROSOMAL ENZYME ACTIVITIES BY POLYCLONAL ANTIBODIES TO TROUT P-450

To investigate the contribution of the individual P-450 isozymes to the microsomal metabolism of xenobiotics and endogenous compounds, polyclonal antibodies to these P-450s, raised in New Zealand rabbits, were used to inhibit the enzyme activities of trout liver microsomes (Miranda et al., 1989). The microsomal incubation mixtures contained 0.1-0.2 nmol of microsomal cytochrome P-450 and purified rabbit antibody (IgG) at concentrations of 10, 20, 40, or 60 mg/nmol of P-450. Microsomes from sexually mature rainbow trout were used in this study because of their higher activity toward the selected substrates compared to that of microsomes from juveniles and mature females. Microsomes and IgG were preincubated at 30°C for 20 min before the addition of other components.

The results of this study showed that testosterone hydroxylase and progesterone 6β-hydroxylase activities of trout liver microsomes were almost completely inhibited by anti-LMC2 IgG and anti-LMC5 IgG, respectively, at IgG concentrations of 20 mg/nmol of P-450. Estradiol 2-hydroxylase activity was markedly inhibited (75% reduction in activity) by anti-LMC5 IgG. Anti-LMC1 IgG and anti-LMC2 IgG inhibited lauric acid hydroxylase activity by 20% and 48%, respectively, at IgG concentrations of 20 mg/nmol of P-450. Anti-LMC3 IgG and anti-LMC4 IgG had no inhibitory effects on any of these enzyme activities.

Using xenobiotics as substrates, we found that the different IgG have varying abilities to inhibit microsomal enzyme activity. Only anti-LMC2 IgG (10 mg/nmol of P-450) was effective in inhibiting the metabolic activation of AFB_1 as measured by the binding of reactive metabolites to DNA. Benzphetamine N-demethylase activity was partially inhibited by anti-LMC2 IgG and anti-LMC5 IgG. Anti-LMC5 IgG inhibited BaP hydroxylase activity by 49% at IgG concentration of 20 mg/nmol of P-450. Increasing the concentration of anti-LMC5 IgG to 60 mg/nmol of P-450 caused no further inhibition of BaP hydroxylase activity, suggesting that some of the P-450-catalyzed metabolism of BaP was insensitive to anti-LMC5 IgG. Antibodies against LMC1, LMC2, or LMC3 had no significant inhibitory effect on BaP hydroxylase activity. The BaP hydroxylase activity of microsomes from BNF-treated rainbow trout was not significantly inhibited by anti-LMC5 IgG, even at concentrations of 60 mg/nmol of P-450. Previously, BaP hydroxylase activity of BNF-induced microsomes was found to be inhibited 90% by anti-LM4b IgG at a concentration of 10 mg/nmol of P-450 (Williams and Buhler, 1984).

The results of these microsomal enzyme inhibition studies suggest that in untreated sexually mature male trout: (1) LMC2 is a major contributor to the hepatic microsomal metabolism of lauric acid, testosterone, and AFB_1; (2) LMC5 functions in the hepatic microsomal metabolism of progesterone, estradiol, and BaP; (3) LMC1 contributes to the microsomal metabolism of lauric acid; and (4) both LMC2 and LMC5 serve as catalysts for the N-demethylation of benzphetamine by trout liver microsomes.

IMMUNOQUANTITATION OF CYTOCHROME P-450

Information on P-450 levels is important in assessing the contribution of individual P-450 isozymes to microsomal enzyme activity in addition to understanding the catalytic activity of the P-450 isozymes. Thus, we have examined the relative concentrations of individual P-450 isozymes in microsomes of trout at various developmental stages. Microsomes were prepared from whole fish or from liver. Individual P-450 isozymes in microsomes were quantitated by the Western blot method (Burnette, 1981). Briefly, the microsomal proteins, separated by sodium dodecyl sulfate polyacrylamide gel electrophoresis, were transferred to nitrocellulose sheets with purified P-450 standards. The nitrocellulose sheets were then treated with the appropriate antibodies and [^{125}I]-protein A to locate the P-450 isozymes. The P-450 bands appearing on the Kodak x-ray film after development were then quantitated by a laser densitometer.

As shown in Table 1, no P-450 isozyme was detected in 21-day-old embryos or newly hatched fish. This finding indicates that the amounts of cytochrome P-450 present in these preparations are too low for detection by the Western blot method. Microsomes from whole-sac fry have trace amounts of P-450 that cannot be accurately quantified. However, if microsomes from the livers of the sac fry are used in the blot, the P-450 isozymes can be readily detected, LMC5 being the most abundant form in these preparations. At 15 mo of age, LMC2 becomes the most abundant form in both males and females; LMC2 remains the dominant form as the male trout reaches sexual maturity (20 mo old). However, in mature females (20 mo old), LMC5 becomes the most abundant form. In general, at 15 and 20 mo, the levels of the individual isozymes are relatively higher in males than in females. Interestingly, the relative proportions of the P-450 isozymes in liver microsomes from sac fry are somewhat similar to those of mature female microsomes. The total P-450 content of the various preparations determined by immunoblotting is ranked as follows: juvenile males > mature males > juvenile females > mature females > sac fry > embryos. These results show that the concentration of P-450 isozymes varies with age and sex of fish. Changes in P-450 isozyme profile with age may have biological significance, because some of these isozymes (LMC2 and LMC5) are involved in the metabolism of xenobiotics as well as that of reproductive hormones.

EFFECT OF BNF ON P-450 ISOZYMES

Previous studies have shown that exposure of rats to chemicals such as polychlorinated biphenyls (PCB) may increase the amounts of certain P-450 isozymes, while the levels of other isozymes are decreased (Dannan et al., 1983). Williams et al. (1984) found that BNF or PCB treatment of rainbow trout decreases the level of the constitutive P-450 isozyme LM2, while inducing the P-450 isozyme LM4b. We now report that BNF treatment of 15-mo-old trout affected the relative amounts of the individual constitutive P-450 isozymes in liver microsomes (Figure 1). In males, the amounts of LMC2 and LMC3 decreased by more than 50% after BNF treatment. (It should be noted that LMC2 may be similar, if not identical, to LM2 isolated by Williams and Buhler because both isozymes are very effective in activating AFB_1 and lauric acid.) In BNF-treated females, LMC2 increased twofold, whereas LMC1 decreased by 66%. Thus, there was a marked sex difference in the response of individual trout constitutive P-450 isozymes to chemical treatment. In contrast, the inducible form, LM4b, which is found in trace amounts in untreated fish, was markedly increased by BNF in both males and females (data not shown).

Table 1. Relative concentrations of cytochrome P-450 isozymes in microsomes from untreated rainbow trout.[a]

Developmental Stage	Cytochrome P-450 (pmol/mg protein)					
	LMC1	LMC2	LMC3	LMC5	LM4b	Total
21-day-old embryo[b]	ND	ND	ND	ND	ND	—
2-day posthatch [b]	ND	ND	ND	ND	ND	—
7-wk-old sac fry [b]	Trace	Trace	ND	Trace	Trace	—
7-wk-old sac fry [c]	13	19	5	30	Trace	67
15-mo-old male [c]	36	91	52	57	Trace	236
15-mo-old female [c]	28	35	33	33	Trace	129
20-mo-old male [c]	28	79	65	34	Trace	206
20-mo-old female[c]	8	24	7	33	Trace	72

[a] P-450 content was determined by the Western blot technique (Burnette, 1981). ND, not detectable.
[b] Microsomes were prepared from whole fish.
[c] Microsomes were prepared from liver.

The incidence of tumors in adult rainbow trout is significantly higher when fertilized eggs from gravid females fed dietary PCB are exposed to AFB_1 (Hendricks et al., 1984). Further investigation is necessary to determine whether constitutive P-450 isozymes involved in AFB_1 activation are modified in young fish when the parent fish were exposed to chemicals before spawning. When parent fish were treated with BNF (100 mg/kg, ip) 2 wk before spawning, no significant increase was observed in the concentration of the BNF-inducible form of P-450, LM4b, in the offspring, although the parent fish showed marked induction of hepatic LM4b. BNF treatment, however, produced an alteration in the relative concentrations of constitutive P-450 isozymes in the offspring (Figure 2): LMC2 decreased, whereas LMC1 and LMC3 increased. Therefore, it is likely that offspring of female trout exposed to chemicals before spawning may have altered ability to metabolize carcinogens and steroid hormones as a result of changes in the relative proportions of P-450 isozymes in the liver.

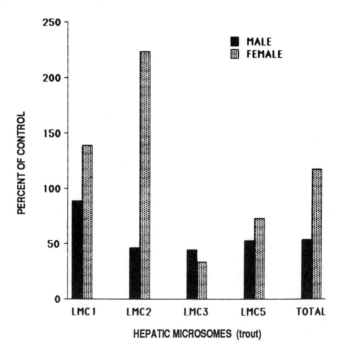

Figure 1. Effect of β-naphthoflavone (BNF) treatment on P-450 isozyme profile of hepatic microsomes from rainbow trout. Microsomes were prepared from male and female trout (15 mo old) fed diets containing BNF (500 μg/g) for 2 wk before sacrifice. Individual P-450 isozymes of treated microsomes were quantitated using Western blot technique. Results are expressed as percent of control values obtained from untreated fish of same age and sex.

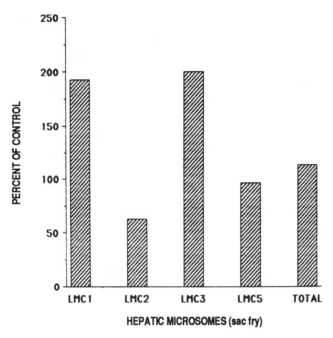

Figure 2. Effect of β-naphthoflavone (BNF) treatment of gravid female rainbow trout on the P-450 isozyme profile of hepatic microsomes of the young (sac fry). Two female trout were injected ip with BNF (100 mg/kg) 2 wk before spawning. Microsomes were then prepared from sac fry (7 wk old after hatching) derived from treated females. Concentrations of P-450 isozymes were determined by Western blot analysis. Results are expressed as percent of control values obtained from untreated fry of same age.

ACKNOWLEDGMENTS

We thank Dr. Jerry D. Hendricks, Mr. Ted Will, and Mr. John Casteel for their valuable assistance. This work was supported by NIH grants ES00210 and ES03850.

REFERENCES

Burnette, WN. 1981. Western blotting: Electrophoretic transfer of proteins from sodium dodecyl sulfate-polyacrylamide gels to unmodified nitrocellulose and radiographic detection with antibody and radioiodinated protein A. Anal Biochem 112:195-203.

Dannan, GA, FP Guengerich, LS Kaminsky, and SD Aust. 1983. Regulation of cytochrome P-450: Immunochemical quantitation of eight isozymes in liver microsomes of rats treated with polybrominated biphenyl congeners. J Biol Chem 258:1282-1288.

Hendricks, JD, TR Meyers, JL Casteel, JE Nixon, PM Loveland, and GS Bailey. 1984. Rainbow trout embryos: Advantages and limitations for carcinogenesis research. Natl Cancer Inst Monogr 6J:129-137.

Miranda, CL, J-L Wang, MC Henderson, and DR Buhler. 1989. Purification and characterization of hepatic steroid hydroxylases from untreated rainbow trout. Arch Biochem Biophys 268:227-238.

Williams, DE and DR Buhler. 1984. Benzo[a]pyrene-hydroxylase catalyzed by purified isozymes of cytochrome P-450 from β-naphthoflavone-fed rainbow trout. Biochem Pharmacol 33:3743-3753.

Williams, DE, RC Bender, MT Morrissey, DP Selivonchick, and DR Buhler. 1984. Cytochrome P-450 isozymes in salmonids determined with antibodies to purified forms of P-450 from rainbow trout. Mar Environ Res 14:13-21.

QUESTIONS AND COMMENTS

Q: Smerdon, Washington State University, Pullman, WA
Do you suspect that the different genes for these isozymes are differentially regulated by the Ah receptor?

A: Miranda
It is unlikely that the genes for the constitutive cytochrome P-450 isozymes (LMC1 to LMC5) in rainbow trout are regulated by the Ah receptor. The only evidence available to date of the involvment of the Ah receptor on cytochrome P-450 regulation in rainbow trout is for trout cytochrome P_1-450 (P450IA1) or LM_{4b}, which is induced by BNF or 3-MC (Heilman et al., DNA 7:379-387, 1988).

Q: Lamartiniere, University of Alabama at Birmingham, Birmingham, AL
You state that anti-LMC2 IgG markedly inhibited the microsomal hydroxylation of testosterone and the bioactivation of aflatoxin. Please comment on the capacity of this antibody to affect the metabolism of dissimilar chemicals, i.e., structure-activity relationships.

A: Miranda
Polyclonal antibodies raised against LMC2 are expected to bind directly to epitopes in LMC2 including the active site of the enzyme. Binding of the antibody to the active site could result in inhibition of enzyme activity. In a reconstituted system, we found that LMC2 catalyzes the hydroxylation of testosterone and the bioactivation of aflaxotin B_1 (Miranda et al., Arch. Biochem. Biophys. 268:227-238, 1989). It is possible that these two substrates of divergent structure fit into the same

active site of the enzyme molecule. Therefore, antibodies binding to the same active site of LMC2 may inhibit the *in vitro* metabolism of these dissimilar substrates. Cytochromes P-450, in general, are known to catalyze the metabolism of a wide variety of substrates with no distinct patterns of structure-activity relationships.

It should be noted also that polyclonal antibodies to LMC2 may cross-react with other P-450 forms such as LMC1 (unpublished data). Therefore, the metabolism of other chemicals that are substrates for LMC1 may also be inhibited by anti-LMC2 IgG.

PHOSPHORUS-32-POSTLABELING ANALYSIS OF DNA ADDUCTS IN LIVER OF ENGLISH SOLE

J. E. Stein, W. L. Reichert, and U. Varanasi

Environmental Conservation Division, Northwest and Alaska Fisheries Center, National Marine Fisheries Service, National Oceanic & Atmospheric Administration, Seattle, WA 98112

Key words: ^{32}P, DNA adducts, English sole, PAH, BaP

ABSTRACT ONLY

The levels of aromatic hydrocarbons in sediments of Puget Sound, Washington State, are positively correlated with the prevalence of hepatic neoplasms in English sole (*Parophrys vetulus*). In a recent study, hepatic lesions, including putative preneoplastic basophilic foci, were induced in English sole treated with the polycyclic aromatic hydrocarbon (PAH) benzo[a]pyrene (BaP) or an organic-solvent extract of a contaminated sediment from Puget Sound.

To further investigate the relationship between the presence of chemical carcinogens in sediments of Puget Sound and the occurrence of hepatic neoplasms in English sole, we have used the ^{32}P-postlabeling assay to estimate the levels of DNA adducts in English sole from contaminated and reference sites.

The autoradiograms of thin-layer chromatography (TLC) maps of ^{32}P-postlabeled hepatic DNA digests from fish sampled at contaminated sites exhibited up to three diagonal radioactive zones (DRZ) radiating from the origin that were not present in autoradiograms of TLC maps of hepatic DNA of fish from reference sites. These DRZ contained several distinct spots as well as what appeared to be multiple overlapping adduct spots. All autoradiograms of DNA from the fish from the contaminated sites exhibited a DRZ that contained DNA adducts with chromatographic characteristics similar to those of PAH-DNA adducts. In reference fish treated with the sediment extract shown to induce hepatic lesions in English sole, the DNA adduct profile was generally similar to that for fish from the site where the sediment was collected. Moreover, in fish treated with BaP at a dosage that induced hepatic lesions, the major DNA adduct detected was derived from the suspected ultimate carcinogen of BaP, BaP-7,8-diol-9,10-epoxide. In neither study was there a significant change in the levels of DNA adducts for at least 60 days after exposure, suggesting slow repair of DNA damage by English sole.

The results of these studies indicate the potential usefulness of the ^{32}P-postlabeling assay as a measure of exposure to genotoxic compounds. The results also support the hypothesis that exposure to chemical carcinogens is an important factor in the etiology of hepatic neoplasms in English sole from contaminated sites in Puget Sound.

CAN CARCINOGENICITY BE PREDICTED FROM CHEMICAL ANALYSIS AND DNA ADDUCTION?

D. D. Mahlum, D. B. Mann, D. A. Dankovic, and D. L. Springer

Pacific Northwest Laboratory, P.O. Box 999, Richland, WA 99352

Key words: *Adducts, initiation, BaP, mixtures*

ABSTRACT

Previous studies showed that the capacity of benzo[a]pyrene (BaP) to initiate mouse skin tumors decreased when the BaP was applied to the skin in a mixture of high-boiling polycyclic aromatic hydrocarbons (PAH). Data on the rate of absorption of BaP in the absence or presence of other PAH did not explain the difference in initiating activity. Other studies indicated that inhibition of BaP metabolism by PAH might explain the decreased initiating activity of BaP in mixtures versus that of BaP alone. We have expanded these studies to examine the effect of other PAH mixtures on BaP initiating activity, binding to mouse skin DNA, and DNA adduct profiles.

Benzo[a]pyrene (25 μg) was applied to the backs of female Charles River CD-1 mice, alone or in the presence of mixtures (5 mg) with various boiling points (300 - 700, 700-750, 750-800, 800-850, and >850°F). In the tumor studies, all mice were promoted with 5 μg of 12-0-tetradecanoylphorbol-13-acetate twice weekly for 24 wk. Tumor incidence and number of tumors were used as end points. For the DNA binding studies, tritium-labeled BaP was administered, as for the tumorigenesis studies. Twenty-four hours after applying the chemicals to the mice, animals were killed, and the skin was removed, treated with proteinase K, and the DNA isolated and purified. The DNA content was determined by absorbance at 260 nm, and the binding was determined by counting the radioactivity.

Of the mixtures examined, only the 300°-700°F distillate failed to affect the tumorigenicity of BaP. The other distillates decreased the number of tumors induced by approximately half. In contrast, even the 300°-700°F distillate decreased the amount of BaP bound to DNA to about half. The other distillates decreased the binding even further: to 10%-20% of the value found when BaP was applied alone. Examination of the profiles of adducts formed by BaP showed that the ratio of *anti*- to *syn*-BaP diol epoxide- (BPDE-) deoxyguanosine (dGuo) isomers was also decreased by approximately 50%. Thus, the binding of BaP to DNA and the production of the *anti*-BPDE adduct were decreased by a substantially greater amount than tumorigenicity was decreased by the presence of the mixtures. If we express potency as the number of tumors per *anti*-BPDE adduct, the potency was increased by the presence of other PAH. Changes in metabolic activation may be associated with the overall decrease in tumorigenicity and DNA binding, since metabolic transformation is necessary for both. However, it would appear that other factor(s) are also involved in increasing the effectiveness of the bound BaP to initiate tumors. Several possibilities exist: (1) The *anti* adduct to dGuo is not the major adduct responsible for tumor initiation. (2) The presence of other PAH may saturate repair mechanisms and result in excess DNA damage. (3) The presence of other PAH may alter the environment around the *anti*-BPDE adduct to dGuo to enhance its effectiveness. Experiments are in progress to evaluate these options.

Tumorigenicity of mixtures is often considered to be a sum of the tumorigenicity of individual components of the mixture. We have presented evidence that this may not be so for mixtures derived from the liquefaction of coal (Mahlum et al., 1984). Tumor initiation is considered to be a genetic event in which DNA is altered by adduction by a carcinogenic chemical or by a physical agent such as ionizing radiation. DiGiovanni et al. (1982) have presented evidence that mouse skin-tumor-initiating activity is closely correlated with the level of DNA adduction. In this article, we examine the relationship between chemical composition of mixtures and their skin-tumor-initiating activity. We also examine the effect of mixtures on the skin-tumor-initiating activity and the adduction of DNA by benzo[a]pyrene (BaP). These studies are directed toward answering the following questions: (1) Can the carcinogenicity of mixtures be predicted from their chemical composition? (2) Is DNA adduct formation a better indicator of tumor-initiating activity than chemical composition?

MATERIALS AND METHODS

Several mixtures with various boiling ranges obtained from a coal liquefaction process were used as source materials for these studies. The major components of these mixtures ranged from two- and three-ring polycyclic aromatic compounds (PAC), their alkylated derivatives, and peri-condensed four-ring PAC for a distillate boiling between 300°F and 700°F, to cata-condensed five- and six-ring PAC with alkylated homologues for a >850°F distillate. Chemical class fractions were prepared from these distillates by the method of Later et al. (1980). Skin-tumor-initiating activities of the various test materials were determined by an initiation-promotion assay using female Charles River CD-1 mice. In some experiments, BaP was added to the test materials before application to the mouse skin.

To study the relationship between skin-tumor-initiating activity and DNA adduction, radiolabeled BaP, by itself or in the presence of one of the mixtures, was applied to mouse skin. After 24 hr, DNA was isolated from skin by a modification of the method of Marmur (1961), and the amount of BaP bound to the DNA was determined by radioactive counting. Adduct profiles were obtained by digesting the purified DNA using the method of Nishimoto and Varanasi (1985).

RESULTS

The mouse skin-tumor-initiating activities for two mixtures (boiling ranges of 800°-850° and >850°F) and their chemical class fractions are shown in Figure 1. It can be seen that the activity of the lower-boiling material is only about one-half to one-third that of the higher-boiling material whether the parent material or its PAH fraction is considered. When the chemical compositions (Figure 2) of the two distillates or their PAH fractions are compared, one would expect that the 800°-850°F material should have the higher activity. For example, both materials have similar levels of BaP, a well-known carcinogen; however, the lower-boiling material also has significant levels of benz[a]anthracene, chrysene, 4- or 6-methylchrysene, and benzo[b + j + k]fluroanthene, all of which have been reported to possess carcinogenic activity (Table 1).

Because the initiating activity of the organic mixtures appeared to be strongly influenced by the overall composition of the mixture, we decided to directly test the effect of some mixtures on the expression of the initiating activity of BaP. We applied 25 μg of BaP to mouse skin in either methylene chloride (50 μl) or in methylene chloride containing 5 mg of organic mixture. In addition to the mixtures used previously, we used two other mixtures with lower boiling ranges that had been shown previously to be carcinogenic (Mahlum et al., 1984). We also tested a mixture boiling between 300° and 700°F that had been shown to be inactive as a skin-tumor initiator. Two weeks later, the mice were promoted twice weekly with 5 μg of 12-O-tetradecanoyl-13-acetate (TPA). The greatest number of tumors occurred when BaP was administered alone (Figure 3). The expression of BaP initiating activity was inhibited by all the mixtures except the 300°-700°F distillate, providing further evidence that these organic mixtures contain materials that interfere with the activity of their carcinogenic components.

Because BaP must be metabolically transformed before it reacts with DNA, we speculated that the decrease in initiating activity observed in the presence of the mixtures might result from competition for metabolism by noncarcinogenic PAH. We therefore tested four chemical class fractions from the 750°-800°F distillate for their influence on BaP initiating activity (Figure 4). The neutral PAH and the nitrogen-containing polycyclic aromatic compound (NPAC) fractions had the greatest inhibitory effect, decreasing initiating activity by about 70%; the aliphatic and the hydroxy-PAH fractions were significantly less effective. These results are consistent with the concept that interference with BaP activation is involved in the decreased tumor response seen when BaP is administered in the presence of other PAH. These experiments also further illustrate that the expression of BaP initiating activity can vary widely, depending on the matrix in which it is found.

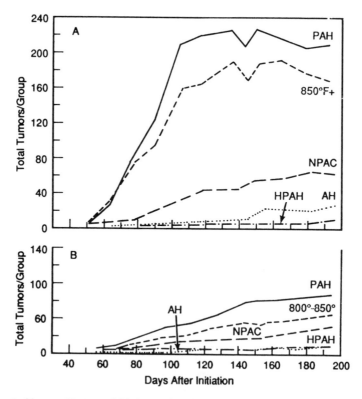

Figure 1. Mouse skin-tumor-initiating activity (total tumors per groups of 30 mice) after initiation (17 mg) with coal liquids boiling at >850° (A) or from 800° to 850°F (B), with the chemical class fractions prepared from them. Abbreviations: AH, aliphatics and olefins; PAH, neutral polycyclic aromatic hydrocarbons; NPAC, nitrogen-containing polycyclic aromatic compounds; HPAH, hydroxy-PAH. Fractions were applied in same proportion as they were found in the distillate.

	Quantity (µg/g)		
Compound	800°-850°	850°+	Structure
Phenanthrene	211	58	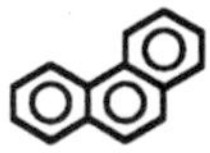
Fluoranthene	232	30	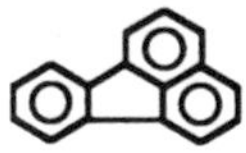
Pyrene	2,375	235	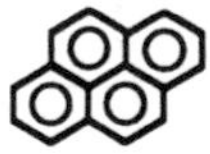
Benz[a]anthracene	2,997	---	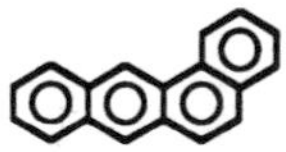
Chrysene	7,324	31	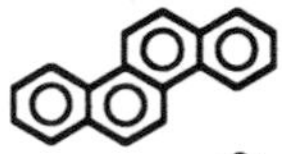
Benzo[k]fluoranthene	3,972	306	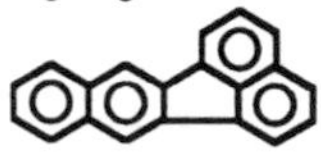
Benzo[e]pyrene	6,135	5,755	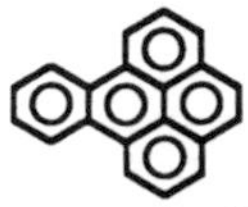
Benzo[a]pyrene	3,530	3,637	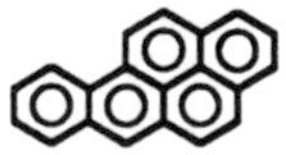
Benzo[ghi]perylene		15,311	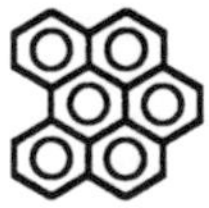

Figure 2. Representative polycyclic aromatic hydrocarbon (PAH) constituents from the 800°-850°F and >850°F distillates.

Table 1. Chemical class fraction content of complex mixtures with boiling ranges 800°-850° and > 850°.

	Percent Composition	
Fraction	800-850°F	>850°F
Aliphatic (A1)	5	2
Neutral PAH (A2)	50	46
Nitrogen-containing (A3) polycyclic aromatic compounds	25	34
Hydroxy-PAH (A4)	18	20

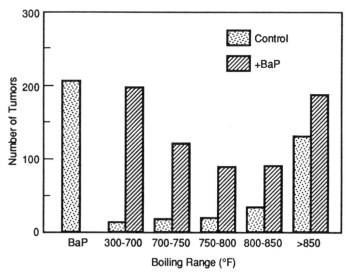

Figure 3. Effect of coal distillates with different boiling ranges on benzo[a]pyrene (BaP) skin-tumor-initiating activity: 25 μg BaP *(stippled bars)* was applied to mouse skin in 50 μl methylene chloride or in 50 μl methylene chloride containing 5 mg coal distillate *(shaded bars).* Activity is expressed as total number of tumors per group of 30 mice.

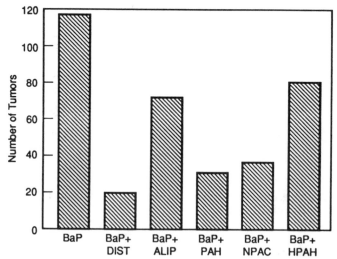

Figure 4. Effect of the 750°-800°F coal distillate and its chemical class fractions on benzo[a]pyrene (BaP) skin-tumor-initiating activity: 25 μg BaP was applied to mouse skin in 50 μl methylene chloride or in 50 μl methylene chloride containing 5 mg distillate, or proportionate amounts of chemical class fractions prepared from 5 mg of distillate. Abbreviations: BaP, benzo[a]pyrene; DIST, distillate; ALIP, aliphatics; PAH, neutral polycyclic aromatic compounds; NPAC, nitrogen-containing polycyclic aromatic compounds; HPAH, hydroxy-PAH.

It is accepted that tumor initiation is the direct result of the interaction of the ultimate carcinogenic form of a compound with DNA. We therefore undertook studies to determine if the skin-tumor-initiating activity of BaP in the presence of other organic compounds was better correlated with DNA adduct formation than with the chemical composition of the mixture. In these experiments, we applied radiolabeled BaP to mouse skin, either alone in a solvent or in a solvent containing 5 mg of one of the distillates used in the tumor-initiation studies. All the distillates used inhibited the binding of BaP to DNA (Figure 5). The 800°-850°F and >850°F distillates were the most effective, decreasing the binding by about sevenfold. Even the 300°-700°F material inhibited binding by about 50%, even though it did not significantly decrease tumor initiation by BaP.

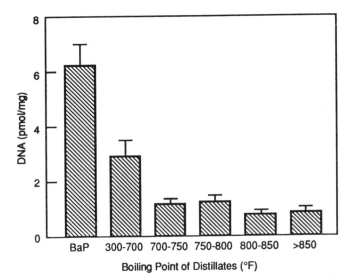

Figure 5. Effect of coal distillates on binding of benzo[a]pyrene (BaP) to mouse skin DNA. ^{3}H-labeled BaP was applied to mouse skin in 100 µl of 1:1 acetone:methylene chloride or in acetone:methylene chloride containing 5 mg of coal distillate; after 24 hr, the skin was removed, and digested with proteinase K, and DNA was extracted and purified. Binding was estimated from amount of radioactivity associated with DNA.

Benzo[a]pyrene adduct profiles were prepared from DNA from mouse skin treated with either BaP alone or with BaP in the presence of one of the foregoing distillates (Figure 6). In all cases the amount of radiolabeled adduct eluting from the high performance liquid chromatography column was decreased when BaP was coadministered with one of the organic mixtures, a result consistent with the total amount of labeled BaP bound to

DNA. The major adducts in all cases corresponded to *anti*-BPDE-dGuo and *syn*-BPDE-dGuo. Interestingly, the ratio of the anti to syn isomer was decreased by about 50% (Table 2).

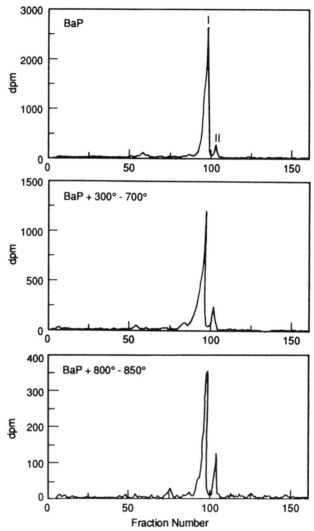

Figure 6. Benzo[a]pyrene (BaP) adducts prepared from mouse skin DNA isolated 24 hr after administration of radiolabeled BaP alone (top) or in the presence of coal distillates with varying boiling ranges. After extensive purification, DNA was hydrolyzed to nucleosides and the adducts separated by high-performance liquid chromatography. Profiles were obtained by determining the amount of radioactivity (dpm) at 0.5-min intervals. Peaks I and II represent the *anti*- and *syn*-BaP diol-epoxide deoxyguanosine adducts, respectively.

Table 2. Effect of complex organic mixtures on the ratio of *anti*-benzo[a]pyrene-diol-epoxide (BPDE) to *syn*-BPDE guanosine adducts from mouse skin DNA after administration of benzo[a]pyrene (BaP).

Test Material	Anti:Syn Ratio
BaP	12.2
300°-700°F + BaP	7.2
700°-750°F + BaP	6.4
750°-800°F + BaP	6.4
800°-850°F + BaP	5.4
>850°F + BaP	5.4

DISCUSSION

Examination of the skin-tumor-initiation data indicates that several of the complex organic mixtures used in these experiments contained tumor-initiating activity. Moreover, the initiating activity tended to increase with increasing boiling ranges of the mixtures. Although chemical analysis indicated that the mixtures contained known carcinogens, the skin-tumor-initiating activity often did not correlate with measured levels of these carcinogens. The results with the distillates alone suggested that the activity of some or all of their carcinogenic compounds was being masked by other components. Direct examination of the tumor-initiating activity of BaP in the presence of the distillates provided support for this conclusion. These data indicate that chemical analysis alone may not adequately predict tumorigenicity of mixtures.

The adduct data obtained in these experiments strongly suggest that there is not a simple relationship between carcinogen binding to DNA and tumor initiation. Although coadministration of mixtures with BaP suppressed both the total binding of BaP to DNA and the number of tumors induced, the effect of the mixtures on binding was substantially greater than their effect on tumor initiation. Moreover, the mixtures decreased the ratio of the *anti*-BPDE-dGuo to *syn*-BPDE-dGuo isomer. If the *anti*-BPDE-dGuo adduct represents the carcinogenic form, as generally accepted, our data indicate that mixtures significantly increase the tumorigenic effectiveness of the BaP that becomes bound to DNA, especially as the *anti*-BPDE-dGuo adduct. Furthermore, these data suggest that measurement of DNA adduction may not be an adequate predictor of the carcinogenicity of materials found in certain mixtures.

REFERENCES

DiGiovanni, J, J Rymer, TJ Slaga, and RK Boutwell. **1982.** Anticarcinogenic and cocarcinogenic effects of benzo[e]pyrene and dibenz[a,c]anthracene on skin tumor initiation by polycyclic hydrocarbons. Carcinogenesis 3:371-375.

Later, DW, M Lee, L Bartle, KD Kong, and DL Vassilaros. **1980.** Chemical class separation and characterization of organic compounds in synthetic fuels. Anal Chem 53:1612-1620.

Mahlum, DD, CW Wright, EK Chess, and BW Wilson. **1984.** Fractionation of skin tumor-initiating activity in coal liquids. Cancer Res 44:5176-5181.

Marmur, J. **1961.** A procedure for the isolation of deoxyribonucleic acid from micro-organisms. J Mol Biol 3:208-218.

Nishimoto, M and U Varanasi. **1985.** Benzo[a]pyrene metabolism and DNA adduct formation mediated by English sole liver enzymes. Biochem Pharmacol 34:263-268.

IRON STORES AND CANCER IN THE NATIONAL HEALTH AND NUTRITION EXAMINATION SURVEY I

R. G. Stevens

Pacific Northwest Laboratory, P.O. Box 999, Richland, WA 99352

Key words: *Iron binding, carcinogens, transferrin, NHANES*

ABSTRACT

Iron status and cancer risk were examined in the first National Health and Nutrition Examination Survey (NHANES I). During the period 1971-1975, a probability sample of 14,407 adults, aged 25 to 74 yr, were given a detailed dietary questionnaire, biochemical tests, and a medical examination. These subjects have been followed prospectively through the period 1981-1984. Among 242 men who developed cancer, the mean total iron-binding capacity was significantly lower (61.4 μmol/L versus 62.0; 342.6 μg/dl versus 351), and transferrin saturation was significantly higher (33.1% versus 30.7%), than in 3113 men who did not develop cancer. These results are consistent with the hypothesis that high body-iron stores increase long-term risk of cancer. The risk of cancer in men in each quartile of transferrin saturation level, relative to the lowest quartile, was 1.00, 1.01, 1.10, and 1.37, respectively (p for trend = 0.02). Serum albumin levels were significantly lower in men who developed cancer than in those who did not.

Among women, those who developed cancer did not have significantly different total iron-binding capacity or transferrin saturation from those who did not develop cancer. However, a *post hoc* examination of 5367 women (203 cancer cases) with a transferrin saturation of 26.8% or greater (highest quartile among men) yielded a relative risk of 1.3 (p = 0.1); in 5228 women with at least 6 yr of follow-up (149 cancer cases), the relative risk associated with high transferrin saturation was 1.5 (p = 0.04).

INTRODUCTION

Results from three previous studies have been consistent with the hypothesis that increased iron stores are associated with increased risk of cancer (Stevens et al., 1986; Selby and Friedman, 1988) and with increased overall death rates (Stevens et al., 1983). Two lines of evidence provide a biological rationale for the hypothesis. First, iron can catalyze the production of oxygen radicals (Halliwell and Gutteridge, 1986), and these may be proximate carcinogens (Cerutti, 1985). Second, iron may be a limiting nutrient to the growth and development of a cancer cell; excess iron may increase the chances that a cancer cell will survive and flourish (Weinberg, 1984).

In the first National Health and Nutrition Examination Survey (NHANES I) cohort, we tested the hypotheses that cancer victims had higher transferrin saturation and lower total iron-binding capacity (TIBC) values than non-cancer subjects when these characteristics were determined appreciably before diagnosis of disease. We then made estimates of the magnitude of the effect (see Stevens et al., 1988).

METHODS

The NHANES I and its epidemiological follow-up have been described by Madans et al. (1986). From 1971 to 1975, a probability sample of the U.S. noninstitutionalized population was identified. A total of 14,407 adults aged 25 to 74 yr were given an extensive dietary questionnaire, a medical examination, anthropometric measurements, and hematologic-biochemical tests. Subjects were traced and reinterviewed between 1981 and 1984. The follow-up period was defined as the time between date of initial examination and the first (1) diagnosis of cancer, (2) death, or (3) follow-up interview. Those lost to follow-up were excluded from analysis.

Determination of cancer was made at the time of follow-up interview with study subjects or proxies and based on hospital record or death certificate. Date of first hospital admission was used as date of incidence. For subjects with only a death certificate, date of death was used as date of cancer incidence. Because preclinical cancer might affect serum chemistries, analyses were restricted to 3355 men who remained alive and cancer free for at least 4 yr after blood was drawn and who had a TIBC determination at baseline examination. Analyses in women were based on 5367 women with a TIBC measurement who had been followed at least 4 yr.

Adjusted means of the variables of interest (e.g., transferrin saturation) at baseline interview were calculated in the subjects who subsquently developed cancer and in the subjects who did not. Relative risks for quartiles of transferrin saturation were estimated by the Mantel-Haenszel procedure adapted to cohort studies. The computer software MOX (Gilbert and Buchanan, 1984) was used for the calculations.

RESULTS

Age- and smoking-adjusted means of biochemical variables at initial examination in subjects who subsquently developed cancer and in those who did not are shown in Table 1. Dietary iron intake was not significantly different between cases and noncases. Iron intake per kilogram body weight (not shown) was also not significantly different. Among women, the differences in hemoglobin, TIBC, transferrin saturation, serum iron, serum albumin, and dietary iron intake between cancer cases and controls were not significantly different from zero (Table 1).

Table 1. Mean value of hemoglobin, total-iron-binding capacity, transferrin saturation, serum iron, albumin, and dietary iron intake in those subjects who developed cancer and in those who did not.

	Men			Women		
Parameter	Developed Cancer	No Cancer	p	Developed Cancer	No Cancer	p
Hemoglobin, mmol/L	9.6	9.6	0.65	8.6	8.6	0.26
TIBC, μmol/L[a]	61.4	62.9	0.01	66.4	66.5	0.91
Transferrin saturation, %	33.1	30.7	0.002	28.2	27.4	0.29
Serum iron, μmol/L	20.0	19.0	0.03	18.2	17.7	0.34
Serum albumin, g/L	43.7	44.3	0.002	43.3	43.4	0.63
Dietary iron intake, mg/day	13.7	14.1	0.34	9.3	9.8	0.19

[a] Total iron-binding capacity.

Table 2 shows the means for the iron variables after adjustment for age and smoking for each cancer site in men. No hypotheses concerning any particular cancer site were stated before examination of the data; thus, this table should be viewed as hypothesis generating. There are few cases. Stomach-cancer patients had lower transferrin saturation and higher TIBC values than noncancer subjects. Persons with cancers of the esophagus, bladder, and colon had very low TIBC and very high transferrin saturation values. Lung-cancer cases showed a modest elevation in transferrin saturation and a modest reduction in TIBC values.

Table 3 shows the relative risks obtained from the Mantel-Haenszel procedure stratified on smoking and age (in 2-yr increments) for each quartile of transferrin saturation relative to the lowest quartile.

Table 2. Mean values of hemoglobin, total iron-binding capacity, transferrin saturation, serum iron, serum albumin, and dietary iron intake by site of cancer for men.

Type of Cancer	n	Hgb[a]	TIBC[b]	Transferrin Saturation	Serum Iron	Serum Albumin	Dietary Iron
Noncancer	3113	9.6	62.9	30.7	19.0	44.3	14.1
Esophagus	6	8.8*	57.4	41.2*	23.8	44.0	10.8
Stomach	8	10.1	67.0	26.4	17.7	44.2	11.4
Colon	12	10.0	61.3	38.6*	22.6*	44.9	19.2*
Rectum	10	9.6	65.3	33.7	21.2	43.9	12.6
Pancreas	11	9.1*	62.9	30.9	18.8	42.8	14.2
Lung	50	9.7	62.0	33.9*	20.7	43.9	13.0
Prostate	52	9.4*	61.4	31.4	19.4	43.1*	12.6
Bladder	9	9.7	55.8*	42.1*	22.4	40.9*	15.3
Other urinary	10	9.6	58.8	26.0	15.6	44.0	13.6
Other	74	9.7	60.9	32.7	19.6	43.9	14.3

[a]Hemoglobin.
[b]Total iron-binding capacity.
*$p < 0.05$; to be used as screening tool, not as test of hypothesis.

Table 3. Relative risk estimates derived from the Mantel-Haenszel procedure for each quartile of transferrin saturation in men: p value for two-sided trend test.[a]

	n	0-22.8	22.9-29.1	29.2-36.7	36.8 +	p
All cancers	232	1.00	1.01 (0.67,1.52)	1.10 (0.74,1.64)	1.37 (0.94,2.01)	0.02
Lung	49	1.00	1.41 (0.49,4.07)	2.04 (0.78,5.33)	2.34 (0.92,5.93)	0.02
Colon	12	1.00	1.76 (0.41,20.4)	3.11 (0.27,35.3)	4.69 (0.45,48.7)	0.10

[a] Numbers in parentheses are 95% confidence intervals for means.

DISCUSSION

Iron is an essential nutrient. It plays a centrol role in metabolism, and severe iron deficiency leads to immune system compromise (Chandra and Newberne, 1977). However, Crosby (1978) has also warned that excessive iron fortification of food may lead to mild hemochromatosis, an effect observed in Swedish males (Olsson et al., 1978). Thus, because the Western diet has a high available iron content and because other diets are becoming more like the Western model, it is important to determine any adverse long-term health consequences of high body-iron stores and high dietary iron intake.

The results of the present study are consistent with results from a previous study that presented evidence of higher cancer risk associated with higher available body-iron stores in men (Stevens et al., 1986). Iron may influence risk for some cancer sites and not others. Cancer of the stomach in men appeared unrelated to markers of iron status; however, cancers of the colon, bladder, and esophagus did appear to be strongly related, and cancer of the lung also appeared to be related to iron status. The relative risks for lung and colon cancers (see Table 3) increase in a dose-response manner. In the Taiwan study (Stevens et al., 1986), lung cancer was strongly related to serum ferritin and transferrin, whereas stomach cancer was not (unpublished data). On the basis of these data, cancers of lung, colon, bladder, and esophagus should be examined specifically in other studies. The relationship of TIBC and transferrin saturation to lung-cancer risk could not be explained by smoking habits in the NHANES I data set.

In conclusion, too little iron is clearly detrimental. However, iron elevated beyond the level necessary to avoid anemia may also have adverse consequences.

ACKNOWLEDGMENT

Work was supported by Public Health Service grant CA-41515 from the National Cancer Institute.

REFERENCES

Cerutti, P. 1985. Prooxidant states and tumor promotion. Science 227:375-381.

Chandra, RK and PM Newberne. 1977. *Nutrition, Immunity, and Infection*. Plenum Press, New York.

Crosby, WH. 1978. The safety of iron-fortified food. JAMA 239:2026-2027.

Gilbert, ES and JA Buchanan. **1984**. An alternative approach to analyzing occupational mortality data. J Occup Med 26:822-828.

Halliwell, B and JMC Gutteridge. **1986**. Oxygen free radicals and iron in relation to biology and medicine: Some problems and concepts. Arch Biochem Biophys 246:501-514.

Madans, JH, JC Kleinman, CS Cox, et al. **1986**. 10 years after NHANES I: Report of initial followup, 1982-84. Public Health Rep 101:465-473.

Olsson, KS, PA Heedman, and F Staugard. **1978**. Preclinical hemochromatosis in a population on a high-iron-fortified diet. JAMA 239:1999-2000.

Selby, JV and GD Friedman. **1988**. Epidemiological evidence of an association of body iron stores and risk for cancer. Int J Cancer 41:677-682.

Stevens, RG, RP Beasley, and BS Blumberg. **1986**. Iron-binding proteins and risk of cancer in Taiwan. J Natl Cancer Inst 76:605-610.

Stevens, RG, DY Jones, MS Micozzi, and PR Taylor. **1988**. Body iron stores and the risk of cancer. N Engl J Med 319:1047-1052.

Stevens, RG, S Kuvibidila, M Kapps, JS Friedlaender, and BS Blumberg. **1983**. Iron-binding proteins, hepatitis B virus, and mortality in the Solomon Islands. Am J Epidemiol 118:550-561.

Weinberg, ED. **1984**. Iron withholding: A defense against infection and neoplasia. Physiol Rev 64:65-102.

QUESTIONS AND COMMENTS

Q: Smerdon, WSU, Pullman, Washington
Sertoli cells in mouse testes are known to produce transferrin, and appear to transport Fe through to developing spermatids. Do you see any enhanced testicular cancer frequencies?

A: There were too few testicular cancer cases to draw any meaningful conclusions from this study.

Q: Eastmond, LLNL, Livermore, California
Are there other factors (particulary dietary ones) within the NHANES I survey that correlated with iron body burden?

A: We used transferrin saturation, TIBC, and serum iron because they were the best indicators of body-iron status available in the NHANES I. No other information in the data base is a very good indicator.

Author Index